LOUISIANA HEALING GARDEN

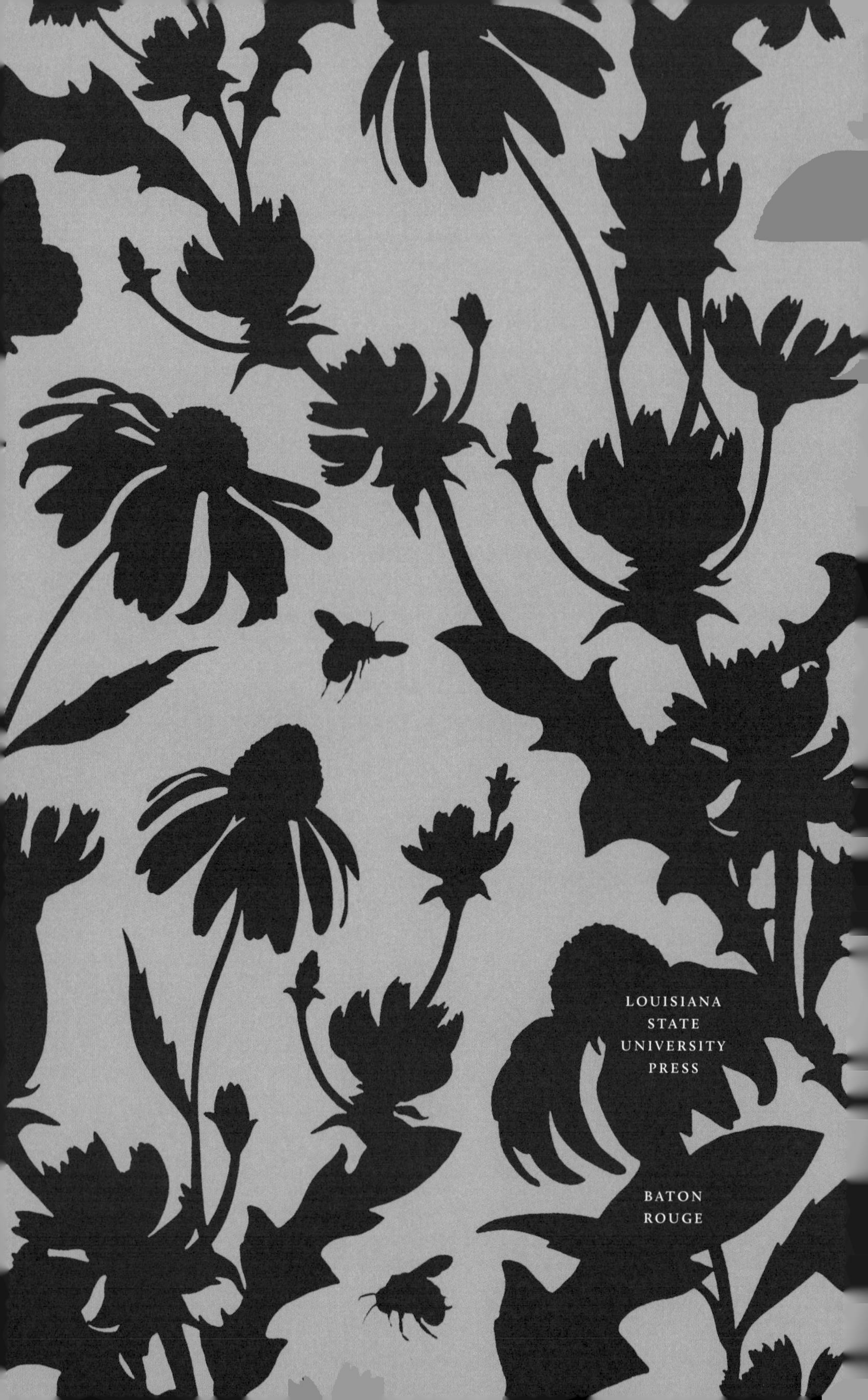
LOUISIANA
STATE
UNIVERSITY
PRESS
BATON
ROUGE

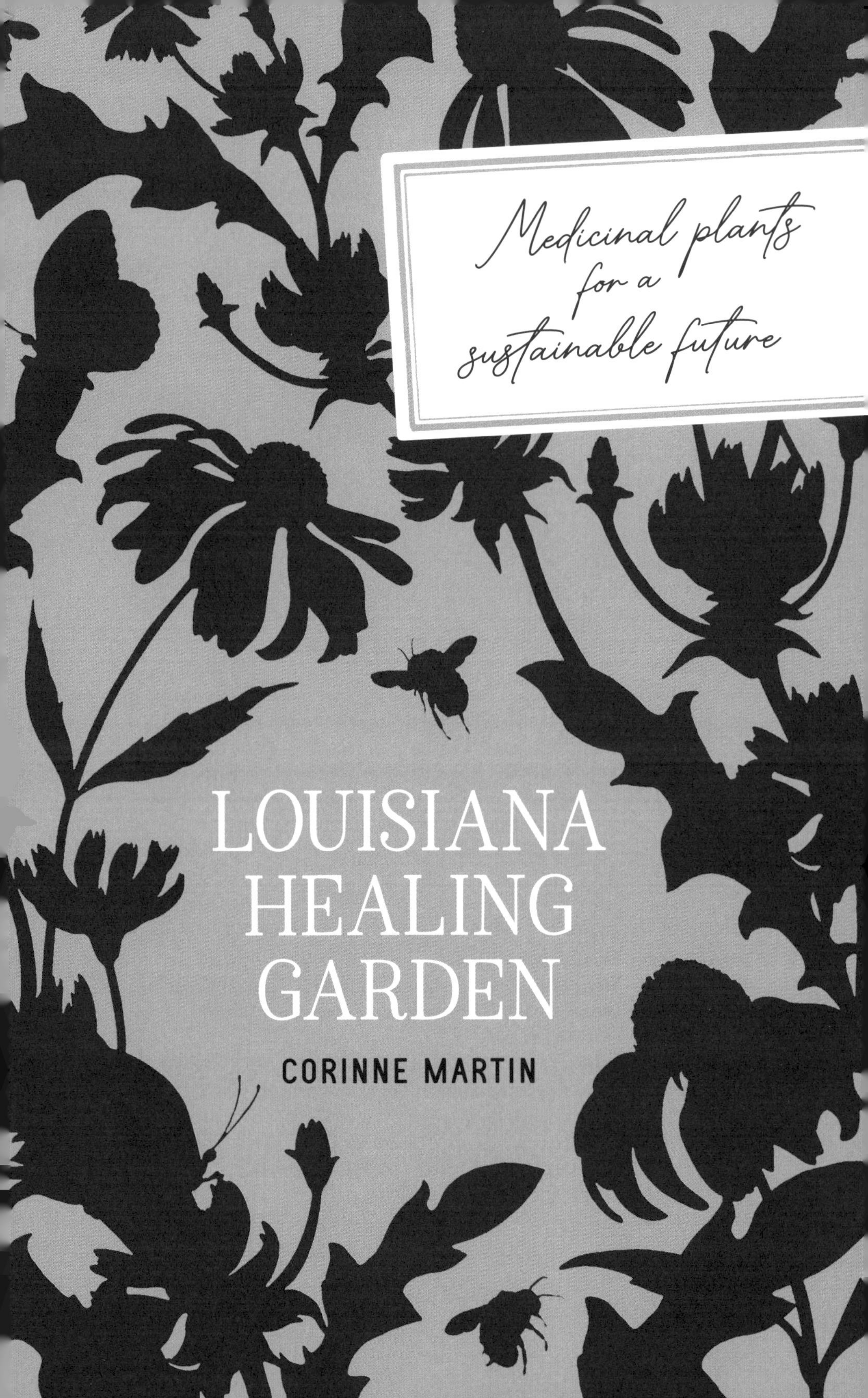
Medicinal plants for a sustainable future
LOUISIANA HEALING GARDEN
CORINNE MARTIN

Published with the assistance of the V. Ray Cardozier Fund

Published by Louisiana State University Press
lsupress.org

LSU Press Paperback Original
Manufactured in the United States of America
First printing

DESIGNER: Michelle A. Neustrom
TYPEFACE: Calluna
PRINTER AND BINDER: Versa Press

Unless otherwise credited, all photographs were taken by the author.
Cover illustrations: Adobe Stock.

The information included in this book is intended for informational, reference, and educational purposes, and should not be used as a substitute for diagnosis and treatment by a licensed health care professional. If you are interested in employing medicinal plants for personal wellness, please consult a health care provider who is familiar with your own health history and is informed about the inclusion of botanical and other natural remedies in maintaining health.

LIBRARY OF CONGRESS CATALOGING-IN-PUBLICATION DATA

Names: Martin, Corinne C., 1947–, author
Title: Louisiana healing garden: medicinal plants for a sustainable future / Corinne Martin.
Description: Baton Rouge, LA: Louisiana State University Press, 2026. | Includes bibliographical references and index.
Identifiers: LCCN 2025045758 (print) | LCCN 2025045759 (ebook) | ISBN 978-0-8071-8530-8 (paperback) | ISBN 978-0-8071-8631-2 (epub) | ISBN 978-0-8071-8632-9 (pdf)
Subjects: LCSH: Herb gardens—Louisiana | Medicinal plants—Louisiana | Sustainable living—Louisiana
Classification: LCC SB351.H5 M314 2026 (print) | LCC SB351.H5 (ebook)
LC record available at https://lccn.loc.gov/2025045758
LC ebook record available at https://lccn.loc.gov/2025045759

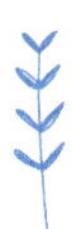

For "Sunny," Leon C. Vial III.
Thanks for carrying on the family garden tradition,
and for showing us the way.

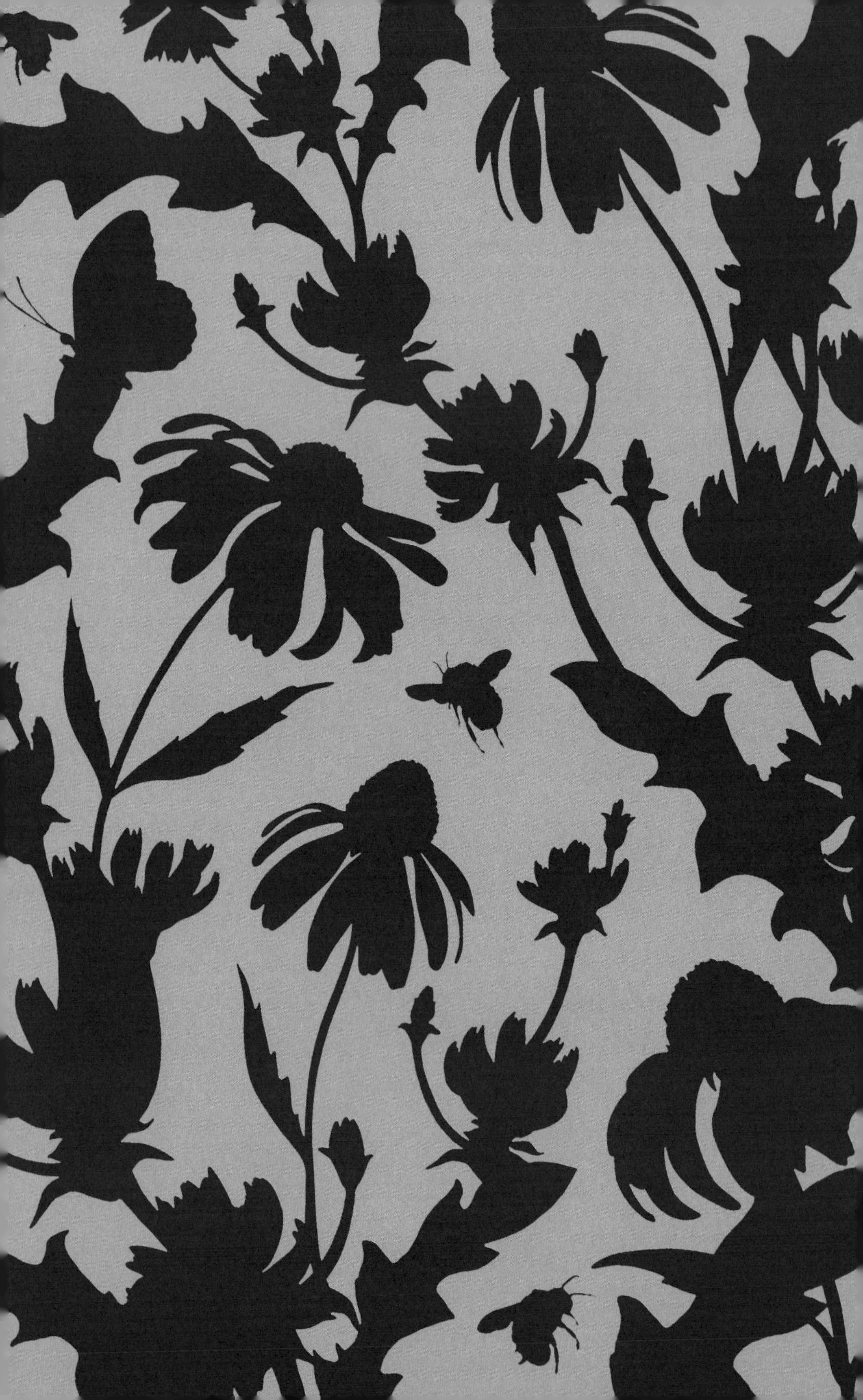

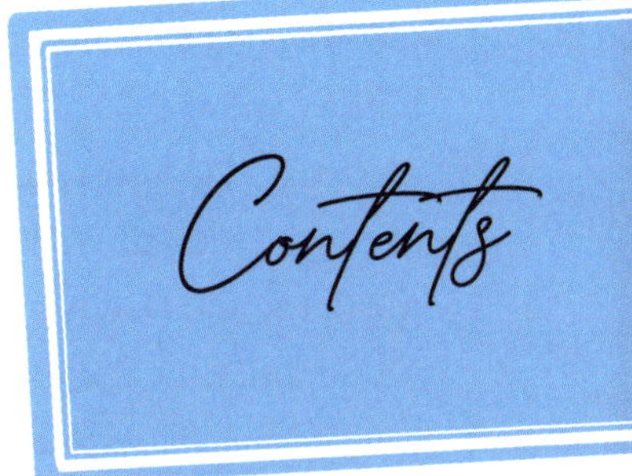

Contents

PREFACE AND ACKNOWLEDGMENTS

A garden is hope. A garden is work, sweaty engagement, a host of lessons, a constant humbling surprise. A promise.

A healing garden is a lively, changeable intersection between the web of wild lives all around us and our own home ground. A garden extends beyond the little plot we've laid out for it and reaches back toward its own feral roots. A garden is the sun and rain and soil, the rascally critters who try to get to the produce before we do, the beetles that nibble holes in our first perfect blooms. A garden is our ancestors—all they've learned, the wisdom they've shared, the world they knew, and all the changes wrought by weather and time and human intervention.

Catholic priest, ecologist, and philosopher Thomas Berry spoke at the turn of the twenty-first century about the state of the Earth's ecosystem and the many threats to its health from human use and misuse. He noted, "The Great Work now, as we move into a new millennium, is to carry out the transition from a period of human devastation of the Earth to a period when humans would be present to the planet in a mutually beneficial manner."

Getting to know the land and plants and animals all around us, and hosting a healing garden where they might thrive, could be one small step in that direction.

Many people have made this book possible. Thanks to Jenny Keegan at LSU Press for all the support, patience, and enthusiasm, to Susan Murray for her sharp eye and edits, and to Min Marcus for helping to polish the final product. Thanks to Dr. Charles Allen for his wild walks and wisdom. Thanks to my cousins Nanette, Jara, Dede, Lennie, Kathi, and others who continue to share wild places, gardens, and family history. Thanks to Jonathan Foret at the South Louisiana Wetlands Discovery Center for his dedication to the preservation of south Louisiana and its bayou culture. Thanks to Jennifer Blanchard for sharing enthusiasm and knowledge in her "Louisiana Medicinal Plants" class in the LSU Horticulture Department. Thanks to the tradition bearers, and to Mary Perrin and Beverly Fusilier, who carry on and share knowledge about Cajun healing and medicinal plants. Thanks to the soggy lands, wild waters, and medicinal plants that continue to offer up healing for our bodies, minds, and spirits. And thanks to Bodi—for all the walks.

LOUISIANA HEALING GARDEN

INTRODUCTION

Louisiana is an extraordinary place. Its landscapes are diverse, hot, steamy, luxurious, unique, and fruitful. The state is wet, unless it's bone dry. Wild, unless it's plowed, mowed, built over, managed, or poisoned. And gorgeous, unless it's beaten by a storm.

And it is host to teeming wildlife and thousands of plants.

Some of the plants growing in the state are native, having evolved over centuries to interact with and mutually benefit other plants, animals, and insects. Other plants have crept in over decades, have become adapted to local conditions, and routinely reseed themselves and attract pollinators. Louisiana is also inadvertent host to numerous invasive plants that are not native and may rapidly outcompete the beneficial native plants that have evolved in the state's habitats. These invasive species are very prolific, are usually not deterred by native insects or diseases, and grow rapidly. For the purposes of ecological balance, natives are "good," invasives are "bad," and the naturalized plants seem to be somewhat benign.

But one commonality of all these plants is that they are composed of hundreds of natural chemical compounds that have a primary benefit for the plants' life cycles and success. They make nutrients available and reproduce to create new life. These plants also produce numerous secondary compounds that increase the likelihood of successful competition for space and resources in their environment. Over fifty thousand secondary compounds have been discovered in the plant kingdom. And these compounds do not just benefit their host plant but have many possibilities for assisting and supporting human life. Medicinal herbs, and many modern medicines, rely on secondary plant metabolites for their actions. Almost one-fourth of pharmaceutical drugs are derived from these botanicals.

Many would argue that these numerous, potentially healing compounds—in thousands of medicinal plants—are worth identifying and saving because they could be the source of healing in the form of future pharmaceutical drugs. But I think they have another use as well. Whether they are welcomed natives, hardy introduced plants, or even pesky invasives, each of these can be an invitation to embark on a journey of healing. Each can also be an opportunity to get better acquainted with the places where we live, and to become coparticipants in the vital great work of helping to mitigate the damage and destruction facing many of Louisiana's low-lying and coastal areas.

These healing herbs may provide essential nutrients, or help to support the function of various body systems, or reduce inflammation and fight infection. But one way or another, working with the herbs engages us in the lands around us. Whether we are discovering or growing, harvesting or weeding or encouraging, we will be learning how to sensitively, wisely, arduously, and gratefully participate in our home ground.

And that is healing work.

I would argue that it is sacred work as well.

USING THE HERBS

HARVESTING GUIDELINES

Plant identification. When in doubt, don't pick or use a plant. There are numerous field guides and phone apps that can help with identification, and local and state native-plant groups can be instructive. In Louisiana, several botanists and online groups are available. Louisiana biologist and a founding member of the Louisiana Native Plant Society (www.lnps.org) Dr. Charles Allen recommends USDA plants (plants.sc.egov.usda.gov/java/) and two in-state files with USDA data, References (www.lnps.org/references) and the Guide to Plants of Louisiana (warcapps.usgs.gov/PlantID/).

Status of plant. Keep in mind that regional abundance doesn't mean that the plant is not at risk in other areas or states. Check with your local conservancies or native plant groups and search the Plants Database (plants.usda.gov) to find out the status of the plant populations in the state.

Where to harvest. One of the most important factors in harvesting plants is the health of the soil in which the plant is growing. Louisiana has one of the lowest standards in the nation for amounts of toxins in air and water that are deemed "acceptable." When harvesting in an area, awareness is key. Even harvesting near apparently barren fields doesn't ensure safety. If you're uncertain about the health and safety of the area where you'd like to harvest, it's best to find another spot, or find a native source of seeds or plants and grow the herb at home.

How much to harvest. A basic rule of thumb in herbalism is to gather no more than 10 percent of the plant population you find. Be aware of population density, not just locally or regionally, but statewide and throughout the country. If the plant is at risk or threatened, it should not be harvested, but you might consider cultivating the plant in your home garden.

Permission. If harvesting from an area that is unknown to you, find out the owner, if possible, and gain permission for harvesting.

Respectful harvesting. Some Indigenous practices include the idea of reciprocity—of giving back to the plant or area when harvesting. You may develop your own practice, or you may just harvest with respect and gratitude, and become an informal steward of the land, keeping an eye on its health and changes. If you determine that harvesting in an area seems appropriate and safe, replace the soil you disturbed while gathering your herb and return the area to its original condition as much as possible.

Harvest timing. Plants have natural chemical compounds in all their parts. But often traditional use has focused on one or more parts to gather. Harvest timing is geared to collecting plant parts when the medicinal compounds in that particular part are highest.

- Flowers/blossoms: Flowers should be gathered when the plant is blooming and has not started going to seed. (Examples: rose, gardenia.)
- Aerial parts: Aboveground parts of plants should be gathered when approximately 10 percent of the plant colony is blooming. (Examples: skullcap, St. Johnswort.)
- Leaves: Leaves should be harvested when they are green and thriving. (Example: mountain mint.)
- Whole plant: If seeds are also to be used, the plant can be harvested when blooming or when beginning to set seed. (Examples: purslane, wild petunia.)
- Fruit: Fruit should be harvested when ripe. (Examples: garlic, okra.)
- Roots: Roots should be dug either in early spring (before blooming) or after colder weather sets in during fall. Some herbalists recommend harvesting in autumn to avoid roots with high concentrations of spring moisture. (Example: burdock.)
- Bark: Bark should be harvested from spring through summer, preferably taken from branches rather than trunk to avoid harming the whole tree. (Examples: hackberry, linden.)
- Seeds, nuts: When the plant has started to set seed, and seeds are ripening, they are ready to be gathered. (Examples: black walnut, burdock.)

MAKING HERBAL REMEDIES

Drying your herbs. Air-drying your herbs in the humid conditions of Louisiana can be challenging, so you might want to purchase a food dehydrator for drying plants, or dry plants slowly in an oven.

For oven-drying, turn the oven to its lowest setting and spread out the plant material on a cookie sheet. Place the cookie sheet in the oven and prop the oven door open several inches to allow any dampness to escape. Dry for an hour or so, then test to see if the plant material is "crispy." Allow to cool before storing.

To air-dry, gather your herb on a dry day (after several days of lower humidity), bundle into small batches, wrap stems with a rubber band, and hang to dry. You can also spread flowers, petals, or leaves on a screen or flat surface and place them in an area where there is good ventilation.

Tea. In making a tea, hot water is used as the medium of extraction, and heat will help leach out the healing compounds from the plants. A tea is a good way to extract plant compounds that are water-soluble, a property shared by many plants. Two basic methods of making a tea include:

- Infusion: An infusion is most appropriate for lighter plant materials such as flowers, leaves, and whole plants. In this process, place the dried plant material in a cup and pour boiling water over the herb. Allow to steep five to fifteen minutes, then strain through a sieve, capturing the liquid and composting or discarding the spent herb. The general guideline for amount of water to plant material is one cup of water to one tablespoon of dried plant material. Slightly more fresh plant material can be used to one cup of water.

- Decoction: A decoction is most appropriate for more dense plant materials such as roots, bark, and seeds. In this process, place plant material in boiling water and simmer gently for five to fifteen minutes, then strain liquid into a cup through a small sieve, and discard spent plant material. Proportions of water to plant material is one cup of water to one tablespoon of herb.

Tincture. A tincture is an extraction of healing plant compounds using an extraction medium other than water. Common extraction mediums include high-proof drinking alcohol, cider vinegar, or plant-based glycerin. Most potent is grain alcohol, which is 190 proof. High-proof vodka can also be used. In these tinctures, the alcohol will preserve plant compounds for up to ten years if properly stored. Glycerin is used for preparations that can be taken by those who wish to avoid alcohol (recovering alcoholics or those sensitive to alcohol, such as nursing mothers or children). It can also be a good tincture medium for plants that contain reproductive hormones (which are fat-based). However, glycerin has a lower potency for extraction and preservation than alcohol, so adults may double the dose of a glycerin tincture. The tincture should be stored in the refrigerator, then discarded after one year.

- Fresh plant tincture: Clean the plant material if necessary, chop into small pieces, and pack down tightly into a clean jar. Pour tincture medium over the herb until plant material is completely covered and add another quarter inch of tincture medium to top off. Replace lid, label jar, and set in a darkened area for two to four weeks. (This will be a 1:1 fresh plant tincture; that is, one part plant to one part liquid.) After two to four weeks, strain liquid through a sieve, discard or compost plant material, replace lid, and label jar with date and contents. Store in a cabinet away from sunlight. (If making a glycerin-based tincture, you should add about 20 percent water to the glycerin, as not all plant parts will be glycerin-soluble. For example, if using an eight-ounce jar that is packed with fresh plant material, measure out six ounces of glycerin and add two ounces of water, stir, then pour mixture over plant material.) Glycerin tinctures need four weeks to set before pouring off, as glycerin is less potent at extraction than drinking alcohol.
- Dried plant tincture: Dried plant tinctures are generally made in proportions of 1:5 (one part plant material to five parts liquid). To set up a dried plant tincture, weigh amount of dried plant material (on postal or diet scale), place herbs in a clean jar, then pour five times that amount of tincture medium over the plant material. (For example, if you have four ounces of dried herb, measure out twenty ounces of alcohol. High-proof vodka works best for this extraction method,

as 100-proof vodka contains approximately 50 percent water and 50 percent alcohol, an ideal mix to extract water-soluble and non-water-soluble properties from plants.) Set jar in a darkened area for two to four weeks, then strain off liquid and plant material through a sieve that is lined with cheesecloth. Bottle the tincture, label the jar, and store. Discard or compost the plant material.

Powder/capsules. Herbs that are most appropriate for use as capsules or powder include the herbs that are commonly used as tea and have water-soluble compounds. Empty gelatin capsules can be purchased in health food stores or online. Powders and capsules have a shelf life of roughly one year. Dried plant material can be powdered in a food processor, blender, or spice grinder.

Oil. An infused oil of a plant is best made from leafy or flower parts of the herb. The herb should be wilted for twenty-four hours or thoroughly dried prior to immersing in oil to reduce the possibility of forming mold. Once plant material is ready, cut or crumble the herbs into small pieces and pack into a jar. Cover the plant material with the oil of your choice. (Organic oils are best, and some popular oils to use include olive, safflower, almond, sunflower.) Make sure that the herbs are completely saturated and covered by an additional quarter inch of oil. Replace lid and allow jar to set on a shelf, out of the sun, for two or three weeks. Then strain the oil through a sieve lined with cheesecloth (to catch small plant bits), discard the herb, and pour oil into a clean jar, replace lid, label with name of herb and date completed, and store.

Salve. A salve can be made from your infused oil. To do this, measure the herbal oil and place it in a saucepan. Then add beeswax. Proportions of wax to oil are 1:4 (one part wax to four parts infused oil) for a solid salve. For instance, if you have eight ounces of herbal oil, you'll add two ounces of beeswax to oil in a pan. Turn heat to a low setting and stir constantly until the beeswax has melted thoroughly. Stir the mixture and pour it into clean jars. Allow jars to set without lids on until they are thoroughly cooled. Don't jiggle or try to stir the salves while they're cooling, as this will result in a grainy texture. (The surface of the salve will seal over before it is completely solidified, so avoid testing it with your finger until the outside of the jar is cool.) Replace lid once salve is completely cooled. Then label and store. For a softer salve, decrease the amount of beeswax you use, so your proportions will be 1:5 (one part wax to five parts oil.)

Syrup. Generally, dried or freshly wilted herbs and honey are the best ingredients for a syrup. Place the herbs in a slow cooker and thoroughly cover herbs with honey. Place lid askew on top of pot and turn heat on low setting. Keep an eye on this mixture, stirring occasionally. Most important in this process is to NOT boil the syrup as it steeps. The mixture should steep for several hours, or overnight, as long as the materials do not boil. When the steeping is finished, pour syrup and herbs through a strainer or sieve into a glass measuring cup and discard the herbs. Then pour syrup into individual jars. Syrups will be stable for six months to a year. If the honey crystallizes, you can simply boil water in a pot, turn off the heat, remove the lid of the syrup jar, and place it in the hot water. Or set the jar of syrup in an oven at its lowest setting (warm).

Compress. Make a simple tea infusion or decoction out of your plant material. Allow the tea to cool, then dip a clean cloth into the tea, wring it out lightly, and place the herb tea–soaked cloth on the affected area.

Poultice. Crush plant material and make a loosely packed ball of herb matter. Place this on a cut, rash, or burn and hold in place for ten minutes or so. Repeat as needed with fresh plant material.

Wash. Prepare an herbal tea, allow to cool, then drip or pour tea over the affected area.

PROLOGUE

All my life, I've been in love with my Louisiana home ground. As a child, nature drew me out on long, aimless walks—through neighbors' yards, abandoned fields, thickets of bamboo, or to any waterside. Those walks were precious. By myself, I could wander and explore and get to know the land of my birth.

Those were the easy parts. How could you not love a flower? An interesting plant? The small fish that swim, like shadows, just beneath the surface of dark water? The heron that squawks as it lifts up huge wings and wrestles away from the Earth? How can you not love winding, ambling roads that go nowhere? Or the end of the land? The flat water? The little lapping waves that nibble at the shore?

But there are hard parts, too, because there's still so much we just don't know.

We don't know how to cherish these gifts for what they offer: Wonder.

We don't know how to use our minds and bodies and hearts toward the same goal: Gratitude.

We don't know how to care for the exquisite Mystery into which we are woven: The Holy.

Our hearts are full.

Our hearts are broken.

We haven't yet figured out how to grow up.

But eventually we have to face consequences.

As it turns out, we are the Consequence.

But so far, we are not the End.

We are also the Hope.

What would it take to nudge this place in the direction of Healing?

Attention—Work—Joy—Hope—Knowledge.

Working with each other, one gritty, soggy step at a time.

This is not just an herb book.

It's an invitation into a place that is complex, wide, wet, shifting, old, and ever-new.

It's a celebration, a lament, an outcry, a rage, a whisper, a plea. A prayer.

Sometimes all we can do is care.

I don't know how the future will play out for Louisiana.

I don't think using herbs will save it. But I do believe that awakening to the many small gifts that surround us and helping them to thrive will at least signal our intentions. Who knows how much impact we can have?

We are living into the Mystery—one hopeful, tender flower at a time.

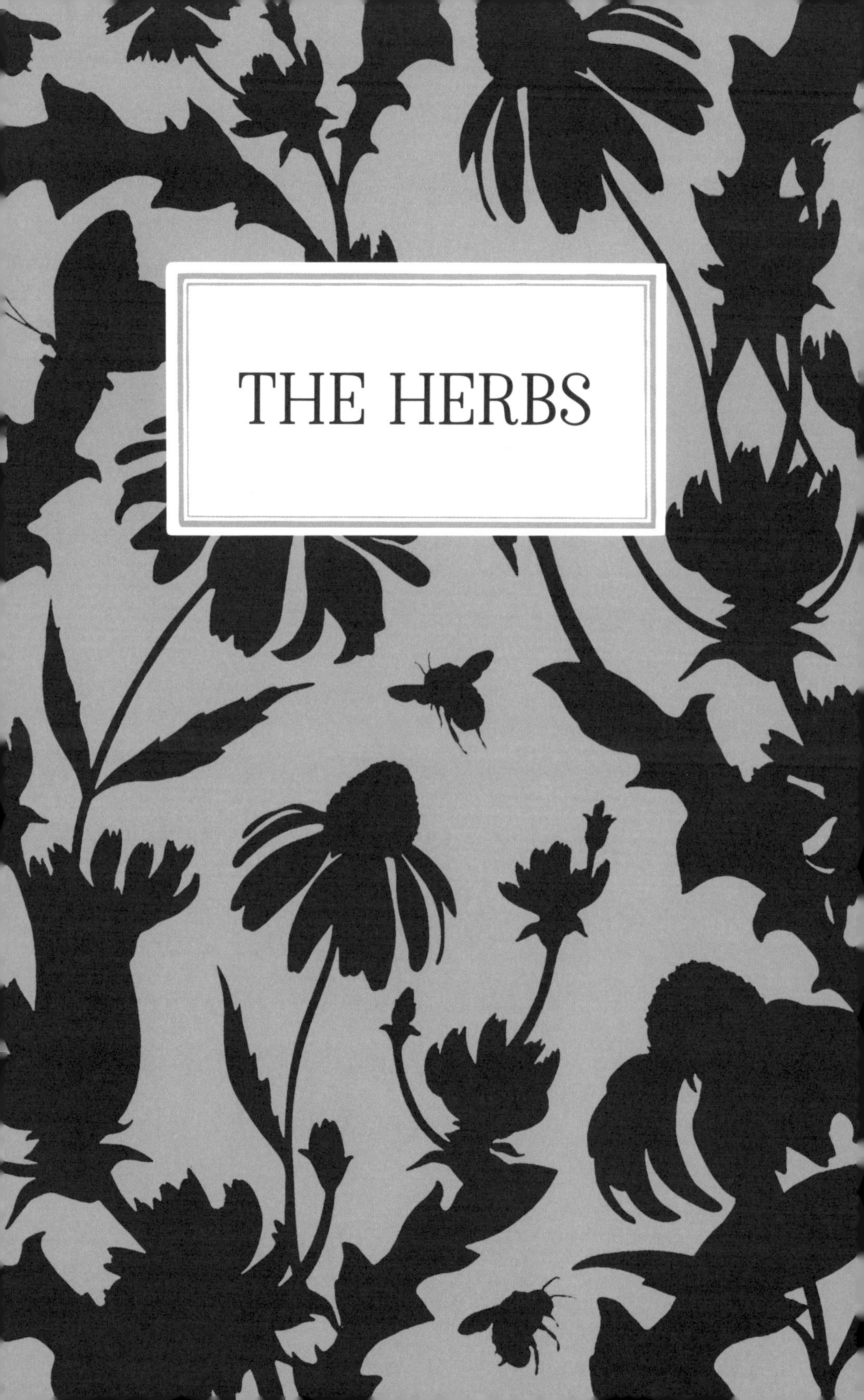

THE HERBS

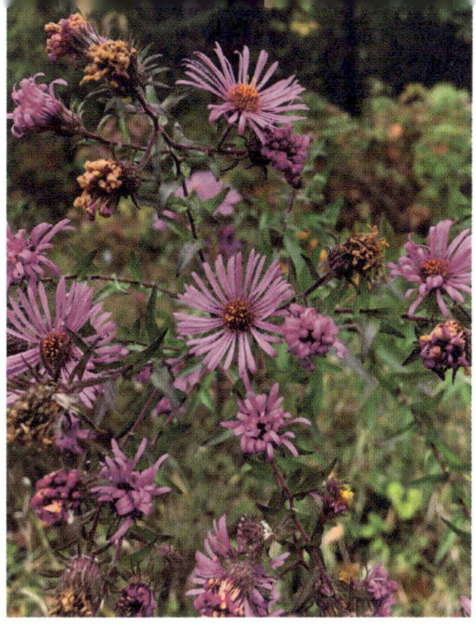

ASTER & LINNAEUS

FALL

Aster
[*Symphyotrichum* sp.]

At the edge of the road in Cocodrie I get out of the car to gaze at the water and end up knee-deep in blooming asters that are thick and bright and . . . everywhere! I'm not alone in enjoying them. Dozens of bees and moths flicker around the flowers, diving in to feast on late-summer nectar. There seem to be different species of the plant—some have lavender flowers, some have white. Some plants are tall, others are short. I'm not enough of a true botanist to tell one species from another, but, fortunately, many species of aster share the same medicinal properties and can be used for similar health issues, so I'm excited to see them all.

In general, the aster relatives have been touted for their anti-inflammatory and antiseptic properties, and for their gentle support of the nervous system. Used for pain and fevers, diarrhea, colds, flu, chest infections, anxiety—there are about as many uses as there are species.

I recently looked up the asters on the Louisiana plant website and was excited to find that twelve species have been identified in the state, and about 350 species worldwide. Some asters in the state are limited to a few areas, and others can be spotted throughout most parishes. Each species, of course, has its own scientific name—which makes me think about Linnaeus, and the botanical naming of plants, and how in the heck anyone keeps all the details straight. Even if a plant has had the same name for decades, botanists might decide to change things around. So, even if I've remembered the formal name for a species, it is very like to change. Some notable changes throughout my years as an herbalist have included black cohosh, formerly known as *Cimicifuga racemosa* and now *Actea racemosa,* and Joe Pye weed, formerly known as *Eupatorium,* now shifted over to *Eutrochium.*

I first became curious about the medicinal properties of aster when its genus name was *Aster!* Pretty simple, or so I thought. It turns out that the genus name has recently been changed to *Symphyotrichum*—not nearly as easy to remember. Fortunately, I have always loved the Latin names of plants. When I first became interested in herbs, I decided to learn their formal names. I figured it is like having an acquaintance versus having a true friend—instead of just the nickname, you learn the official name instead. Turns out that it can be very helpful, since sometimes different plants can have the same common name.

But where did all this naming practice start? With Swedish botanist, physician, and zoologist Carl Linnaeus (1707–1778), it turns out. Apparently, his father was a botanist, and when little Carl was upset, his father would just place a flower in his hand, and he would become calm. Some sources call Linnaeus the first environmentalist. He believed in the balance of nature and felt that each species had an important place in our surroundings. Linnaeus created a system for naming all living things—plants and animals and even minerals. That system, known as binomial nomenclature, is used to this day.

His original system of genus and species identification was formalized in 1867 to what is now known as the International Code of Nomenclature (ICN). With ongoing, thorough examination of the history and identification features of various plants, a plant's assignment to a new genus or species may shift over time.

With so many species of asters, it makes sense that they are associated with multiple healing properties and that they may be reassigned occasionally to a new genus. But I'm still a little irked by the changes that drag us poor herbalists and "plant people" along with them. Despite my irritation about plants' name changes, there's something I like about the process. It signifies for me that plant study (and the study of all of nature) is never stale or static but an ongoing exploration that delves ever more deeply into the miracles and mysteries of natural life forms.

And, whatever they're called, I'm happy to see the asters so lush and abundant and glad to be able to harvest some in the wild to take home. In fact, I should probably seed a few native species in my own home garden sometime soon. For now, I gently break off flowering stalk after stalk, while the bugs rise up and shift to another plant. On this gorgeous day, here we are, doing our work side by side, grateful for the sun and warmth and for all the gifts that the asters offer up.

Species: Twelve species of *Symphyotrichum* grow in Louisiana and share similar healing properties. These include:

Symphyotrichum concolor

Other Names: Eastern silver aster.

Medicinal Uses: Used for fevers and pain by Indigenous tribes.

Description: Hairy stem, up to 3 feet tall, flowers lavender to bluish-purple ray florets surrounding creamy-white disk florets. Leaves linear, covered with a silky, silvery pubescence, alternate and slightly appressed. Bracts pubescent with purplish uppers and green undersides. Fruit is an inconspicuous achene.

Habitat: Woodlands, thickets, old fields, prairies, and dry, sandy places.

Distribution: A few eastern, central, and northern parishes.

Plant Status: Native.

Cultivation: Plant grows in low-nutrient soils and is very drought tolerant.

Symphyotrichum drummondii

Other Names: Drummond's aster, Michaelmas daisy.

Medicinal Uses: Anti-inflammatory, antiseptic.

Description: Plant has small, white, daisy-like flowers with yellow centers. The seeds are small, black, and oval shaped. The seedlings are thin and have long, narrow leaves. Up to 4 feet in height.

Habitat: Rocky or dry openings in wooded areas.

Distribution: Mostly northern and central parishes, a couple of southern parishes.

Plant Status: Native.

Cultivation: Grows best in average, dry-to-moist, well-drained soils in partial shade. Stems may be pinched back in late spring to early summer if shorter plants are desired. Plants can spread aggressively by self-seeding.

Symphyotrichum dumosum

Other Names: Bush aster, rice button aster, American aster, white bushy aster, long-stalked aster.

Medicinal Uses: Used by some Indigenous tribes for nervous system support or insomnia.

Description: Grows 2–4 feet in height. Flower color varies—white, pink, blue, lavender. Many-flowered, but each tips a separate branch with its own leaflets that are spread along branches, not clustered at major branch ends.

Habitat: Sandy, open sites, occasionally marshy ground. Also in loamy prairies, old fields, woodlands, meadows, and pastures.

Distribution: Top two-thirds of the state, a few southern parishes.

Plant Status: Native.

Cultivation: Can be propagated by seed and division; likes full sun to partial shade. Adaptable to a variety of conditions.

Symphyotrichum lanceolatum

Other Names: Panicled aster, lance-leaved aster, white panicled aster, eastern lined aster.

Medicinal Uses: Used by various Indigenous tribes for fevers, wounds, nosebleeds.

Description: Grows up to 5 feet tall or more. Lance-shaped leaves are generally hairless but may feel slightly rough to the touch. Flowers grow in clusters and branch in panicles. They have sixteen to fifty white ray florets that are up to 0.5 inch long and may be tinged pink or purple. Disk florets begin as yellow and become purple as they mature.

Habitat: Moist, low places, damp or drying meadows.

Distribution: Spotty throughout the state.

Plant Status: Native.

Cultivation: Prefers well-drained sandy, loamy, and clay soils that are rich, but can tolerate nutritionally poor soils. This species prefers sun but can succeed in partial shade.

Symphyotrichum lateriflorum

Other Names: Calico aster, farewell summer, side-flowering aster, starved aster, white woodland aster.

Medicinal Uses: Some Native American tribes use it for headaches and venereal diseases.

Description: Small white flowers are 0.5 inch across and bloom in clusters along the branches. Each flower has eight to fifteen white to purple-tinged rays which surround a disk; flowers mature to purplish-red. Leaves turn coppery in late summer and grow to 1.5 inches wide by 6 inches long. Leaves significantly decrease in size as they ascend the stems.

Habitat: Fields, sandy and moist boggy areas, thickets.

Distribution: Most of the state.

Plant Status: Native.

Cultivation: Prefers moist, semishaded woodland areas. Tolerates periodic flooding. Stems may be pinched back in late spring to early summer if shorter plants are desired.

Symphyotrichum oolentangiense

Other Names: Sky-blue aster, sky blue American aster.

Medicinal Uses: Used by some Native American tribes for skin ailments and constipation.

Description: Plant grows 1–5 feet tall with flower head arranged in an elongated, spreading cluster. Each flower has ten to twenty pale-lavender rays surrounding yellow disk flowers (that turn reddish with age), and blossoms are 0.5–0.75 inch wide. Lower leaves are elongated, up to 4 inches long, and somewhat heart-shaped, with a roughish surface.

Habitat: Edges of woods, open woods and prairies, and along roadsides. In rocky, sandy, open sites. Also grows well in rock gardens or perennial borders. It is valuable for prairie restoration projects.

Distribution: A few northern and central parishes.

Plant Status: Native.

Cultivation: Prefers full sun and is adaptable to a variety of soils if it is well drained. Requires average watering.

Symphyotrichum patens

Other Names: Late purple aster, spreading aster, spread-leaf aster, sky-drop aster.

Medicinal Uses: Internal—Respiratory conditions including asthma, allergies, colds, coughs, fevers, infections, laryngitis, and for anxiety. External—Rash from poison ivy, poison oak, poison sumac.

Description: Leaves clasp and surround the stem and are rough textured. Distinguished by light-purple blooms with bright-yellow centers. Grows 1.5–2.5 feet tall.

Habitat: Open, dry areas, rocky soils in open woodlands and fields, pastures, woodland borders.

Distribution: Top two-thirds of the state.

Plant Status: Native.

Cultivation: Seed germination improves with cold/moist stratification. Prefers open, sunny areas and medium to fine textured soils. Somewhat drought-tolerant.

Symphyotrichum praealtum

Other Names: Tall aster, willow leaf aster, veiny lined aster.

Medicinal Uses: Respiratory issues, immune health, digestive discomfort, antioxidant.

Description: Leaves are simple, narrow, alternate, slightly toothed and willow-like, up to 5 inches long and 0.75 inch wide, with pinnate major veins. Flowers are in heads, and the heads are in densely crowded panicles. White to lavender ray flowers and yellow disk flowers. Grows 2–5 feet tall. Small veins in a reticulated pattern are very noticeable on the whitish-green leaf undersides.

Habitat: Savannas, wet woods, meadows, prairies, and old fields.

Distribution: Much of the state, more heavily concentrated in bottom two-thirds of the state.

Plant Status: Native.

Cultivation: Easily grown in rich, moist loams in full sun to partial shade.

Symphyotrichum pratense

Other Names: Barrens silky aster, meadow aster, western silver aster.

Medicinal Uses: Skin irritations, edible.

Description: Distinguished from other asters by its appressed, whitish-looking leaves covered with fine appressed hairs, blue flower heads, and leaves that are not reduced on the flowering branches.

Habitat: Prairies, plains, meadows, pastures, savannas, ditches, ravines, depressions, open woods, and sandy soils.

Distribution: Spotty in western-central half of the state.

Plant Status: Native.

Cultivation: Seed germination improves with cold/moist stratification. Western silver aster self-sows and can also be divided in late fall or early spring. Cuttings can be taken in spring when shoots are 1.5–2 inches tall, and rooted in sand.

Symphyotrichum subulatum

Other Names: Eastern annual saltmarsh aster, hierba del marrano.

Medicinal Uses: Diarrhea, general health, inflammation, ulcers.

Description: Blossom has white to lavender ray flowers and bright-yellow disk florets, and are 0.5 inch wide. Leaves grow 1–2 inches long on a single erect stem that can reach up to 3 feet in height. Stem and thin green leaves are hairless. The top of the stem extends into a raceme.

Habitat: Brackish marshes, old fields, ditches, and occasionally in new restorations.

Distribution: Found in about a dozen southern parishes.

Plant Status: Native.

Cultivation: Prefers moist soil, shade to partial shade, and can tolerate a variety of soil types.

Symphyotrichum subulatum var. *ligulatum*

Other Names: Southern annual saltmarsh aster, lawn American-aster, white wood aster, saltmarsh aster.

Medicinal Uses: Diarrhea, inflammation, ulcers.

Description: Plant has smooth, slender, wiry stems that grow 1.5–5 feet tall.

Leaves are narrow, linear to subulate; lower-stem leaves grow 0.75–2 inches long, up to 0.5 inch wide. Few to many small white composite flowers in open panicular arrays, each less than 0.5 inch across, with sixteen to thirty white to lavender or purplish rays and four to ten yellow disk florets.

Habitat: Dry woods and clearings, ditches, swales, roadsides, and lawns.

Distribution: Most of the state.

Plant Status: Native.

Cultivation: Prefers moderate moisture, shade to partial shade, and alkaline soil that may be sandy, loam, clay, or limestone-based clay.

Symphyotrichum tenuifolium

Other Names: Perennial saltmarsh aster, saltmarsh aster.

Medicinal Uses: Like most asters, useful for asthma, congestions, spasms, seasonal allergies, cold, and flu.

Description: Blue ray flowers, occasionally white. Zigzag stems. No leaves on flowering branches, and leaves that grow 1–1.5 inches long.

Habitat: Salt or brackish marshes.

Distribution: Extreme southern parishes, often coastal areas.

Plant Status: Native.

Cultivation: May be propagated by seeds, cuttings, or division.

For All Species, Parts Used: Whole plant.

Medicinal Properties: Anti-inflammatory, antioxidant, antimicrobial, antispasmodic, anxiolytic, astringent, decongestant, diuretic, emmenagogue, immunomodulary, prebiotic, and wound healing properties. Significant nutritional content including Na, K, Ca, and Mg, vitamins A, B, C, and D, and some protein.

Uses: Internal—Asthma, colds, coughs, fevers, flu, respiratory infections, seasonal allergies; diarrhea, gastrointestinal disturbances; stress, occasional insomnia. External—Abrasions, cuts, minor burns or wounds, insect bites, poison ivy, poison oak, poison sumac rashes.

Risks: Avoid during pregnancy; avoid if allergic to daisy family members (Compositae).

Animal Uses: Many species are eaten by deer, rabbits, wild turkeys, and are visited by pollinators, including butterflies and native bees.

Natural History: Genus name comes from the Greek *symph,* meaning "coming together," and *trich,* meaning "hair," in possible reference to the flower anthers. Many species of *Aster* aka *Symphyotrichum* have been used by various Native American tribes and by Indigenous and cultural healers.

Designation: Folkloric herbal medicine in U.S. and other countries, Indigenous and Native American plant remedy, traditional Chinese medicine herb, Ayurvedic herbal remedy, homeopathic remedy.

Cultivation: Propagation may be done by seed or division in spring. For division, cut into a clump, dividing it into two or more parts, and promptly plant them in their new location. Or seeds may be collected and sown shallowly in moist potting soil. Keep soil moist. Transplant seedlings to the garden once they have their first true leaves and are large enough to handle. See above for preferences of individual species.

Remedy Form: Internal—Tea, tincture. External—Compress, poultice, steam.

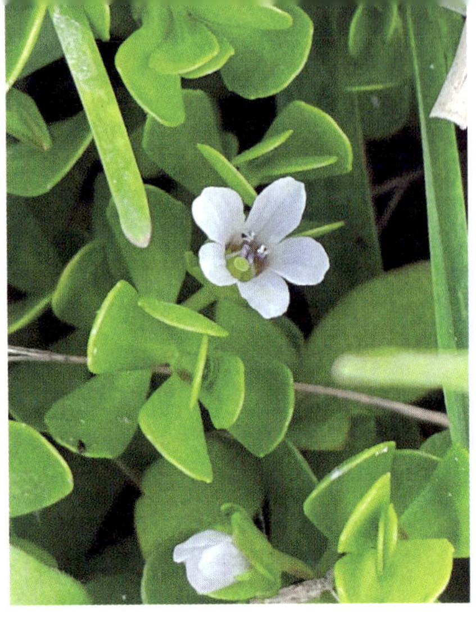

BACOPA & LIVING IN PLACE

LATE SPRING

Bacopa
(*Bacopa monnieri*)

On an early April day, the air is warm and close, the sky is patchy with fast-moving clouds, and the ground is damp underfoot. Today, I'm in search of bacopa—an herb I've heard about but had not spotted here until yesterday. At first, I thought what I'd found was another of the recently abundant blackberry flowers, but I soon figured out I was wrong. I took a photo of the little white flower and, using my phone app, was able to identify *Bacopa monnieri.* I was so excited! I've heard about bacopa's important medicinal properties, especially in Ayurvedic medicine, but have never been able to find it. And suddenly, there it was.

But now I can't remember exactly where I saw it, so I'm prowling over the levee and batture, bent down and peering close. I find the usual treasures, of course—the bur clover and black medic, the dependable and prickly cleavers, the hearty cranesbill still blooming even after being whacked down by the town mower crew. The lyreleaf sage is still flowering, sow thistles are starting to seed, the little blue veronicas are bright and hearty. And down near the batture pond, at the back of a battered house that has been empty since the latest hurricane, the limbs of several loquat trees are bending under the weight of ripe fruit. I trek down to taste a few, keeping my eyes on the ground while I walk. I stop to take a few photos of field madder and betony on the way down to the trees. I taste a few of the sweet loquats and then round off my treat with a few nibbles of corn salad—all in all, a lovely wild breakfast.

A cyclist passes by while I'm searching and feasting, and I imagine he wonders what I'm up to. It makes me reflect on what I do every day—

walking along, looking to see what's blooming or fruiting or seeding. This watchful meandering is so much a part of my life. It's how you know a place, I guess, how you find your own spot in the thatch of wild and tamer things, and how you make a home.

When I was in herb school decades ago, *Bacopa* wasn't really talked about much in Western herbalism. In the last decade, though, there has been more understanding of its healing properties, many of those gleaned from the Ayurvedic healing tradition of India. Recent research has proven the plant to be useful as an adaptogen—an herb that helps the body to handle stress. It has also been recognized as a nociceptive, which helps to nourish and protect the nervous system and to enhance cognition and memory. And bacopa has also proven to be useful for anxiety, attention deficit hyperactivity disorder (ADHD), and even for symptoms of Gulf War syndrome.

Before researching bacopa, I had seen it in garden centers sold as an ornamental plant. Now I know that it offers more than beauty and am eager to find it again. After a while, though, I give up and head for home. I check to see how the fruit trees are doing, and then—right in my own messy backyard—finally spot the bacopa again! Around the base of my fig tree, the plants are growing in a thick mat, interspersed with grass. Almost every stem is topped with a small pinkish-white flower. I am so happy to find it that I decide to make a small tincture of the plant before the lawn gets mowed. I run inside to grab a clean jar and am soon bending low again to start my harvest.

I break off a small leaf and taste it. Dewy-damp, and very slightly fleshy, the leaves are faintly bitter but not bad, and the flowers are a little sweet. Apparently, the plant parts used in making commercial preparations are stems and leaves. But all parts seem to have medicinal value, so I'm going to make a tincture out of whatever parts are aboveground.

At first, the picking isn't so easy—I have to separate each tiny stem from the blades of grass that grow along with it, then trace each stem down to its base and pluck it carefully. Sometimes the small flowers that decorate each stem drop off just as I touch the plant, so I learn how to nip the stems with my fingers while holding the flower in place. I imagine that this is going to be long and tedious work, but soon enough the little jar fills up. I pack the plant parts down so more will fit, add a few more bacopa stems into my jar, and head into the house. There, I pour grain alcohol over the plants, replace the lid, and label the contents. Now I just have to wait a couple of weeks for the healing properties to be leached out by the alcohol. In the meantime, I'm so happy to have found bacopa and can't wait to try my teensy tincture when it is ready. I'm happy, too, to have discovered so many healers in my raggedy lawn—so many more things to love.

I had an anatomy teacher once who told us that we are made of all the elements that surround our bodies in nature—in the air and water. We are made of stardust, she said—siblings to the whole universe—the stars and planets and moon. And I think she was right, because here I am, tasting the bacopa and corn salad, the black medic and loquats, and they taste like home.

Other Names: *Bacopa monnieri,* coastal waterhyssop, herb-of-grace, water hyssop, brahmi, three-leaf granola, Indian pennywort.

Parts Used: All parts have healing properties, though commercially only stems and leaves are used.

Medicinal Properties: Adaptogen, anticancer, antidepressant, antioxidant, anxiolytic, astringent, cardiotonic, cholinergic, cognition enhancing, diuretic, mild laxative, neuroprotective, refrigerant, sedative, vasoconstrictive.

Uses: Alzheimer's disease, anxiety, attention deficit hyperactivity disorder (ADHD), Gulf War syndrome, and to improve intellect, memory, and concentration. Used preventively for seizures. Also used as a wild edible. In Ayurvedic medicine, bacopa's healing properties are thought to be absorbed best if taken with a fatty food.

Risks: Though probably safe for most people, bacopa should be avoided by pregnant women and those with stomach ulcers, thyroid disease, intestinal blockages, urinary obstruction, a slow heart rate, or a lung disease. If taking certain drugs (including fluoxetine, thyroid hormones, or drugs to treat Alzheimer's disease, glaucoma, high blood pressure, or diabetes), seek a physician's guidance before taking bacopa.

Description: Leaves are succulent, oblong, opposing, slightly thick, 0.2 inch wide and 0.5 inch long, and one-veined. Flowers are small and white, with four to five petals, one petal often larger than the others. The plant often grows in fresh or brackish waters. (Two other *Bacopa* species can be found in Louisiana—*B. caroliniana* and *B. rotundifolia,* both of which have been documented to have some medicinal properties, though *B. monnieri* is the most often used in commerce.)

Habitat: Sandy margins of fresh or brackish marshes, freshwater tidal marshes, riparian areas, streams, pools, and muddy shores.

Distribution: Throughout most of the state.

Plant Status: Native.

Animal Use: Bees, butterflies, and possibly deer, cattle, and rabbits.

Natural History: The Acadian French name for water hyssop is *pourpier de marais,* which means "marsh purslane."

Designation: Important Ayurvedic herb, herb of commerce, edible.

Cultivation: Bacopa requires a sunny or partially sunny location and protection from drying winds. Should be watered daily when summer temperatures rise. If allowed to dry out, bacopa will stop blooming, and it will take a week or two for it to send out a new crop of flowers.

Remedy Form: Edible, tea, tincture, powder, capsules.

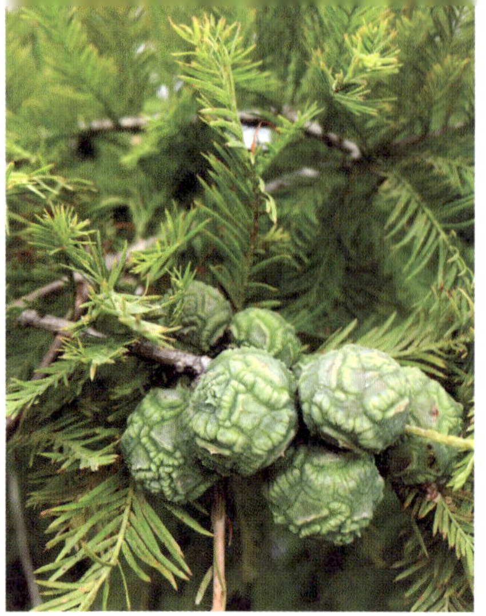

BALD CYPRESS & THE END OF BAYOU GAUCHE

WINTER

Bald cypress
(*Taxodium distichum*)

After a busy day of house chores, my little labradoodle, Bodi, and I are ready for a change. Though it's kind of late to head out for a trek, I drive to Bayou Gauche as the sun sinks in the sky. It's not too far from home, and the little island is one of our favorite places to walk. I remember hearing my dad talk about fishing out there when he was young, and I know that the island has an interesting history. Today, though, instead of fish, I've come for the quiet, the slow-moving water, and the birds and wildlife. And Bodi loves the scent trails and the chance to be off leash, with so few people and pets around.

But I have some worries for this place. Always a little ragtag spot, it's at high risk these days, being surrounded by so much water. The most recent hurricane took a big toll. Some of the damage on the island has been fixed, but many houses are still draped with blue tarps that flap in the constant wind. Some places have just been abandoned. I recently heard that about half the people who had houses in Bayou Gauche have left for good—no longer able, or willing, to keep up the fight. A few of my cousins are among those folks. Their homes were wrecked by the storm, so they have settled farther inland for now. Even though they loved living there, it's just too risky, they say.

Lately, I come here as often as I can. Sometimes the road is iffy, flooded after a heavy rain. Today it's not too bad. With no recent deluge, the road is passable, and a few folks wave as we drive by. A couple of boat trailers are parked at the launch. Bodi and I check out an old wrecked boat tucked at the edge of a little marsh and spot two glossy ibis in winter plumage fishing in the shallows. They squawk at us and sail up to a nearby tree as we start our walk. In a small wind, the water lifts and sinks and ripples just as the sun drops into the horizon, another gorgeous day's end in Bayou Gauche.

As lovely as this spot is, though, it is also broken. Some of the piles of house debris left over from the big storm have been removed, but the bayou side is still a mess of battered trees. One of my favorites, a tall bald cypress, has lost much of its height. All that's left now is the lower trunk and a few hardy limbs that stretch out just below the spot where the tree snapped off in 150 mph winds. In today's cooler temps, the cones hang from branches like dull ornaments on a Christmas tree, dangling in the breeze.

I wonder if this bald cypress will survive—and how long it can stand as the rising bayou water drags soil from its roots. I've always loved cypress trees—especially the scent of their feathery "leaves" and the sticky resin that clings to the green cones. My interest in this broken tree prompted me to research its possible uses for healing, and I found quite a few medicinal properties listed for the plant. Apparently, it has antibacterial, antifungal, antitumor, antispasmodic, antiviral, and bronchodilator activities. Cypress trees—members of the genus *Cupressus*—have documented historical uses for more than four thousand years. And though not a true cypress, *Taxodium distichum* does share many of its cousin's properties and uses. It has reportedly been used internally to treat bronchitis, diarrhea, gout, and heart disease, as well as malaria and liver ailments. And various parts of the tree have been used to prepare ointments for hemorrhoids, ulcers, and wounds. Some research has proven its use for the treatment of viruses, an important potential, given recent worldwide health concerns.

The tree has important environmental uses as well. In low-lying areas, it can gather sediment, soak up floodwaters and slow their onset, and trap pollutants and prevent them from spreading. The tree has wildlife uses, too. It's not too finicky about moisture, can tolerate both wet and dry periods, and offers habitat and hunting opportunities for ducks, cranes, eagles, and other birds, and for small mammals and even some insects. Grown in home gardens, it can provide cover for beneficial wildlife and offer shade and autumn color, while also helping to soak up floodwaters. I'm not sure how many folks here would use the tree for healing, but it's fun to know its history. And maybe if we begin to appreciate how much benefit the bald cypress provides to this waterlogged land, we can all keep an eye on how the trees are doing and somehow contribute to their healing and thriving.

I don't know what we can do for the island, though, or for places like it. It's such a hard and sad choice to have to make—stay or leave. Fight or give up. Find solutions or just figure we'll have to get used to the bustle of everyday life without living close to nature's low-lying areas. I do know that I need places like this—quiet, set aside, and away from the fractured fray of everyday modern life. Bayou Gauche and the cypress trees offer something constant, even when they're broken—a healing not only for our bodies but also for our exhausted minds and our deeper, tender, and most sensitive selves.

For now, for as long as we can, Bodi and I will trek out here to Bayou Gauche, park down at the boat launch, and amble around in the waterlogged quiet, soaking it all up. And maybe what's left of this broken tree will still produce enough sap and resin for me to make a small batch of salve, or I can find another cypress nearby that's still tall and whole. But I look forward to using bald cypress for healing, and for a sweet and poignant reminder of a place that may only exist in memory years from now.

I take a few photos of the sun sinking into the water and of the flaming sky it leaves behind and then pack Bodi into the car and head on home.

Other Names: *Taxodium distichum,* southern cypress, swamp cypress, Gulf cypress, yellow cypress, red cypress, white cypress.

Parts Used: Cones, seeds, leaves, bark, resin.

Medicinal Properties: Antibacterial, antifungal, anti-inflammatory, antispasmodic, antitumor, antiviral, bronchodilator, carminative, diuretic, vulnerary.

Uses: Internal—Benign prostatic hyperplasia (BPH); circulatory abnormalities including phlebitis, varices (ulcers), varicose veins; coughs, colds, bronchitis; diarrhea; heart disease; gout; hemorrhoids; liver support; nosebleed; tumors; ulcers. Historically used for malaria. External—Hemorrhoids, burns, wounds, fungal and bacterial infection, eczema and psoriasis, chest rub for colds. In Ayurvedic medicine, cypress helps alleviate stress, depression, and grief and is used to help regulate female hormones and relieve ovarian cysts.

Risks: Those with sensitivity to cedar, peaches, or adhesive bandages might have allergic reactions to cypress. Cypress might increase the risk of bleeding during and after surgery. Stop taking cypress at least two weeks before a scheduled surgery.

Description: A large, deciduous evergreen tree with a tapering trunk, buttressed at its base with knee-like structures arising from the roots. Young branches are green, becoming brown the first winter and bearing feathery, compound leaves that are alternate, linear, and flat. Needles point upward. Tree can be up to 120 feet in height and 3.5 feet in diameter. The tree has a taproot with horizontal roots that can expand horizontally for up to 50 feet before bending down.

Habitat: Swamps, near rivers and streams, in brackish water, and sometimes cultivated in upland areas.

Distribution: Throughout most of the state.

Plant Status: Native.

Animal Use: Seeds are eaten by several species of ducks, cranes, swamp birds, evening grosbeaks, wild turkeys, and small mammals. The trees provide shelter to wildlife like owls, squirrels, raccoons, and birds, and catfish spawn beneath logs. Fishing spiders fish from the base of the trees, and bass may hunt among the roots. The height of the trees offers a safe haven for birds of prey like osprey and bald eagles.

Natural History: *Cypre* is the Acadian term for the bald cypress, and *Boscoyos* or *boscoillots* is the French term for cypress knees. The slow-growing, long-lived trees regularly live up to six hundred years. The rot-resistant heartwood of mature trees is highly valued and has been widely used to make fence posts, doors, flooring, caskets, houses, cabinetry, and boats. The name "bald cypress" comes from their tendency to be among the first trees in the South to lose their leaves in the fall. Historical cultures that employed the tree for medicinal uses include the Aztec, who used resin or pieces of burnt bark topically to treat burns and sores, and many Indigenous groups.

Designation: Indigenous healing traditions, Ayurvedic medicine; essential oil is used in aromatherapy.

Cultivation: Tree can tolerate full sun to partial shade and requires moderate water and maintenance. Growth is moderate to fast. Often 50–70 feet tall and 2.5 feet wide, but older specimens can be much taller. Provides wildlife habitat, fall color, and adapts to dry or wet conditions. Cypress "knees" should not be cut down.

Remedy Form: Tincture, tea, syrup, salve, essential oil.

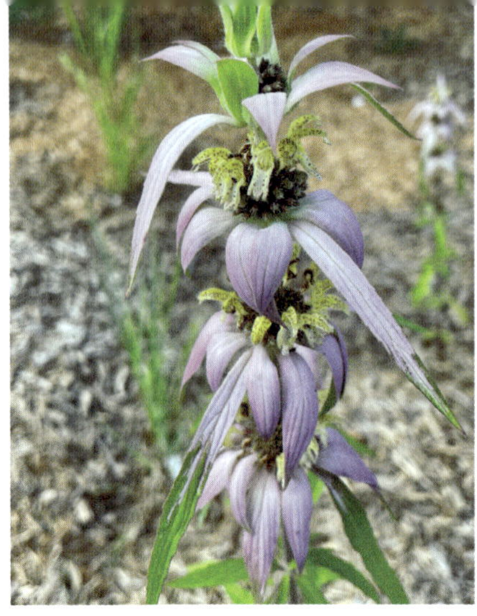

BEEBALM & THE AFTERMATH

SUMMER

Beebalm
(*Monarda* sp.)

It's a crazy time. So many things are awry. Sometime today, the tiny house next door will be moved back in the field where more of the hurricane damage can be repaired while a new foundation is laid. Later, a crew of workers will tear apart my mold-beleaguered laundry shed, rip off what is left of the carport roof, and take the first steps in healing my poor little home. Everywhere Bodi and I walk these days—months after the latest hurricane steamed through the town—we pass by devastation. More than half the roofs in town are still covered by blue tarps. The trees on the batture that once made a tall, wild fence between the river and the levee have been battered, broken, left in ruins. Every yard has a pile of debris waiting for the town to have the resources to pick it all up. Where it goes after that, I don't know yet. But we have gotten used to mowing around the piles.

And about every fourth house has a FEMA trailer in the yard, where residents are living until their place can be repaired. Some houses have collapsed, some just blown away. And, oddly, some places seem just fine. But that doesn't mean they are—140 mph winds, sustained for over twenty-four hours, take a toll. Foundations undermined, interior walls cracked, and the inevitable mold forming behind walls, around electrical outlets, in attics. And then there's the crazy circus of trying to navigate between low-balling insurance companies and high-balling contractors and the shortage of construction and repair workers. And the garden is a wreck—whatever potted plants didn't get blown away are ragged or just plain dead. It all makes for a pretty depressing time.

But this place is nothing if not resilient. And despite the mess, some signs of hope are emerging. The beebalms and the new monarch caterpillar chrysalis hanging under one wrinkled leaf are a couple of those signs. Like the people in Louisiana, beebalm adapts, survives, is flexible, gentle in its nature, strong in its constitution. Traditionally, beebalm flowers have been thought to signify sympathy, clarity of thought, prosperity, and protection. We could certainly use all of that.

Historically, beebalm was an important plant in sweat lodge ceremonies of East Coast Native American tribes. It also played a valuable role when colonists needed a drinkable substitute after the Boston Tea Party. Some say the plant was named for its ability to soothe bee stings. And it turns out that beebalm has so many healing compounds that it can help relieve a number of problems and is gentle enough to use on a daily basis.

Quite a few of the beebalms that grow in the wild in Louisiana have a history of medicinal use, and others can be easily cultivated. Louisiana botanist Charles Allen gifted me with several *Monarda* species when I visited him at Allen's Acres in Pitkin a few years ago. Since then, I've learned some of the medicinal properties of the plant and am eager to harvest some of the *Monardas* to use for tea and syrup. The beebalms are most commonly used for colds, flu, fevers, whooping cough and other upper respiratory problems, or for gastrointestinal illnesses including diarrhea or nausea. They are also said to support the nervous system, and they tend to be pretty hearty.

When Dr. Allen gave me the plants, I brought them home, tucked them into a corner of the garden, and then basically ignored them. Now, despite the messy, storm-battered yard, the beebalms are doing fine and have just started to bloom. I'm happy to have them in my garden and happy to be hosting plants that will offer nutrition to important pollinators.

I'm pretty sure that beebalm won't alleviate all—or any—of the problems that need to be solved in order for this area of the state to recover from the storm. But knowing that they have survived and even thrived despite the weather challenges gives me a little hope. If the beebalms can make it, who knows what we humans can do? Together, maybe we can make a stab at starting over again. Together, maybe we can heal.

As Bodi and I wrap up this morning's walk, sun rises through what's left of the batture woods. The church bells chime loudly, over and over. And suddenly the coyotes, who have taken refuge near the river now that the trees are down, begin to howl. I guess everything is hearing and answering the call. Together, they seem to say, we can weather anything. We are still here; we can rise again. And I believe.

At home, I check on the little monarch chrysalis, pick some sprigs of beebalm to use for tea, and get ready for the day.

Species: There are several *Monarda* species in the state. Those with medicinal properties and a history of use for healing include:

Monarda citriodora

Other Names: Lemon beebalm, purple horsemint, lemon mint, plains horsemint, lemon horsemint, horsemint, purple lemon mint.

Medicinal Uses: Internal—Coughs, colds, fevers, respiratory ailments; intestinal parasites. External—To repel fleas and mites. According to botanist James Duke, the plant has almost two hundred medicinally active compounds.

Description: Plant grows 12–30 inches tall and has tubular, scented, two-lipped, light-lavender to pink to white flowers that bloom in dense, globular, headlike clusters from May to August. Plant has a distinctive citrus or lemony scent when the leaves are crushed.

Habitat: In pastures, often with sandy loams or rocky soils on slopes and hills, or in prairies, meadows, and savannas.

Distribution: Spotty, found in about a dozen parishes throughout the state.

Animal Use: Acceptable to cattle as forage. Bees, butterflies, insects, and hummingbirds visit the plant for its nectar.

Cultivation: Prefers limestone-rich, rocky, or sandy soils, but tolerates other soils. Prefers full sun to partial shade. Plant seed in fall or early spring. This plant self-seeds and may form large colonies in optimum growing conditions.

Monarda fistulosa

Other Names: Bergamot, wild bergamot, horsemint, Oswego tea, mintleaf beebalm, wild bergamot, long-flowered horsemint, beebalm.

Medicinal Uses: Internal—Colds, congestion, headaches, fevers, sore throats; gastric disorders. External—Skin eruptions, cuts, sore eyes.

Description: Grows from slender creeping rhizomes and occurs in large clumps. Plants may grow up to 3 feet tall, with a few erect branches. Leaves are 2–3 inches long, lance-shaped, and toothed. Flower clusters are solitary at the ends of branches. Each cluster is about 1.5 inches long and contains about twenty to fifty flowers. Flowers from June to September.

Habitat: Dry, open fields, old fields, wet meadows, ditches, edges of woods and marshes, wooded slopes and meadows, sandy and dry soils.

Distribution: Top two-thirds of the state, spotty in a few central and southeastern parishes.

Plant Status: Native.

Animal Use: Acceptable cattle forage. A good hummingbird plant. Attracts clearwing sphinx moths and many butterflies.

Cultivation: Seeds may be harvested 1–3 weeks after flowering. Fruiting heads should be cut into paper bags and shaken to remove seed. The vegetable matter can then be removed by sieving. While seeds germinate well (1–2 weeks) without treatment, germination improves after cold/moist stratification. Tip cuttings may be taken May to August. Sections of rhizome root easily when taken during the summer and planted horizontally about 1 inch deep. Clumps are best divided in early spring before new stems appear. Responds well to pinching and fertilizing.

Monarda lindheimeri

Other Names: Lindheimer's beebalm.

Medicinal Uses: Flowers used as diaphoretic; leaves and flowers used as a gargle or tea for sore throats, fevers, colds, respiratory complaints. In general, contains the same medicinal compounds and has the same uses as other *Monarda* species.

Description: Grows 2–5 feet tall, 1–2 feet wide. Flowers occur in single terminal cluster of creamy-white flowers.

Habitat: Sandy soils usually on edges of woods and meadows, and slopes and flats.

Distribution: Acadia, Calcasieu, Jefferson Davis, and St. Landry Parishes.

Animal Use: Nectar for bees (especially bumblebees), butterflies, and a variety of other insects.

Plant Status: Native.

Cultivation: Propagate from cuttings of stem or root. Prefers full sun to partial shade, and average to well-drained soil, with even moisture. Similar propagation to *M. fistulosa,* and cold/dry stratification gets best results.

Monarda punctuata

Other Names: Spotted beebalm, spotted horsemint, dotted beebalm, horse mint.

Medicinal Uses: The herb has been used traditionally for gastrointestinal and respiratory ailments.

Description: Clump-forming, features branching or simple, square stems, 1–4 feet tall. Rosettes of yellowish, purple-spotted, tubular flowers occur in whorls, forming a dense, elongated spike at the end of the stem or from leaf axils. Each whorl is subtended by large, conspicuous, whitish, purple-tinged, leaflike bracts.

Habitat: Full-sun areas with dry soil in prairies, sandy areas, old pastures, rocky woodlands, coastal plains, and roadsides.

Distribution: Much of the state.

Animal Use: Good forage for cattle, and attracts a number of specialist bees, bumblebees, predatory wasps, hummingbirds, and hawk moths.

Plant Status: Native.

Cultivation: Fairly adaptable to various temperatures, dry conditions, and poor soil. Susceptible to powdery mildew and rust, especially in crowded gardens. Prune stems to increase airflow, pinch buds to encourage branching, and deadhead spent flowers. If the soil is allowed to dry out, the stressed plants become increasingly susceptible to disease.

For All Species, Parts Used: Aerial parts.

Medicinal Properties: Antifungal, analgesic, anti-inflammatory, antimicrobial, antiseptic, antispasmodic, bitter tonic, carminative, decongestant, diaphoretic, digestive stimulant, diuretic, emmenagogue, expectorant, local anesthetic, mild sedative, nervine tonic, nutritional.

Uses: Internal—Anxiety, stress; gastrointestinal ailments including nausea, vomiting, indigestion, and intestinal gas; coughs and respiratory tract symptoms including colds and flu, immune system support. External—Cuts, rashes, insect stings, fungal infections, minor burns, inflammation, pain. Gargle for gingivitis, sore throat, toothache.

Risks: Generally recognized as safe. Consult a health care provider if pregnant or lactating.

Animal Use: Many *Monarda* species provide important food for bees, hummingbirds, and other species.

Natural History: Seventeen species of *Monarda* are found throughout North America, and five of those occur in the wild in Louisiana. *M. didyma* and *M. fistulosa* are two of the most popular species, though over fifty cultivars of the plant exist. The *Monarda* plant was named for the Spanish physician and botanist Dr. Nicolas Monardes of Seville, Spain (1493–1588). Monardes authored the book *Joyful News—Botany of the New World (North America)* and attempted to keep the new plants' native names when reclassifying them. He never actually visited North America but had people bring the plants to his gardens in Spain. His book was translated into English in 1577.

Designation: Indigenous/Native American herb, Ayurvedic remedy, herb of commerce, Cajun traiteur remedy, flower essence, magical remedy.

Cultivation: See above for individual species.

Remedy Form: Internal—Tea, tincture, syrup/oxymel, flower essence, homeopathic remedy. External—Liniment, poultice, compress, salve.

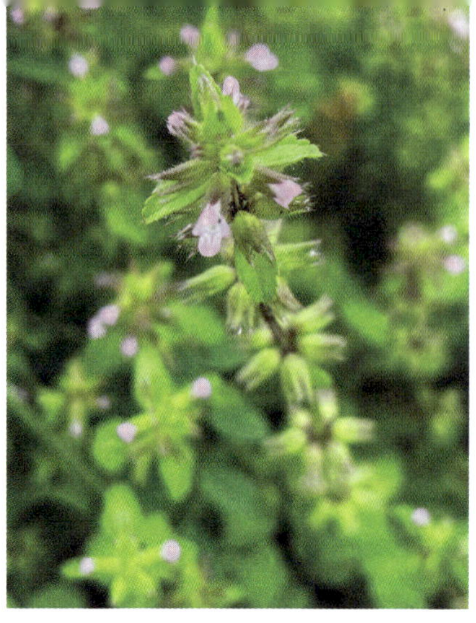

BETONY & THE CRANE FLIES

SPRING

Betony
[*Stachys* sp.]

One of the things I love about Louisiana is the lushness—the lands, the waters, creatures underfoot and overhead, the scents and sounds and textures that make a throbbing backdrop to my days and nights. A friend once told me that she wasn't surprised to find out I was from Louisiana—that the sensuous lushness of my home ground showed up in my language, in my house, in my love of land and waters and creatures. It's a southern thing, I guess.

This morning I'm out for a walk before light seeps into the sky. My little labradoodle, Bodi, is still snoozing when I leave, and I let him rest. The air is close and damp, and a thick fog blankets the yard, the batture, the woods, the river. It's a warm morning, in the high sixties, with a gray day predicted, and rain to come later. Layers of dark and lighter clouds—some fast moving, some motionless—crowd the sky. What's left of the full moon hangs in the west and gets covered over quickly by the fog.

Nearby, seven egrets sit in one small tree, and a little blue heron feeds in a shallow batture pond. And with every step I take, the newly born crane flies flit up out of the grass. They flick in loopy circles all around me and then settle on my head and arms. I'm learning more about them lately—how short their lives are as flies (one to two weeks), how long their larval stage lasts (up to two years), how helpful they are to the ecology of a place (eating leaf debris and helping to recycle nutrients), and what a bad reputation they have for being "giant mosquitoes." But, actually, they cannot bite and are only interested in mating and laying eggs in their short, winged lives.

I take a few photos of the sky as light begins to break through clouds and then head toward home. As I walk, I keep my eyes on the ground, eager to spot whatever plants are emerging in these warming days. Henbit, cleavers, violets, yellow dock, speedwell, and the many clovers have sprouted up all around. At the edge of the batture woods, I spot something new to me—a small, low-growing, thickly leaved plant, with pretty lavender flowers. It looks like a mint family member, with a squared stem and opposing leaves, and reminds me of something I've seen before.

Curious as to whether it is a medicinal herb, I check my field guide and find that it is a form of betony I've heard about but not seen. *Stachys arvensis,* the guide says. But that's kind of odd, because, according to the Plants of Louisiana website, this species doesn't occur in the state. Apparently, there is high variability among these species, which makes correct identification tough for an amateur botanist. Well, at least I was able to recognize one species in the past. Last year, I found what I am sure was Florida betony, *Stachys floridana,* growing alongside ditches. But that plant was a bit more delicate and was tucked into grass and clovers, whereas the plant here is taller and more sturdy looking. I decide to do some research on this species when I get home.

I know that *Stachys floridana* is useful for a number of minor health concerns, and I wonder if this species is as well. Apparently, many plants in the *Stachys* genus contain a wide variety of bioactive chemicals. And in ancient times, several species were collectively known as "woundwort" and were used for healing injuries. Seeds of the plant were scattered by Roman soldiers and reportedly continue to mark the lines of Italian roads. And even though Florida betony is considered an invasive weed in Louisiana, it is also known as a prized wild edible with very tasty roots. I guess one woman's invasive weed is another woman's healing treat!

I pick a few sprigs of this morning's *Stachys* and taste a small leaf—it is a bit fuzzy, tender, immediately astringent, then a little bitter, but not too bad. I can't say I'd want a whole salad of the leaves, but since the roots of Florida betony are a forager's delight, maybe that's true for this mystery species, too. I'm not ready to dig up these roots to try them, though. Since they're growing close to the road, I'm concerned about pollutants in the soil. But I'll know now what to look for when I get a chance to hike back into a cousin's field. And at some point, maybe I can seed these into a little patch of my flower garden to have my own supply.

Arriving home, I tie my betony bundle to dry and boil some water for tea. While I work, a "passenger" crane fly—having ridden in on my jacket sleeve—lifts up into the kitchen. I gently clasp a few fragile spindly legs, open the back door and let it flit up into the air outside where it can enjoy the rest of its very short life. And I'm happy. Today I've gained more knowledge about crane flies, discovered another of the quirky *Stachys* species, and am grateful for the wildlings outside my door—all offering their own gifts.

Species: There are several *Stachys* species in the state, and some have medicinal properties and a history of use for healing. These include:

Stachys crenata

Other Names: Shade betony, mouse-ear.

Medicinal Uses: Colds, pneumonia, pain.

Description: Plant is an annual or biennial with hairy stems that are usually branched at the base. Leaves are ovate to oblong with rounded teeth along the margins. Pink to lavender flowers are two-lipped and borne in small clusters both terminally and in the leaf axils. Leaves have blunt or rounded teeth (crenate). Leaf blade is acutely apical.

Habitat: Grows in mostly shaded, rocky, or gravelly soils in woods, ravines in prairies, and stream banks.

Distribution: Found throughout most of Louisiana and East-Central and South Texas.

Animal Use: Flowers are a favorite nectar source for small bees and other insects

Stachys floridana

Other Names: Chinese artichoke, Florida betony, Florida hedgenettle.

Medicinal Uses: Headaches, anxiety, nervous system support; edible.

Description: Plant has a hairy, erect stem that grows up to about 18 inches from a network of rhizomes with tubers. Tuber is typically 0.5 inch wide and 1–4 inches long but can grow to 8 inches or longer. New tubers are formed in late spring, as the temperatures begin to increase, and are segmented, resembling the rattle on the tail of a rattlesnake. Leaves are opposing, about 2 inches long. Trumpet-shaped flowers grow in clusters of three to six from the upper leaf axils. Tubular, hairy calyx has pointed lobes. The two-lipped corolla is white to pink with purple spots or darker lines.

Habitat: Wet, sandy soils, roadsides, thickets, shrub borders.

Distribution: Scattered throughout three dozen parishes, concentrated more heavily in southwestern areas.

Animal Use: Nectar source for some insects.

Stachys tenuifolia

Other Names: Smooth hedgenettle, slender betony, thinleaf betony, slenderleaf betony.

Medicinal Uses: Gargle for sore throat; poultice or wash for boils, sores, earaches, wounds.

Description: Leaves with serrate edges, petiole is one-third as long as the leaf blade, and leaf blade is rounded apically. Plants have hairy, erect stems reaching 19 inches high and are square in cross-section with flowers in long clusters, heads, or interrupted whorls on the stem. Plant grows from a network of rhizomes with tubers. Pale-colored tuber is segmented and resembles the rattle on the tail of a rattlesnake. The oppositely arranged leaves have blades up to 2 inches long. Flowers grow in clusters of three to six from the upper leaf axils. The tubular, hairy calyx of sepals has pointed lobes. The two-lipped corolla is up to 0.5 inch long and white to pink with purple spots. The fruit is a schizocarp less than an inch long that splits in half.

Habitat: Bottomland hardwood forests and batture areas.

Distribution: Found in most parishes in the state.

Animal Use: Long-tongued bees pollinate the flowers. Butterflies and hummingbirds use the flowers for nectar. Checkerspot larvae will use the foliage for food.

For All Species, Parts Used: Aerial parts, roots.

Medicinal Properties: Anxiolytic, analgesic, anti-Alzheimer's, antidiabetic, antifungal, anti-inflammatory, antimicrobial, antioxidant, anticholinesterase, antidepressant, hepatoprotective.

Uses: Stress relief, skin inflammations, gastrointestinal disorders, asthma and respiratory symptoms. Genital tumors treated in many herbal traditions. Some in vitro studies suggested that at least one *Stachys* species was helpful in relieving polycystic ovary syndrome (PCOS).

Risks: Use during pregnancy should be monitored by a health care practitioner.

Natural History: About three hundred *Stachys* species can be found in temperate regions of the Mediterranean, Asia, America, and southern Africa. Long revered throughout ancient Europe for healing and magical properties, *Stachys* was the most prized medicinal plant of Anglo-Saxons and Romans. Several species of this genus are extensively used in various traditional medicines, and many share similar chemicals. The genus name is derived from the Greek word *stachys,* which refers to the type of the inflorescence that is characterized as a "spike of corn."

Designation: Native American remedy, prized healing plant of ancient Europe.

Cultivation: Most *Stachys* are unfussy about the soil and growing conditions but prefer full sun and soil that doesn't become soggy in winter. Plants should only need watering until they are established. Otherwise, they are fairly drought-tolerant and only need watering if they show signs of wilting in prolonged spells of dry weather. Feeding isn't normally necessary.

Remedy Form: Internal—Edible, tea, tincture. External—Poultice, compress, wash.

BETONY PICKLES

Several good-sized tubers, cleaned and sliced

One medium onion, sliced thinly

1 1/2 cups white sugar

1/4 cup brown sugar

2 cups apple cider vinegar

3 teaspoons mustard seeds

1. Place sliced tubers and onions in clean jar.
2. Combine sugars, vinegar, mustard seeds. Place over medium heat.
3. Cook until sugar is dissolved.
4. Pour brine over tubers and onion, then let cool.
5. Seal and label. Place in refrigerator and let sit at least 12 hours.

(www.holisticlivingschool.org/2019/03/14/april-plant-of-the-month-fl-betony/)

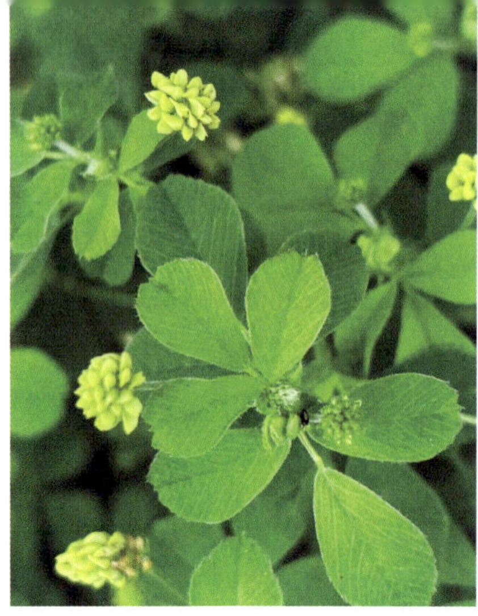

BLACK MEDIC & BODI'S PAWS

SPRING

Black medic
(*Medicago lupulina*)

In mid-February, Bodi and I take a short walk along the levee and then through town. It's a blustery day, and egrets are hanging out in the marshy woods, trying to escape the wind. The air is cool, but there is sun, blue sky with multilayered clouds, and much plant growth. The lyreleaf sage is getting lush, violets are abundant, and the loquat fruits are starting to ripen. Patches of clover-type herbs are spreading out all over the batture, coming into flower. White clover colonies are humming with bees, some red clover blooms are starting to open, and the white and yellow sweet clovers crowd the path near the river.

But today it's the black medic that I'm tracking down. When I first arrived in Louisiana, I was intrigued with the vining, yellow-flowered plants I saw all along the levee, and I did some research. It turned out that these belong to the *Medicago* genus and aren't just one species but several. And two of them—black medic and bur clover—are so similar that only recently have I learned to tell them apart. And that's important, because one species is a great healing herb, and another is downright pesky.

As the two related clovers—black medic and bur clover—begin to bloom, they look very much alike, with cloverlike leaves and small yellow flower clusters. To confuse the picture, they grow side by side and often intertwine. But later in the season, black medic blooms and then sets small innocuous seeds, whereas the bur clover begins to develop "Bodi's nemesis," the sharply prickled seed pinwheels that plague his curly hair. By midspring, with every walk we take, Bodi ends up limping along, and I end up bent over trying to pull out the painful prickles from his hairy paws. One morning, after a walk, I pulled out thirty burs from just one foot. And his tail is often matted with the seeds. He's learned to chew them out from wherever he can reach, but he just spits them on the floor, where I'm constantly stepping on them when I walk around the house barefoot.

The most well-known of the medicinal *Medicago*—alfalfa, or *Medicago sativa*—is a highly revered healing plant. That purple-flowered herb is appreciated by the herb community for its antioxidant and anti-inflammatory properties. And the flowering tops contain vitamins A, C, E, and K4, as well as calcium, potassium, phosphorous, and iron. Alfalfa has been proven to reduce cholesterol absorption in the digestive tract and has a history of use for such issues as high cholesterol, asthma, osteoarthritis and rheumatoid arthritis, and diabetes. It has also been used supportively for kidney and bladder problems, prostate issues, and digestive upsets. It has been proven to stimulate the immune system and to have weak estrogenic effects. And it turns out that at least several of its cousins have some of the same effects. But there's still the problem of knowing which ones to pick.

Just lately, though, I've found some identification clues. It turns out that the flowerheads of black medic, or *Medicago lupulina,* bear eight to thirty buds, whereas the bur clover has only three to eight. A third species, *Medicago persica,* or Persian clover, is easy to identify—each of its cloverlike leaves are marked with a black spot. Another challenging fact about these *Medicago,* though, is that while they share so many characteristics, the black medic has a history of many medicinal uses, whereas both bur clover and Persian clover have apparently shown to have few healing properties. Some vague references are made to bur clover's use in Chinese and Korean medicine, and research studies hint at its potential for relieving diabetes. But black medic has been well researched, so for now I'm hoping to limit my harvesting to that species. If I find it, I can use it for tea, and maybe for tincture or salve. So far, I've discovered that the herb is rich in essential minerals and has antibacterial and antifungal properties. It's also known to support the body's blood-clotting process, which could make it helpful as an external application for small cuts and scratches. And due to its fiber contents, the herb can help promote healthy digestion and has a mild laxative effect, making it a great natural remedy for constipation. The herb has also been used as an effective green manure cover crop, gradually improving the fertility of the soil where it grows.

Inspired by all this information, I kneel down to peer more closely at the clovers around our feet. I try to remember what features go with which *Medicago* species, and then, finally, I think I've got it. One thick clump of *Medicago* has the usual lush clover leaves and yellow flower buds, but these unfolding buds are so numerous I realize that this is what I've been looking for—black medic! I'm so excited that I decide to make a small harvest of the herb. While I pick small lengths of the herb, Bodi continues to sniff and discover, and we both keep an eye on the red-shouldered hawks that sail overhead as nearby crows squabble over a found tidbit.

At home, I chop up my little bundle of black medic, boil water, pour it over the herb, and then let it steep while Bodi settles into his post-walk snooze. I'm eager to see if this herb makes a difference in my irritating arthritis. I'll also want to keep it on hand to use in salves for cuts and scratches, since it is known to help with blood clotting. And I'll want to make another harvest soon, before the prickly pinwheels on bur clover develop. Still, I'm glad that these plants are good at protecting themselves and at spreading their seeds. In the future, they can help to stabilize sandy banks and eroded soil—an important quality as the state wrestles with subsidence and land loss. I might even try to transplant some of the black medic species and encourage its growth on a newly turned plot of soil where I'd like to introduce more native plants. That way, the herb can do double duty—enhancing my soil and going into medicinal preparations I'll use for my health.

As pesky as the bur clover can be, I'm developing a greater gratitude for the *Medicago* tribe of plants that offer both healing and nutrients wherever they grow. And Bodi and I will just try to avoid walking around the bur clover plants when they are getting ready to seed.

Species: Several species of *Medicago* grow in the state and have documented healing properties. These include:

Medicago arabica

Other Names: Spotted medick, southern burr clover, spotted burrclover, calvary clover, hogweed.

Medicinal Uses: Inflammation, attention deficit hyperactivity disorder (ADHD), erythema, edema, hypothermia, chills.

Description: A prostrate or sprawling herb that grows about 1–2.5 feet tall. Leaves alternate along the stems and are pinnately compound, with three leaflets. Margins are toothed toward the tips. Upper surface is hairless, usually with a dark patch near the middle. Flowers are pale yellow. This plant differs from its more frequently found cousin, black medic, not only by its trefoil leaves having one dark spot in the center of each heart-shaped leaflet but also by its seed pods. These are twisted, spiny pods with little hooks on them.

Habitat: Moist stream banks, grasslands, thin pasture, lawns, meadows and fields, and disturbed areas including waste lots and roadsides.

Distribution: Throughout the state.

Plant Status: Native.

Cultivation: Prefers light, sandy, and gravelly soils.

Medicago lupulina

Other Names: Black medic, black medic clover, black medick, hop clover, hop medic, nonesuch, yellow trefoil.

Parts Used: Whole plant.

Medicinal Uses: Internal—Mild bacterial infections, nutritious edible, constipation. External—Minor wounds.

Description: Distinguished from other species by its entire stipules (not spiny) and eight to thirty flowers. May be confused with *Medicago polymorpha,* which typically only has three to five flowers and has stipules that are deeply toothed, and from *Medicago arabica,* which has dark spots on its leaves.

Habitat: Fields, lawns, pastures, streams, prairies, roadsides, waste places, and other disturbed areas.

Distribution: Throughout most parishes in the state.

Plant Status: Introduced.

Cultivation: Plant clumps in direct sunlight. Soil should drain well, though the plant likes to remain moist. Loamy soil with a pH of 6.0–6.8 is optimal. Seed can be sown any time of year except late fall and winter. Soak seeds in warm water for at least 12 hours before planting. Space 12 inches apart, cover seeds lightly in soil, and tamp down gently. Water well, but don't soak the soil.

Medicago polymorpha

Other Names: Burr clover, bur medick, toothed medick, California burclover, smooth bur-clover.

Medicinal Uses: External—Skin placques, rheumatic pains, wounds.

Description: An annual sprawling broadleaf legume that grows about 6–22 inches in many areas. Stem is weak but may become erect. Leaves have a characteristic cloverlike shape, appearing alternately on the stems, and have slightly serrated edges. Flowers are cloverlike, small, bright yellow, and cluster into flower heads of two to ten flowers at the stem tips. Fruit is a prickly, flattened, and coiled pod, about 0.15–0.4 inch in length. Pod prickles often end in tiny hooks and cling to animal fur/wool. The pods contain several kidney-shaped seeds.

Habitat: Common lawn weed, in fields, roadsides, and waste places.

Distribution: Most of the state.

Plant Status: Introduced.

Cultivation: Prefers well-drained, neutral to slightly alkaline soils, and requires regular irrigation in drought conditions. Thrives in full sun.

For All Species, Parts Used: Whole plant.

Medicinal Properties: Analgesic, antidiarrheal, anti-inflammatory, antifungal, antioxidant, anthelmintic, immunomodulary.

Uses: Various internal and external uses including ADHD; bacterial infections, chills; constipation, dysentery; edema; edible; erythema, pain, minor wounds (external). See above for specific uses of individual species.

Risks: Should not be used by pregnant women or children, or by those taking pharmaceutical anticoagulants. Should be heated before use; that is, in tea or as a steamed green.

Animal Use: Numerous species utilize the foliage in daily diets. Many wild herbivores including deer, mice, woodchucks, bees, flies, and small butterflies will nibble the plants, and many classes of livestock (except horses and mules) will eat it as forage.

Natural History: *Medicago* is a genus of flowering plants that includes over eighty species, which are distributed mainly around the Mediterranean basin. The best-known species is alfalfa (*M. sativa*), but numerous species are important forage crops and are utilized in local areas for healing. The genus name originates from the Greek *medica*, which translates roughly to "medicinal grass."

Designation: Native American edible and medicinal herb; seeds and leaves are edible. In Europe and Asia, the foliage is cooked much like collards or spinach. Also used in Ayurvedic, homeopathic, and naturopathic medicine.

Remedy Form: Internal—Edible, tea. External—Compress, poultice, wash.

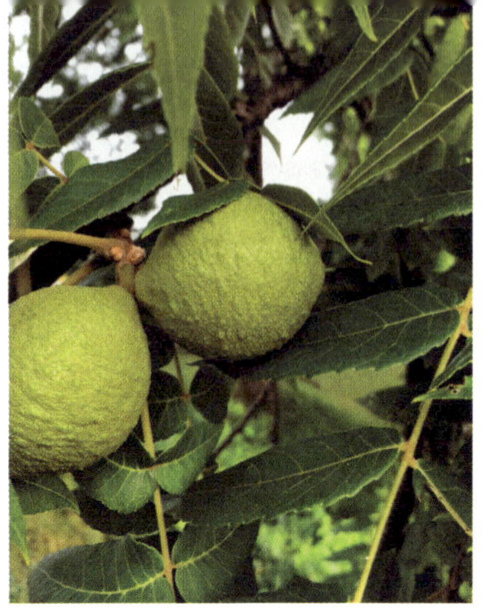

BLACK WALNUT TREE & THE BROKEN HOUSE

WINTER

Black walnut
(*Juglans nigra*)

When I was a child, my sister and I walked to school. I loved to take the "wild" way there—trekking into some neglected place that was so much more interesting than the street. I'd push my way through tall bamboo or slip down to the intracoastal canal to see what floated by. Shaking the grasses for snakes, I'd check to see what was growing around me. I'd sniff up damp air, and search for anything interesting. One of my favorite things to find in autumn was the huge fruits of the black walnut tree that grew not too far from the water. If I managed to pry the hulls open, my fingers would be stained dark brown, and the penetrating scent of the walnut's oil would waft around me for much of the day. I liked that smell and liked my time away from the well-traveled road. Little did I know then that this tree had so many healing properties and nutrients, in addition to its potent scent.

A native plant in much of Louisiana, the tree has a number of historical and medicinal uses, but I haven't really employed it much so far. Recently, I was reintroduced to the tree by a neighbor and did a little research on some of its benefits.

This morning, I walk down the road and past my neighbor's house. M is an interesting guy—a would-be holdover from the 1960s and sort of reclusive. We've become neighborhood friends, and he often sees me before I spot him. Today he's perched high in a tree, secured by some old ropes he's tied around himself, his limb-cutting gear lugged up and tied close by. He's trimming the tree, he says, because his new neighbor, a woman who loves her yard and has planted roses and other shrubs, wants more sun for her garden. And since the tree is on his property, he's doing the work, grudgingly but surely. Day by day, step by lofty step.

He's a grizzled kind of guy. I've never seen him in anything other than a raggedy pair of gray overalls. He's often barefoot, no matter the season. His hair is shoulder length; his beard and mustache mostly cover his face. He has an old, grayish truck tucked near a rattletrap shed. And his house, falling down and broken, rests under a lowering tunnel of trees. The whole back has folded in on itself, the roof caved in. I worry about him and his fusty-messy home, and whether he's safe there.

But his woodpile is tidy. Every day he works at the bits of tree limbs he's taken off. The foot-long lengths are lined up, leading out, in two even lines, to the street. I ask him if he is going to use them for firewood, now that they're neatly cut and lined up. He is eager to tell me about it. The tree is a black walnut, he says, and it burns well. He's also heard that the green hulls of the nuts can relieve indigestion and constipation.

I recall what I've heard from healer friends—that black walnut hulls make an excellent digestive tonic, especially for heartburn, intestinal gas, and stomach ulcers, and I know that the nut has numerous nutritional benefits. Research has proven that some of the natural compounds in the plant have anticancer, anti-inflammatory, and antioxidant properties, and that parts of the tree can support cardiac health and protect nervous system tissues. Some Native American tribes and Asian cultures have used the various tree parts for fevers, kidney ailments, toothache, snakebites, syphilis, and colic. The nut hulls have been proven to stimulate the flow of bile, inhibit bacterial and fungal growth, and can help control skin, mucosal, and oral infections.

So it turns out M is right—the tree parts do have numerous healing properties. But I'm pretty sure that cutting a few branches won't help his neighbor's rose bushes. I also remember hearing that the tree produces an organic compound in the soil that negatively impacts plants that grow within thirty feet of it, often severely diminishing growth if not actually killing them—a process called allelopathy. But I'm guessing that if it turns out to be the case in this instance, it will take a while, and neither M nor his neighbor will make the connection. In the meantime, he's doing his best to help out his friend.

And as for me, now that M has reintroduced me to black walnut, I'll be keeping an eye out for it and might come over to harvest some of the fallen nuts for their hull. Maybe I can get M to cut off some bark so I can try that, too. In the meantime, I'll be keeping an eye out for him, to make sure he's okay. Snarky and feisty and independent, wise in the ways of the land, my neighbor and the walnut trees have deep roots in this ragtag place. And they are two great examples of spunky resilience close to home.

Other Names: *Juglans nigra,* black walnut, noyer noir, eastern black walnut.

Parts Used: Fruit/nut, nut hull, bark, roots, leaves, oil.

Medicinal Properties: Highly nutritious edible, containing many vitamins and minerals including magnesium, phosphorus, potassium, iron, zinc, copper, manganese, and selenium, as well as fiber and omega-3 and omega-6 fatty acids. Additional healing properties include: alterative; anodyne; anti-aging; anticancer for mouth, esophagus, breast, liver, lung, skin, pancreas, cervix, and colon; anthelmintic; antidiabetic; antifungal; anti-hypertensive; antimicrobial; antinociceptive, memory booster; antioxidant; astringent; gastroprotective, hepatoprotective, liver and kidney protective; lipid-lowering; laxative/vermifuge.

Uses: Bacterial and fungal infections of skin and oral mucosa, *Candida* yeast infections; colic, diarrhea; herpes, eczema; toothache; headache; hypertension; decrease or cessation of milk production in nursing mothers trying to wean infants (use under direction of a health care practitioner). External—Athlete's foot, ringworm, wounds.

Risks: Bark should only be used internally for short periods of time. Avoid if allergic to tree nuts. Skin contact with hull or oil may cause local irritation. Walnut preparations contain high concentrations of tannins. If taking pharmaceutical medications, take walnut preparations at least one hour before or after medications. If pregnant, use only under the guidance of a health care practitioner.

Description: Mature tree height is 70–100 feet. Leaves are alternate, compound, and deciduous, and have twelve to twenty-four leaflets along a stout, light-brown twig. Leaf is aromatic when crushed. Fruit is a nut that measures 1.5–2.5 inches around and is covered by a fleshy, thick, light-green husk. Buds are pale, silky, and covered in downy hairs. Catkins (male, tassel-like flowers) and small female flowers, both found near tip of stem, are yellowish-green and brown. Bark is gray-black and deeply furrowed into thin ridges that give the bark a diamond-shaped pattern. Pith of the twigs is chambered and light brown.

Habitat: Rich, moist bottomlands, fields.

Distribution: Northwestern parts of the state. Cultivated in other areas.

Plant Status: Native.

Animal Use: A favorite food for red and gray squirrels. Preferred host for the luna and regal moths. Deer browse on buds, mice and rabbits nibble young tree stems, and eastern screech owls roost in the tree.

Natural History: Tree is native to the Himalayas, Kyrgyzstan, and Central Asia and was cultivated in Europe as early as 100 BC. Black walnut is an important tree commercially, as the wood is a deep-brown color and easily worked. Walnut seeds (nuts) are cultivated for their distinctive and desirable taste, and the trees are grown both for lumber and food. Many Native American tribes used parts of the tree for fevers, kidney ailments, digestive upsets, ulcers, snakebites, and other illnesses. Found to have over seven hundred medicinal properties.

Designation: Highly nutritious edible, African American home remedy, Native American medicinal plant, important herb of commerce, Ayurvedic healing plant, traditional Chinese medicine herb.

Cultivation: To grow from seed, gather black walnut seeds in late autumn after husks ripen to a bright, yellowish-green color. Collect fruit from the ground, avoiding any fruit with large holes and black spots, and stratify in refrigerator over several months. Can also be propagated by budding, grafting, and layering.

Remedy Form: Internal—Edible, tea, tincture, powder. External—Compress, poultice, powder, wash.

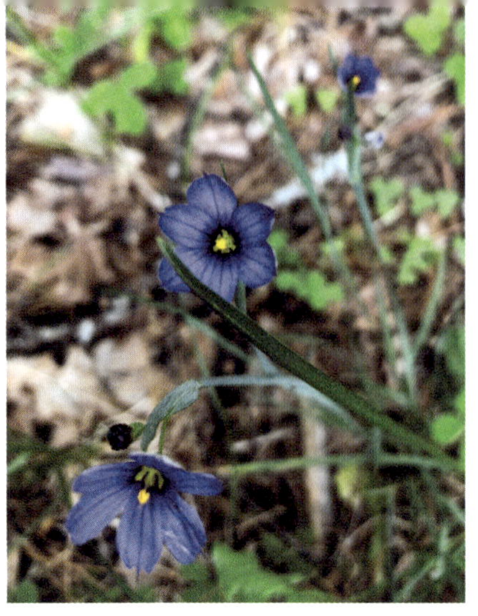

BLUE-EYED GRASS & THE CRAWFISH TRAIL

SPRING

Blue-eyed grass
(*Sissyrinchium* sp.)

Just about the time the crawfish chimneys get tall and the shellfish tastes yummy, blue-eyed grass shows up in the lawns. I've been seeing it everywhere lately. Tiny and delicate, with bright-blue flowers, the plant crowds all along the levee and batture and roadsides, its long grasslike stems appearing wherever the mowers have missed. I've read that there is a yellow version, too, though I haven't seen that yet. But I love seeing this tiny herb for a couple of reasons—for the medicinal uses that I'm learning about, and also because I know I'll soon be sampling what has turned out to be my favorite shellfish.

Lately, my cousin Nanette and I have been trekking around the southern part of the state on what we're calling the "crawfish trail." It's a great excuse to eat out and to spend time catching up on what's happening with our families. Sometimes, we take my sister or a couple of friends along. We all look forward to chatting and feasting, and we keep a mental list of our favorite spots. A few we've visited in the last month or so include Seither's in Harahan (where we order their Cajun street corn, too). Salvos in Belle Chase is high on our favorites list. In Houma, 1921 is good, and they also have fabulous "after the boil soup," if it's not already sold out when we get there. And there's Cajun Critters, and we can always go to Kenner Seafood just outside of New Orleans. We keep discovering more good places to go.

On this particular Good Friday morning, Nanette calls to see if I'm up for another trek along the crawfish trail, and, of course, I am. It's a stormy kind of day, and Bodi has fallen back to sleep after a wet walk, so I'm free to be off on a crawfish adventure. Today we might check out a place we've heard about in Breaux Bridge, but if anyone is short on time, another visit to Seither's is always a good bet.

Sometimes, though, we decide to cook up the crawfish ourselves. There's nothing like a family crawfish boil. It takes hours; there are many "batches" to boil up and lots of preparation chores, but it's so much fun. Everyone pitches in, either bringing ingredients or helping with the work. The tables get covered with newspapers or paper tablecloths. A few people take charge of the kettles and tend to the fires, while another couple of folks work at tweaking the seasonings. Little kids chase down the live crawfish "escapees," while some nutty cousin (not any of mine, of course) attempts crawfish "earrings" by allowing a crustacean to grab onto an earlobe or two. And we get to see folks who don't get out and around as often as they used to and visit for a while. The whole process adds up to hours—which reminds me of what Nanette said once when I complained about sitting for so long just to eat. "It's the difference between eating and dining," she said. Eating is just putting food in your mouth. Dining is the whole mix of things: the food and who's cooking it, catching up with loved ones, telling family stories, and the sweet blend of generations coming together. A few years ago, Mary Alice peeled and tasted and loved her first crawfish. Now she's fifteen, singing in the church choir, dancing in the city ballet corps, and learning to cook.

Which brings me back to blue-eyed grass. Though it is known to be edible, I've never tried cooking it up as a dish. Mostly, I just grab a few sprigs of the herb as I'm walking along the levee or wandering down to the river and nibble it along the way. If I think about it, next crawfish boil, I'll see if I can talk a cousin or two into steaming a bit of the herb and try it as a side dish to the shellfish that shares its season. I imagine it will take quite a handful of the herb to add up to anything, but its flavor is pleasant and mild, and I'll be getting a bit of healing while I eat.

But I won't want to eat too much of it. I'm aware that it has laxative properties, and a little goes a long way. Still, I feel pretty safe eating it. The herb is not a particularly strong or widely used plant. Some Indigenous tribes used it especially for digestive upsets like constipation or diarrhea. And a few species were found to have anti-inflammatory properties and could be helpful for the first stages of a fever or cold. It was also employed for hay fever, and externally, it was felt to help soothe and heal minor wounds. But I don't mind that it's not a "super herb." I love the blue flowers and the fact that blue-eyed grass signifies the arrival of spring. And I'm especially grateful that it reminds me of our crawfish trail adventures and where I might sample the shellfish again this year. It's yet another reminder of how many of our needs nature meets, which is a pretty cool thing to keep in mind.

Species: Several species of *Sisyrinchium* grow wild in Louisiana, and all have been reported to have similar uses. Those with documented medicinal properties include:

Sisyrinchium angustifolium

Other Names: Narrow-leaf blue-eyed grass, common blue-eyed grass, Bermuda blue-eyed grass.

Medicinal Uses: Diarrhea, regulating bowels.

Description: A clump-forming perennial with a tuft of narrow, grasslike, flattened leaves that are 0.25–0.5 inch wide. Generally grows 12–20 inches tall. Clusters of violet-blue flowers that are up to 0.5 inch wide bear six pointed tepals and a yellow eye.

Habitat: Meadows, grassy places, damp woods, deciduous woods, moist prairies, low wet areas, sandy or rocky acid soils.

Distribution: Scattered throughout the state (except for south and central eastern areas).

Plant Status: Native.

Sisyrinchium atlanticum

Other Names: Eastern blue-eyed-grass.

Medicinal Uses: Diarrhea.

Description: Grows up to 20 inches with dense tuft of narrow grasslike, light-green leaves. Clusters of violet-blue, star-shaped flowers are borne on short stalks and are 0.5 inch wide, with yellow centers.

Habitat: Wet areas, fields, meadows, open woods, and edges of salt marshes.

Distribution: In a few parishes in northern half of the state, more widely spread (though patchy) in southern half.

Plant Status: Native.

Sisyrinchium langloisii

Other Names: Langlois' blue-eyed-grass, roadside blue-eyed grass, dotted blue-eyed grass, southern blue-eyed grass.

Medicinal Uses: Scurvy.

Description: Up to 12 inches tall, flowers around 0.5 inch, and may be blue, violet, or white.

Habitat: Roadsides and open areas.

Distribution: Sparsely patchy throughout the state.

Plant Status: Native.

Sisyrinchium rosulatum

Other Names: Yellow blue-eyed-grass, annual blue-eyed grass.

Medicinal Uses: Gastrointestinal complaints; colds, fevers; eye infections.

Description: Leaves are bright green and flat with smooth edges that taper into rounded tips. Leaves grow in tight clusters, forming a basal rosette. Flowers grow singly on zigzag-like stems that extend from basal clusters. Flowers are typically white to light purple with a dark-purple ring around the center of the petals. Fruit is spherical and reddish-brown. Annual blue-eyed grass has a bunch-like growth habit

Habitat: Lawns, meadows, roadsides, old fields.

Distribution: Much of the state.

Plant Status: Introduced.

For All Species, Parts Used: Whole plant.

Medicinal Properties: Astringent, anti-inflammatory, anodyne, edible, laxative.

Uses: Internal—Diarrhea, gastrointestinal upsets, regulating bowel function; fevers, chills, colds, hay fevers; pain. External—Compress/poultice for minor wounds.

Risks: Generally safe in small amounts. Avoid if using prescription or over-the-counter laxatives.

Description: All *Sisyrinchium* have clumps of stiff, upright, sword-shaped leaves that occur in a fan shape. Individual leaves are usually narrow, and many species have the general appearance of grass. Flowers are relatively simple and often grow in clusters and resemble irises, to which they are closely related. Flower color may be blue, white, purple, or yellow, often with a contrasting center.

Habitat: Wet areas, fields, meadows, open woods, and edges of salt marshes.

Animal Use: Various species are visited by pollinators including sweat bees, bumblebees, bee flies, sylphid flies, and blue azures. Seeds are eaten by cardinals, song sparrows, wild turkeys, and bobwhite, among other species.

Natural History: The genus name *Sisyrinchium* is derived from the Greek *sys,* which means "pig," and *rynchos*, or "snout," referring to the roots that are consumed by swine. It was named by Linnaeus in 1753; despite the common name, the plant is not a grass but is instead a member of the Iris family.

Designation: Appalachian folk medicine, Native American remedy, homeopathic preparation, flower essence remedy.

Cultivation: The herb can be used as a border plant or a groundcover. Propagation is best when done from seed. Collect the capsules when they become wrinkled but before they fall from the plant. Capsules should be dried and then crushed to release the seeds. Fresh seed should be planted in fall into cool soil. Cold/moist stratification improves germination.

Remedy Form: Tea, tincture, edible, compress. Some species have been used as a homeopathic remedy (for snakebites) or a flower essence preparation (to help release stuck or rejected emotions).

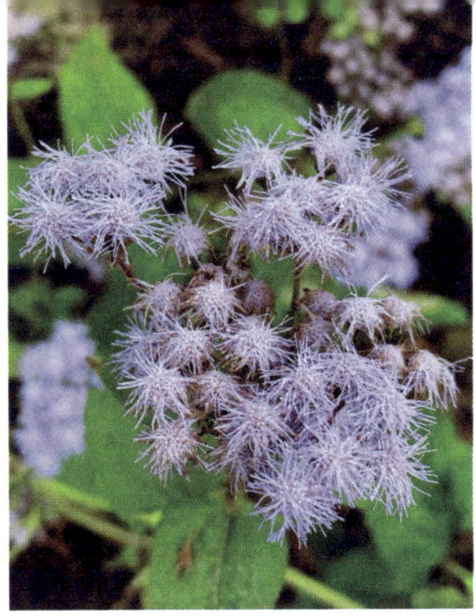

BLUE MIST FLOWER & THE IBIS

FALL

Blue mist flower
(*Conoclinium coelestinum*)

In Houma for a visit, I wake up early and trek down to the intersection of the bayou and the intracoastal canal, trying to catch the sunrise. Suddenly, I am taken far back in time to all those childhood mornings when I was up and out of bed before school and headed out for my morning "rounds." I'd wander through empty streets, just wanting some time to be alone before the day and school and parents and chores claimed me. Then, I loved the early quiet, the damp bayou-scented air, the heavy fog that pressed down over the slow-moving water, and the little ripples of early fish that were up to taste the air. Across the canal today, fishermen are out early, hoping for a breakfast catch.

On the boardwalk, I trek past old bald cypress trees whose branches droop toward the bayou. A few turtles stir the water as their heads poke up. They are hoping for treats, probably used to having food tossed into the water from nearby cafes. The usual leftover flowerings of autumn surround my feet. Goldenrod is heading toward seed, a few weathered clumps of beggar's ticks are still blooming, and I spot a pretty surprise—a stand of blue mist flowers still bright and heavenly blue despite the late season.

Someday soon I'm hoping to harvest blue mist flower plants to use for healing. Related to boneset and its other cousins, I've recently discovered that it also has many medicinal properties. Apparently, all parts of the plant can be used for treating respiratory problems and menstrual cramps, for boosting immune system function, and for helping to relieve anxiety and stress. I'd like to get to know this herb and to better understand its uses.

I'm impressed with what I've read so far, and I figure that if it is anywhere near as helpful as its herbal relatives, it will find an important spot in my herb cabinet. It also turns out that this plant has a respected place as both a flower essence remedy and as a magical healing herb. Its spiritual or "energetic" effects are said to include a calming effect on the mind and spirit. It is also believed to be protective against negative influences. And it is said that a bath including infusions of the herb may be used to ground and center one's energy.

As the sun slides up over the arc of the bridges, I head toward my car, still grateful for this wet and fertile and sinking land and these slow, dark waters. But I wonder how the future will unfold here. Parts of the town look rejuvenated and lovely. The boardwalk is decorated with sculptures depicting wildlife or First Nations peoples and bordered with native plants. And a new outdoor seating area around small cafes is now covered with a well-lit canopy. The little theater is attractive, and a new gazebo has been set up in front of the courthouse, inviting performers. But then there's the mess. Old business buildings are half crumbled and empty, and deserted parking lots surround abandoned stores. The bayou is peaceful in some areas but used as a trash dump in others.

I remember this same scenario from childhood—the general malaise that seemed to afflict the place. I am still not sure what's at the heart of it, but it seems pretty depressing to me, and sad. A couple of friends talked recently about people who've just moved there and how their ideas of what the place should be like are "unrealistic." This is Louisiana, after all, they say. You can't expect too much. But where does that leave the residents, if status quo always reigns?

I pull into the motel parking lot, gather my things, and open the car door. Then I notice movement near the front fender and see—just slipping up out of a trash-littered ditch—two ibis that are graceful as a dream, shy and beautiful. One is an adult, with white plumage, the other a juvenile with its darkish-brown feathers. I am so glad to see them—so glad that even in this relatively crowded area, they can make a home. But I'm also sad. Here they are, living, maybe even nesting, in a garbage dump. I wish they had a better place. I wish people would care enough to pick up their garbage instead of slinging it into a ditch. More apathy, I guess. They do what's easy instead of what could make a difference, no matter how small. How does the state pull itself up out of so much apathy and despair and begin to treat itself with dignity and attention? How do any of us, I wonder?

Well, for right now, I can do something. As the ibis flicker away into the underbrush, I step down the little slope and into the ditch to pick up trash. And I find another surprise! Here in this mucky, messy spot stand more tall clusters of blue mist flower, getting ready to seed. I grab a few stalks of flowering tops to take home, then pick up as much damp and decaying trash as I can hold, and head back to get a garbage bag. Maybe the area won't stay clean for long, and maybe the ibis will eventually figure out there might be a nicer place to stay. But I have to try to make a difference.

And maybe the blue mist plants here will shed enough seeds to make the area seem more like a stand of wildflowers than a garbage drop-off spot, and people will stop throwing trash out their windows. For now, I can take a few seeding tops of the herb and start some at home in my little garden where there's no trash. Then I can have my own patch of the beautiful herb, and maybe someday the ibis will visit there and find a cleaner spot in which to nest and thrive. And if, as I've read, it turns out that blue mist flower has some magical uses, well, all the better. With all the work we have ahead of us in trying to stabilize and heal and rebalance the lands and waters of the state, we could probably use a little magic! For now, I head in with my load of garbage and my treasure of blue mist seeds and get ready for the day.

Other Names: *Conoclinium coelestinum,* blue mistflower, wild ageratum, blue boneset.

Parts Used: Leaves, flowers, roots.

Medicinal Properties: Muscle relaxant, immune system support, anti-inflammatory, mild sedative.

Uses: Digestive upsets; respiratory conditions including coughs and congestion, boosting immunity; menstrual cramps, anxiety, and stress. Historically used by the Cherokee people of the southeastern United States to treat snakebites. Essential oil from blue mistflower has been used to alleviate headaches, migraines, and other types of pain.

Risks: Contact may cause redness, inflammation, and itching of skin. If prone to skin allergies, handle with gloves and avoid direct contact.

Description: The perennial plant will grow 1–2 feet tall on downy purplish stems. Leaves are coarsely toothed, ovate-deltoid, and up to 3 inches long. Flowers lack rays and occur as numerous small, fluffy, tubular, blue-purple flowers up to 0.5 inch wide, with discoid heads in dense, flat-topped terminal clusters, or corymbs.

Habitat: Wood margins, stream banks, low woods, wet meadows, ditches.

Distribution: In most of the state.

Plant Status: Native.

Animal Use: Pollinators that visit flowers for nectar include monarchs, swallowtails, queens, soldiers, pearl crescents, white peacocks, little yellows, and many other butterflies and native long- and short-tongued bees, flower flies, moths, and beetles. Caterpillars, such as the clymene moth and lined ruby tiger moth, will eat the foliage. Seeds are eaten by birds.

Natural History: Blue mist flower was described and named by Linnaeus in 1753 as *Eupatorium coelestinum.* Swiss botanist A. P. de Candolle determined it was worthy of its own genus and named the plant *Conoclinium coelestinum* in 1836. The name was not widely accepted, and various botanists used *Eupatorium coelestinum* well into the 1900s. More recent genetic analysis supports the separate genus *Conoclinium,* and manuals and floras now use that name. The species name *coelestinum* means sky blue or heavenly.

Designation: Native American remedy, Indigenous Oriental medicine plant.

Cultivation: Seeds may benefit from cold/dry stratification. Plant prefers moist, humus soils that do not dry out, and will thrive in full sun to partial shade. Once established, taller plants may be cut back in spring to prevent flopping. The plant does especially well around pond borders as long as spreading roots will not affect other plants. Not recommended for smaller planting areas as it can spread aggressively. A good plant for habitat restoration within its native range, especially in wet soils. Propagate by clump division in early spring. Home gardens and fields can become important habitats for this plant. Moderately resistant to damage from deer.

Remedy Form: Tea, tincture, capsules, poultice, steam.

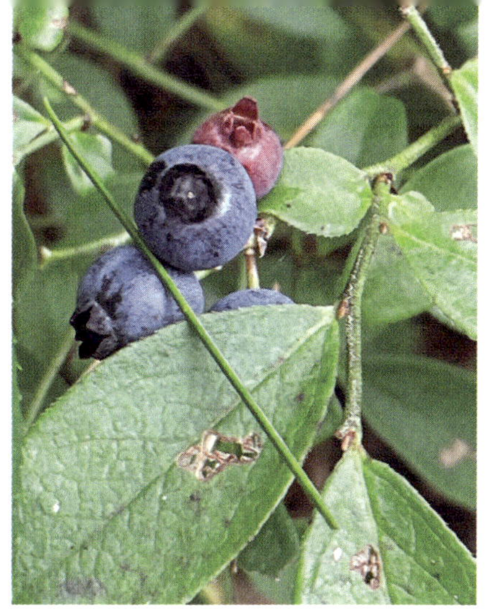

BLUEBERRY & HEALING THE WORLD

SUMMER

Blueberry
(*Vaccinium corymbosum*)

On a hot, early summer morning, I am half wild and in love with the world. I am grubby, itchy, thirsty, and I don't care. I cram a handful of wild blueberries into my mouth. They are tangy, sweet, gritty with sandy soil. And perfect. What more could I want?

Some of the things I love about this wild harvesting are the quiet, the tedious creeping along on hands and knees, the minuscule choices as I pick up just this perfect berry and not that squishy one. I swipe at my sweaty brow and swat at the amazingly shiny green bee that keeps buzzing around my head.

In this chore of one small plucking after another, again and again, I slip back into my animal self. I am nothing but skin and muscle and bone, inching forward, searching for food. My body leans this way and that, arms reaching, while all the crows yell and the hummingbirds joust with each other over the heat-ragged flowers and the mosquitoes try to find the inch of skin I haven't sprayed with bug repellent. Nearby, the ants are busy at their little army parade, and all around me the scent of coming rain hangs in the air. Leftover dewdrops roll down the dark fruit I pick.

But as much as I love this quiet work, all is not well.

Lately I wake up in the middle of dreams, trying to figure out how to make sense of things that don't make sense. I worry about the world. I worry about this place. I had thought that surely, after all the decades I've lived, we humans would have made some gains. That we, as inhabitants of this great, mysterious hodgepodge, would have broken through layers of self-centeredness and fear and misunderstanding to take our truly rightful place.

In this collective journey toward the Absolute, we are not the "leaders," not the top of the heap. Instead, maybe we are just another possibility, just another blessing, just another tiny but essential part of loving and healing the world.

I guess we never get to know—in any concrete way—what we've actually been "for." Maybe, for as long as we live and move and fail and rise again, we can only hope to love, to give, to breathe, to care. And somehow that will make a difference.

I don't know if this is healing, this little chore. But I have to trust my body and my joy. And I trust the blueberries to do their part. For all my years as an herbalist, I've been impressed with their healing potential. And I'm not the only one! For as many folks who love the fruit, there are hundreds of scientists who have been trying to figure out why they are so good for us. It turns out that many different species of *Vaccinium* not only contain dozens of nutrients but also are filled with natural chemical compounds that have some amazing effects. Both the fruits and the leaves have healthful nutrients, and significant biological activity as well. Using blueberry on a regular basis can help to prevent serious eye conditions, shore up our heart health, battle some life-changing inflammatory conditions, or help to balance blood sugar.

I feel so lucky to live in a place where the wild berries are pretty abundant. But for those who can't harvest the fruit in the wild, the berry bushes are pretty easy to grow and not too demanding for a home gardener. I might consider trying to introduce a couple of bushes into my yard as I get older. But I don't think I want to stop my wild harvesting just yet. I depend on the fruit and leaves for healing, and I depend on this simple chore of picking berries one grateful inch at a time, on a quiet summer day.

Species: Five species of *Vaccinium* grow wild in Louisiana, share many of the same medicinal compounds, and can be used interchangeably. Species with documented medicinal use include:

Vaccinium arboreum

Other Names: Tree huckleberry, farkleberry, tree sparkleberry, whortleberry, gooseberry, winter huckleberry.

Medicinal Uses: Internal—Diarrhea, sore throat, tonic. External—Chronic eye inflammations, swellings.

Description: Large shrub or small tree with flaking grayish-brown to reddish bark and a crooked trunk with twisted branches. Grows 5–25 feet tall, 4–15 feet wide. Leaves are oval or elliptic, 1–3 inches long, 0.5–1 inch wide. Upper surface is dark, glossy green; lower surface is dull green and often sparsely pubescent. Leaves alternate along stem, are late deciduous to evergreen, and turn pink to maroon during winter months. Flowers are white to pink, bell-shaped, about 0.375 inch long. Fruit is a long-stemmed and shiny blackish berry, 0.25–0.5 inch long.

Habitat: Sandy soils, pinelands, open mixed forests, thickets, clearings, fields, coastal scrub forests, sandy rocky woods, along wooded streams.

Distribution: Northern and western parishes, with a few eastern and central areas.

Plant Status: Native.

Vaccinium corymbosum

Other Names: Highbush blueberry, New Jersey blueberry, southern blueberry, smallflower blueberry.

Medicinal Uses: Blood sugar balance, cardioprotective, supports collagen production, boosts immunity, cancer protective.

Description: An upright, multistemmed deciduous shrub that grows 5–8 feet tall with an equal spread and a dense, rounded habit. Leaves are glossy, dark green, elliptical, and up to 2 inches long. In autumn, leaves turn brilliant red or orange. Flowers are bell-shaped, white with pink tinges, and 0.3 inch long. Fruit is a blue, sometimes dusky, berry, 0.25–0.5 inch in diameter.

Habitat: Open swamps, bogs, upland woods, old fields, pocosins, pine barrens.

Distribution: Bienville, Evangeline, Jackson, Lincoln, Morehouse, Natchitoches, Tangipahoa, Union, and Winn Parishes.

Plant Status: Native.

Vaccinium darrowii

Other Names: Darrow's blueberry.

Medicinal Uses: Fevers, eye problems, chronic fatigue syndrome, constipation, fevers, hemorrhoids, multiple sclerosis, poor circulation, urinary tract problems, varicose veins.

Description: Shrub may grow approximately 1–3 feet tall and 2 feet wide. Leaves are small, simple, ovoid to acute, and grow in whorls up the stem; size is approximately 0.5 inch and appear to be blue-green with occasional pink-violet overtones. Flowers are bell-shaped, white-pink in color, and grow at ends of stems in bunches. Berries are round, bluish-black.

Habitat: Pine flatwoods, sand hills, scrub, dry sandy soil along open banks of creeks.

Distribution: St. Helena, St. Tammany, Tangipahoa, and Washington Parishes.

Plant Status: Native.

Vaccinium elliottii

Other Names: Elliott's blueberry, southern high bush blueberry.

Medicinal Uses: Colic, diarrhea; sore throats and mouth inflammations; chronic fatigue; eye diseases; immune system support.

Description: Shrub is 6–13 feet tall, with multiple trunks. Leaves are small, simple, ovoid-acute, 0.75–1.5 inches long with finely serrated margin. Flowers are small bell/urn-shaped, white-pale pink, 0.3 inch long, and occur in clusters on bare twigs.

Habitat: Open flatwoods, ravines, dry uplands along river valleys, along streams and in swamp forests, cleared river bottoms that are subject to periodic flooding.

Distribution: Top two-thirds of the state and some central and eastern parishes.

Plant Status: Native.

Vaccinium stamineum

Other Names: Deer berry, squaw huckleberry, squaw berry, gooseberry, buck berry.

Medicinal Uses: Cancer chemopreventive.

Description: Low-growing shrub with alternate leaves that are elliptic or oval, 0.75–2.75 inches long and 0.3–1 inch wide. Upper surface is shiny green; lower surface is dull and pubescent. Margins entire and ciliate. White, bell-shaped flowers occur in racemes in spring along with leaves. Berries are green to yellow, 0.4 inch in diameter.

Habitat: Dry open woods, floodplain thickets, sand or clay soils in pinelands, mixed forests, savannas, and bottomlands.

Distribution: Top two-thirds of the state (except for extreme east coastal parishes), some eastern and central parishes.

Plant Status: Native.

For All Wild Species, Parts Used: Fruit, leaves.

Medicinal Properties: Highly nutritious edible containing vitamins B6, C, E, K1, and manganese, copper, iron, and fiber. Also antioxidant, anticancer, cardioprotective, astringent, antidiarrheal, antibacterial, improves cognitive function, protects against dementia-related diseases, anti-inflammatory (more than thirty anti-inflammatory compounds are found in the fruit), blood sugar balancer.

Uses: Blood sugar regulation in type 2 diabetes; eye problems including prevention against retinal detachment; diarrhea and other inflammatory bowel diseases including colitis; cardiovascular disease prevention, poor circulation; cognitive impairment, memory loss, dementia-related diseases; arthritis; kidney stones and urinary tract infections; varicose veins, wounds, and skin diseases. Research has proven blueberries to have anticancer properties against breast, cervix, colon, esophagus, liver, lung, mouth, pancreas, throat, skin, and stomach cancers.

Risks: If taking antidiabetic medications while using blueberry, have blood sugar levels monitored closely. Dose of medication may need to be changed. Interactions with certain blood sugar medications may occur, including glimepiride (Amaryl), glyburide (DiaBeta, Glynase PresTab, Micronase), insulin, pioglitazone (Actos), rosiglitazone (Avandia), chlorpropamide (Diabinese), glipizide (Glucotrol), tolbutamide (Orinase), and others.

Animal Use: Important nectar source for pollinators; fruit eaten by deer, rabbits, and other mammals and numerous species of birds; shrubby thickets provide cover. Adult butterflies gather nectar from the blooms, and caterpillars of many butterfly species eat the leaves. Fruits are eaten by songbirds, small mammals, ruffed grouse, wild turkeys, deer, and black bears.

Natural History: The origin of the genus name *Vaccinium* may have come from a precursor to Greek or early Latin. Various species of the berries have been eaten for several thousand years, and the oldest specimen was found in a Bronze Age grave in Denmark. About 450 species of the plant exist and can be found in many areas of the world. Wherever they are found, they have been used over time for both food and healing. In the U.S., many Native American tribes used the fruit and leaves for relaxing muscles and aiding in childbirth. Some believed that in times of starvation "the Great Spirit sent the star berries down from the night of heaven to feed the children."

Designation: Important herb of commerce in the U.S., Europe, and Canada, Native American remedy, African American home remedy (*V. myrtillus*).

Cultivation: Apparently, wild blueberries are difficult to cultivate, though they are the best to use for medicinal properties. One source recommends using stem cuttings and seeds if attempting to grow wild species. For cultivated varieties, full sun is best for good fruit production but can tolerate up to 50 percent shade. Soil pH should be 4.0–5.3 for best production. (Soil sample can be submitted to parish extension office so amendments can be made prior to planting.) *Vaccinium* like plenty of organic material and good drainage and cannot tolerate excessive moisture. Water if rainfall is not adequate. Fall and winter planting work best.

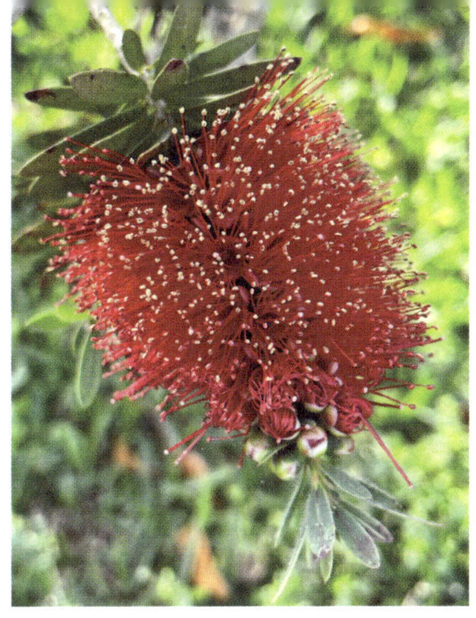

BOTTLEBRUSH & THE GARDEN CLUB

SPRING

Bottlebrush
[*Callistemon* sp.]

Every single day, I start out with a walk. Often I'm on a well-trodden trail, but sometimes I take a ramble into unknown territory. And every single day, I'm entranced. But no matter what twisty trail I take, every walk ends up back at home, in the garden. Some of my first memories are of trailing after my mom or grandmother to check their yard, see what was blooming, what was not doing so well, where there might be an empty spot to fill with something new. For me, the garden has always been the connection between my tame, "inside" life and my "into the wilds" life. It is often where I feel most at home.

There's something about Louisiana that is so sensual—the air thick with moisture, the heat, the thriving liveliness—that I think it becomes part of our identity. For all our insistence that humans are somehow separate from and superior to nature, we are, in fact, just one more expression of it—along with the flowers, the trees, the hummingbirds, and even the pesky possums.

Lately, I think a lot about the land that surrounds us and how we care for and interact with it. I've come to the conclusion that a garden isn't just something we create; it is also something we discover. All around me, all around each of us, is a thriving, hearty, interwoven meeting ground between humans, creatures, and plants that make up this astounding life on Earth.

Of course, all those joyful feelings about gardening don't exactly mean I'm good at it. I guess you could say I'm a casual gardener—which basically means that I'm kind of messy. I've finally begun to realize that (a) my enthusiasm for gardening far outweighs my skill and (b) even though I get so excited about having a variety of plants, I can't keep up with them all. But

I've come to a certain peace with that—because it turns out that having imperfect rows and lots of raggedy weeds and lots of visiting bugs actually means my garden is healthy. Many pollinators, a variety of weeds, and lots of neighborhood critters seem to feel right at home there. And that, I guess, is kind of the point.

Which leads me to garden clubs. Gardening is often a solitary pursuit. We relish the time to be outdoors by ourselves, to create just exactly what we envision, and to break away from the routine of taking care of a home, a life, a family, a job. But sometimes we just need to share both the many small joys and the grueling and often frustrating work. And garden clubs can be a perfect solution. Together, we get to experience wonder, excitement, and woes. We get to be revitalized, to work and sweat and get dirty—and it's all okay. We're moving in the direction of making things beautiful and lovely and lush. As we participate with others in our home ground, we learn gratitude, wonder, humility, and persistence. And we can make a contribution not only to our own and our neighbors' gardens but to the community in which we live. I think that's what garden clubs are all about.

Which leads me to bottlebrush. I don't remember seeing *Callistemon* when I was growing up. But discovering it on my return to Louisiana has been a joy. I saw it first a few years ago in a cousin's yard, and of course I had to look it up to see if it had any potential medicinal uses. It turned out that bottlebrush is a close relative of an internationally respected medicinal tree—*Melaleuca alternifolia,* better known as tea tree. Like its famous kin, bottlebrush has many healing properties. The flowers, leaves, and stems can help to protect the liver, heart, and nervous system and assist in treating bronchitis and cough, gastrointestinal disorders, arthritis, and numerous other conditions. And some folks use it for spiritual or energetic properties as well. In its native Australia, the flowers are sometimes used to signify abundance, laughter, joy, and birth. Once I discovered all of that, of course I had to have my own.

It wasn't so easy to find seedlings, though. It turns out that there are trends in horticulture, and bottlebrush is a bit passé. But I finally found two tiny trees and gave them a sweet spot on either side of the front steps to my house. Then I had to find out how to take care of them. Since the plant isn't native to Louisiana, I needed to find out what kind of habitat it likes. I decided to check in with some of my garden club buddies. In Ama, Marie Ann invited me over to see and photograph her healthy, well-established shrubs. She has two species—the "normal" *Callistemon citrinus* and the "weeping" *Callistemon viminalis.* They look quite similar to me, but Marie Ann says her husband insists that he knows which is which. She doesn't really care—just loves them because they're so beautiful and draw so many bees and butterflies. She is an ardent member of her local garden club, and she and my cousin Jara often share plants with each other or consult over a new discovery or a longed-for addition to either of their gardens.

And in Houma, I know several folks who are members of the Terrebonne Garden Club (TGC). A couple of years ago, I was invited there to talk about medicinal plants and was astounded by how many members arrived for the presentation. The club, perhaps the oldest in the country, had just celebrated its ninety-fifth anniversary, and locally it has a rich history and a significant presence. In monthly meetings, many programs and speakers address a wide range of topics related to not only the garden but also the local ecology. An important theme in the past few years is the use of native plants in landscaping and the benefits that can bring. Each month, members are invited to share interesting plants from their own gardens and to help plan field trips to historic gardens or homes several times a year. According to current garden club president, Gail Aycock, the club's commitment isn't just to plants grown in home gardens but also to education, community engagement, and helping to support the local environment. One recent project has been filling and maintaining large planters with colorful flowers in Houma's downtown. And interest in the TGC is rising. The group has had so many folks joining that they've recently had to cap the number of members. But there are still a few spaces, and the process for joining is pretty simple.

Gail explained that if someone is interested, a couple of introductory meetings will help to make sure that the club and the potential member are a good fit. After that, if someone wants to continue, they will make a pledge to the garden club's mission—to "protect and conserve the natural resources of planet Earth, and . . . to promote education so that we may become caretakers of our air, water, forest, land, and wildlife."

So even though it's a garden club, it's not all about gardens. In a way, it's about the larger garden all around us—yards, flower beds, trees, bayous, woods—and the people and fellow creatures who inhabit them.

Which leads me back to bottlebrush. This year, after nursing them along, my tiny trees have dozens of blossoms, and I've already harvested some of the flowers and dried them for tea. Even if bottlebrush isn't currently trending, I'm excited to have it close to home. And if I have any questions about how to care for my little shrubs, I'll know right where to turn.

One thing is for sure—no matter what the future holds for the state, as long as there is land here, there will be gardeners. And for that we are all very glad.

Other Names: *Callistemon citrinus, Melaleuca citrina,* common red bottlebrush, crimson bottlebrush, lemon bottlebrush. (Another species, *C. viminalis,* aka "weeping bottlebrush," has also been associated with many healing properties and is equally easy to cultivate in a home garden.)

Parts Used: Flowers, leaves, stems.

Medicinal Properties: Antibacterial, anticholinesterase, anticough, antidiabetic, antiflu, antifungal, antioxidant, antinociceptive, antiplatelet aggregation, hepatoprotective, cardioprotective, neuroprotective, relaxant, antiaging, anti-inflammatory, antimicrobial, anticancer, prostaglandin inhibitor, relaxant. External—Insecticidal, wound healer.

Uses: Bronchitis, cough; diarrhea, gastrointestinal disorders; infectious diseases caused by bacteria, fungi, viruses, and other pathogens; pain, rheumatism; skin infections; urinary tract infections, incontinence; hemorrhoids; heavy menstruation; insect repellent. (Essential oil can apparently be used to harmonize a room or house and can bring tranquil healing vibrations.)

Risks: None known.

Description: Grows 3–10 feet tall and wide. Bark is hard, fibrous, or papery, and young growth is often covered with soft hairs. Leaves are evergreen, aromatic, alternate, lanceolate with entire margins, and narrow (with narrow end near the base), and with a tinted end. Leaves are 1–4 inches long and 0.2–1 inch wide. Many veins are clearly visible on both sides of leaf, with many oil glands visible on both surfaces. Flowers are red, arranged in spikes on ends of branches, and continue to grow after first flowering. Blossom spikes are 2–3 inches in diameter and 2–4 inches long, with numerous individual flowers. Fruits are woody, cup-shaped capsules, 0.2–0.3 inch long and 0.3 inch wide in cylindrical clusters along the stem. Fruiting capsules remain unopened until the plant, or the part bearing them, dies.

Habitat: Native to Australia and commonly found in swamps and near rivers and rocky streams in wild areas of New South Wales. In cultivation, plant is very adaptable and can tolerate various conditions as long as drainage is good.

Distribution: Widely cultivated in the state.

Plant Status: Introduced.

Animal Use: Especially attractive to hummingbirds, butterflies, and bees. Deer resistant.

Natural History: The genus name *Callistemon* is a blend of two Greek words, *kallis,* meaning "beautiful," and *stemon,* referring to "stamen." The species name, *citrinus,* means "like citrus," indicating its flavor. During their exploration of the east coast of Australia in 1770, scientists Joseph Banks and Daniel Solander collected the first *Callistemon citrinus* specimen for examination. The genus name was created by Robert Brown (1773–1858), a Scottish botanist who made significant contributions to the field.

Designation: Australian Aboriginal medicine, traditional Chinese medicinal herb, a flower essence remedy, Jamaican and other Caribbean islands folkloric healing plant.

Cultivation: Adaptable to many soil conditions, though needs good drainage. Prefers full sun and once established does not need irrigation and has few pest or disease problems. A weeping version of the bottlebrush tree (*C. viminalis*) can also be found in the nursery trade. Both are drought, frost, and deer resistant. Can be easily propagated from seed or cuttings.

Remedy Form: Tea, tincture, oil. (In preparing tea, pour boiling water over plant parts and then cover the cup immediately with a small plate or lid in order to prevent volatile oils from evaporating.)

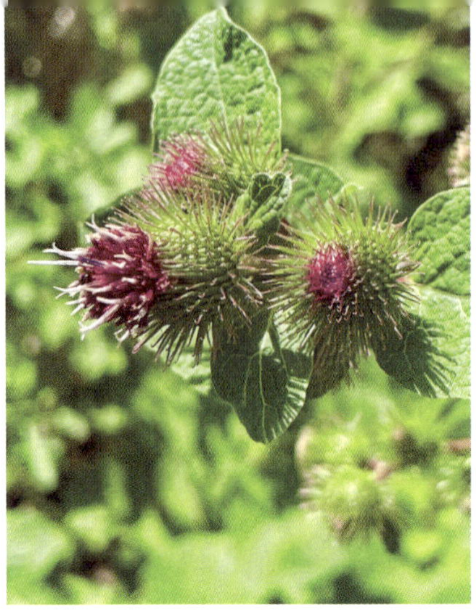

BURDOCK & THE SEEDS

EARLY WINTER

Burdock
(*Arctium* sp.)

This morning, I'm photographing seeds. In late autumn, all the plant life is headed toward its resting season. A few bright leaves hang on until the next big wind, but many plants have already hunkered down as they get ready for the season's shift. Queen Anne's lace seedheads have tucked into themselves and look like wiry little bird's nests. Goldenrod seeds, left over from the bright-yellow blossoms, look like gray fluff. St. Johnswort leaves are faded already, but the seed capsules are dark, deep red with remnants of the powerful anthocyanin compounds in the herb. And the wild crabapples are shrinking, their gift of new life tucked inside soft flesh the deer will nibble at in the coming months as they do their part in recycling the seeds. And the burdock leaves are fading, but its seed cases are prickly and strong. As I walk around taking photos, I think a lot about seeds—and about nature, our great home, and how brilliant she is at celebrating today and preparing for her future. I think, too, about how central a love for this land and these waters is to my life.

But there's also the terrible tension—the great conundrum—of loving this world and, at the same time, of being part of the species that is rapidly destroying it. Inadvertently, mindlessly, sometimes systematically without realizing the dire consequences. According to a recent report on the future of the planet, humans might just cause the "next great devastation" of the Earth. In the past, the most destructive ecological events were triggered by natural occurrences. But now, we humans are likely to have the most disastrous effects on the future of the planet. I'm not sure how to live with that.

Even if I did all that I possibly could to change my habits, those would only be a paltry stab at a remedy to all that's awry.

Today, though, burdock gives me hope. No matter how rugged and challenging the climate conditions become, I'm pretty sure that this herb will weather the changes. And while it is pretty darn impossible to love it from a gardener's point of view, and hard to imagine anyone wanting to grow it in their flower bed, it has a lot to offer.

The common burdock that is found in Louisiana (*Arctium minus*) is a close relative of greater burdock (*Arctium lappa*), which is one of the most well-known and respected plants in the international herb trade. Recognized in much of North America, Europe, and Asia for their valuable healing properties, the burdocks offer compounds that affect and support important body systems and also contain much nutritional value. In fact, the root is an important food item in many Asian countries. One nutritionist noted that, even if we are using burdock for its medicinal properties, the best way to ingest it is in our daily diets. The nutritional components of the roots include inulin, which is a dietary fiber that aids in digestion and may also lower LDL cholesterol. In addition, burdock can help stabilize blood sugar and may even help reduce the risk of colon cancer. It has also been recommended for helping to relieve chronic skin conditions like psoriasis and eczema and to stimulate immunity, fight infection, and relieve arthritis.

In my wild food foraging days, I tried many plants I wouldn't have normally included in my diet. Queen Anne's lace roots, which were supposed to taste like carrots, tasted—at least to me—like wood! Daylily buds that were reported to be a great substitute for green beans tasted weird and slimy. Rose hips were pretty good, though it took a lot of work to cut open the red fruity "hips" and scoop out all those seeds. I have to admit, though, that burdock roots—once I wrested them up out of their earthy home and cleaned and peeled them—were pretty tasty.

One of my favorite homemade nutritional and medicinal tea blends is burdock root, nettles, red clover, and licorice root. As I age into my senior years, I encounter some of the health challenges that occur in this phase of life, and lately I am thinking it might be time to revisit my favorite herb blend. Reintroducing burdock and a few other herbs will offer me not only nutritional benefits but the healing anti-inflammatory and antioxidant support my body will find helpful.

With that in mind, I do a little research on using the various parts of burdock for healing and read up on harvesting the seeds. It sounds a little intimidating. One herbalist reports on trying to get the seeds out of their very prickly burrs, and notes that he crushed the burrs (wrapped in a heavy-duty plastic bag) by driving over them with his car! And he notes that the challenge of separating seed from chaff involves wearing a mask to provide protection from very tiny hairs that can irritate mucous membranes if they're inhaled during the process. For now, I guess I'll stick to using the root for my tea and adding it to stir-fry dishes as a food. And while I'm not sure I want to grow the herb in my flower beds, I might consider allowing some of the burdock that pops up in my back garden to stay in place instead of removing it along with the other "weeds." Then I'll have my own crop of the herb instead of having to forage for it.

Which leads me back to seeds, and to the ways we will move forward in these challenging times on planet Earth. I have to hope that caring matters, and that speaking up might matter. And that staying informed and changing habits might add up to something. Who knows what we can do if we work together?

In the meantime, I can do my part. I can learn more about how to help. And I can collect the burdock's prickly burrs and scatter them lightly over disturbed soil, where they can stabilize the land. Because seeds are a way forward. They are the future, packed up and ready to sprout. In this small way, I can play my own part in the tender, hopeful unfolding of the future, even as the land slips away under my feet. And I can pray, inspired by Christian mystic Julian of Norwich during the Black Death plague many hundreds of years ago. "May all be well. May all manner of things be well."

Other Names: *Arctium minus,* lesser burdock, little burdock, louse-bur, common burdock, button-bur, cuckoo-button, wild rhubarb, bardane.

Parts Used: Roots, leaves, stems, seeds.

Medicinal Properties: Adaptogen, alterative, antifungal, antimicrobial, antioxidant, antipyretic, astringent, cholagogue, choleretic, circulatory, diaphoretic, diuretic, expectorant, laxative, liver stimulant and hepatoprotective, lymphatic tonic. Edible and contains prebiotic compounds, inulin, vitamin B6, iron, and manganese.

Uses: Internal—Skin conditions including acne, eczema, impetigo, psoriasis, and dry skin; blood sugar imbalances including type 2 diabetes; sore throat and infections; arthritis, rheumatic pain; colds with sore throat and cough, pharyngitis, acute tonsillitis and abscesses, chills; measles; high cholesterol/triglycerides. May help prevent colon cancer. External—Alopecia, burns, boils, bruises, fevers, herpes, impetigo, insect bites, ringworm. Oil extract (bur oil) is used in Europe as a scalp treatment. Used in both Chinese medicine and in Ayurvedic healing practices for eliminating toxins, providing liver and gastrointestinal support, treating skin disorders, and managing chronic inflammation.

Risks: Should be avoided by those who have allergies to members of the daisy family (*Compositae/Asteraceae*). If taking pharmaceutical diuretics or diabetes medications, check with a health care provider before taking burdock. Avoid if pregnant or nursing.

Description: A shrubby, leafy plant that grows up to 6 feet in height and forms multiple branches. First year's growth forms a short, dense rosette of leaves. Leaves may be up to 2 feet long, are oval with wavy margins, and are dark green above and wooly underneath. Taproot may grow up to 1 foot deep in soil. Flowers are prickly, pink to lavender, and flower heads are up to 0.75 inch wide. Disk florets and globular bracts terminate in fine, sharp hooks forming prickly burs that aid in seed dispersal by latching onto animals, birds, or other hosts.

Habitat: Roadsides, near old dwellings, pastures, feed lots, stream valleys, and waste places. Often grows in partial shade.

Distribution: Ouachita and West Carroll Parishes.

Plant Status: Introduced.

Animal Use: Pollen from blossoms is collected by bumblebees, honeybees, miner bees, and leaf-cutting bees, who also feed on the nectar. The foliage is a food source for the caterpillar of the painted lady butterfly.

Natural History: According to some reports, burdock burrs and seeds were the inspiration for the invention of Velcro in the 1940s by George de Maestral, who was intrigued with the powerful attachment of the burrs that he pulled out of his dog's fur. Over centuries, the burdocks have been used in numerous healing traditions including Native American tribes, traditional Chinese medicine, Ayurvedic medicine, and North American, European, and Asian healing practices. It is also used by many traditions as a magical or spiritual healer, thought to ward off the evil eye. It is believed to bring prosperity, vitality, and virility. In Turkish Anatolia, the plant is believed to symbolize abundance, to nourish the spirit at its deepest level, and to be a reservoir of spiritual energy.

Designation: Important herb of commerce in numerous countries, traditional Chinese medicine remedy, Ayurvedic medicinal plant, Native American herb.

Cultivation: Adaptable to most soils and likes moisture. Prefers sun or partial shade.

Remedy Form: Internal—Edible, tea, tincture, powder. External—Compress, poultice, powder, wash.

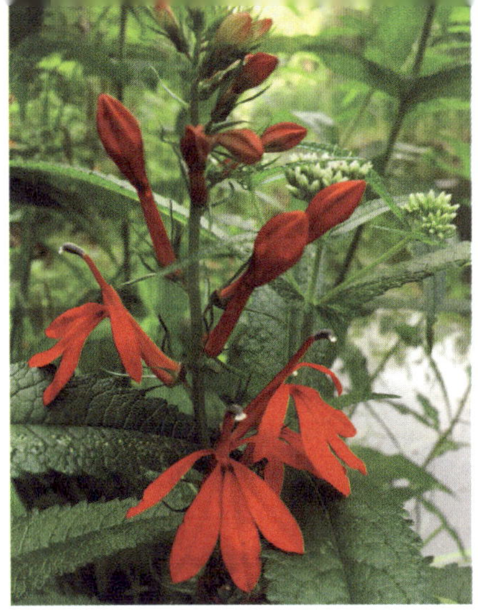

CARDINAL FLOWER & THE PEACE OF WILD THINGS

LATE SPRING

Cardinal flower
(*Lobelia cardinalis*)

This morning, the first sunrise we've had for a week or more is gorgeous. Orange and coral colors spill through the windows and over the yard. Bodi is still asleep, so I leave him to his dreams and head on out. I'm on a mission today. Last year, I spotted a little stand of cardinal flower near an old beaver dam beside the river, and today I want to check to see if it has come up again. Outside the sodden ground has my feet sopping wet within minutes, but I'm happy to be under way.

It's a quiet morning except for the chatter of whistling ducks who feed at the edges of puddles, and a couple of hawks who are sparring overhead. I tramp back through the batture tangles and then stop at the little pond. I look out at the calm water and drink in the stillness of this early-spring day. And I think about how precious the silence is—and how much I relish it.

It's been said that silence feeds the soul, and that nature heals. I know this to be true. It reminds me of a poem I love by Wendell Berry, entitled "The Peace of Wild Things." Its last line reads, "I rest in the grace of the world, and am free." I'm pretty sure I know what he means. And for me, one of the graces is the many healing plants that surround us.

At the little beaver dam, I can't spot the residents, but they're probably out scavenging for breakfast. Then I discover just what I was hoping to find. The clutch of bright *Lobelia cardinalis* is tall and seems to have spread since I saw it last. Many stands of the herb are topped now with bright-red flowers that sway in a little breeze. I'm always so happy to see it—not just for its beauty but because I know it offers healing and also shares nectar with so many visiting pollinators

Lobelia is one of the first plants I found, and tried, when I was studying herbs. Decades ago, a friend mentioned that medicinal plants might help with my daughter's health, and she began to introduce me to some of the local herbs. I was enthralled. It was such a miracle to me to realize how many of the plants I passed by every day had these secret lives as healers. There were some simple herbs that were easy to harvest, free of side effects, and didn't taste too terrible. Dandelion, self-heal, and several different clovers were familiar and dependable.

There were other herbs, though, that should only be used with caution. *Lobelia* was one of those. A powerful group of herbs, various species have long been used by Indigenous and Native peoples for such conditions as asthma, bronchitis, pneumonia, and cough. In modern medicine, *Lobelia* continues to be the subject of ongoing scientific research for its potential as a remedy for neurological conditions such as dementia and other serious health conditions. However, the herb is not to be taken lightly. Side effects of some species include vomiting, the source of one of the plant's nicknames—"pukeweed!" And the herb has external uses as well. Cardinal flower has been safely crushed and applied to cuts, minor wounds, and skin infections with helpful results.

One of the species that has turned out to be the most powerful is tiny *Lobelia inflata,* also known as Indian tobacco. It earned this common name because the herb contains lobeline, a compound that is very close to nicotine in its effects. Folks trying to stop smoking cigarettes might smoke the dried herb instead.

The first time I tried tasting little *Lobelia inflata,* I was amazed. For a delicate plant, it had a dramatic, very spicy, peppery taste—maybe a hint to its powerful effect. I've only used this species a few times in the last decades, and on those occasions, mostly for its effect on the respiratory tissues in an asthma attack when a pharmaceutical preparation was unavailable. Over the years, I've sampled other species of *Lobelia* and found that not all of them taste as strong. But I'm still very cautious with the genus even though I love seeing them in the wild.

Lately, I've tucked a few cardinal flower transplants into my garden and am happy to see them blooming there. Now I'll just have to make sure they get enough water, since cardinal flower seems to like the edges of streams or ponds. In my garden so far, the newly introduced plants look pretty happy.

They're blooming and seeding, and the hummingbirds and bees seem to love it. I'm recommending the plant to neighbors for their wildflower gardens—it will add beauty, offer a sweet meal to visiting pollinators, and bring just a little bit of that "peace of wild things" closer to home.

Species: Several *Lobelia* species grow in the state, and some have a history of medicinal use. These include:

Lobelia appendiculata

Other Names: Pale Lobelia, earlobe Lobelia.

Description: The slender stem is erect, 14–24 inches tall, usually unbranched. Leaves are 1–1.5 inches long and occur below the flower spike. Flowers are pale blue to white, about 0.5 inch long, growing directly on stem. They are two-lipped, tubular, and arranged loosely on the spike that is 6–15 inches long.

Habitat: Prairies, pinelands, and old fields.

Distribution: Western two-thirds of the state, and some eastern and central parishes.

Plant Status: Native.

Lobelia brevifolia

Other Names: Shortleaf Lobelia.

Description: Plant height is 2–3 feet. Stems are single or multiple from a taproot, pubescent, erect, unbranched, and from 0.5–3 inches in length. Stems have a milky sap when broken. Leaves are alternate, 1–2 inches in length, 0.275 inch wide, with sharply toothed margins. Leaves are numerous and reduced in size up the stem. Flowers occur in terminal racemes. Flowers are pale lavender to blue. Upper lip is two-lobed and lower lip is three-lobed. The fruit is a capsule containing many small seeds

Habitat: Wet prairies, savannas, and pinelands.

Distribution: St. Helena, St. Tammany, Tangipahoa, and Washington Parishes.

Plant Status: Native.

Lobelia cardinalis

Other Names: Cardinal flower.

Description: Plant height is 1–6 feet. Leaves form a basal rosette, and are either entire or serrated, and may contain milky sap. When serrated, small and large teeth alternate at edges of leaves. Erect stems produce racemes of brilliant red flowers. Each flower has three spreading lower petals and two upper petals, all united into a tube at the flower's base. Fruit is a small capsule, containing many tiny, oval, semitranslucent seeds.

Habitat: Ditches, ravines, depressions, woodlands edge, openings, stream banks, roadsides, prairies, plains, meadows, pastures, savannas, near lakes or ponds, swamps, wet or moist soils.

Distribution: Much of the state, with exception of the extreme southeast.

Plant Status: Native

Lobelia inflata

Other Names: Indian tobacco.

Description: Plant height is 6 inches–3.5 feet, with stems covered in tiny hairs. Leaves grow approximately 3 inches long, and are ovate, toothed, and alternate. Stems have several tiny lavender or blue-violet to white flowers in terminal, leafy, elongated clusters. Flower has two-lobed upper lip and three-lobed lower lip.

Medicinal Uses: Medically the most important variety of the *Lobelia* genus. Traditionally used for asthma, bronchitis, pneumonia, and coughs.

Habitat: Plants prefer partial sun and can be found in fields, open woods, roadsides, meadows, gardens, rich soils, woodlands.

Distribution: East Feliciana, St. Helena, and West Feliciana Parishes

Plant Status: Native

Lobelia puberula

Other Names: Downy Lobelia.

Description: May grow 3–4 feet tall. Leaves are alternate with small teeth that are irregularly spaced and have a fuzzy underside. Blue flowers with white-pink centers mature in late summer and continue into mid-fall.

Habitat: Wet soils, bogs, meadows, woodlands, swamps, prairies, open fields, strongly acid soils, partial shade.

Distribution: Western two-thirds of the state, and some central and eastern parishes.

Plant Status: Native

Lobelia spicata

Other Names: Pale spike Lobelia.

Description: Stem bears a delicate spike of small, pale-blue, two-lipped flowers that occur on an elongated, slender spike. Leafy stem is often reddish and hairy at base, smooth above.

Habitat: Moist native prairies and meadows, open woodlands.

Distribution: Central and northern parishes.

Plant Status: Native

For All Species, Parts Used: Flowers, leaves, roots.

Medicinal Properties: Analgesic, anthelmintic, antispasmodic, emetic, expectorant, febrifuge, nervine, stomachic.

Uses: Internal—Respiratory conditions such as asthma, bronchitis, pneumonia, and cough. External—Poultice on sores, minor inflammations.

Risks: Potentially toxic if used in large quantities. Symptoms include nausea, vomiting, diarrhea, salivation, exhaustion and weakness, dilation of pupils, convulsions, and coma. It contains the alkaloid lobeline, which has a similar effect upon the nervous system as nicotine. Sap of the plant may cause irritation in those with sensitive skin.

Animal Use: Plant is pollinated by bees, butterflies, and hummingbirds. Slugs and snails may feed on the plant, but it is generally deer- and pest-resistant. *Lobelia* is toxic for dogs.

Natural History: The *Lobelia* genus is named for the Flemish botanist Mathias de l'Obel (1538–1616), who anglicized his name to Matthew Lobel. He was apparently the first person to attempt to classify plants by attributes other than their medicinal uses. *Lobelia cardinalis* was introduced to Europe in the mid-1620s, where it was given the common name cardinal flower, supposedly because the flowers are the same color as the vestments worn by Roman Catholic cardinals.

Designation: Folkloric healing plant, Cajun traiteur remedy, homeopathic remedy, Native American medicinal plant.

Cultivation: Propagation can be done by cuttings, division, or seeding. For cuttings: Take two node stem cuttings (4–6 inches) before the flowers open and remove the lower leaf and half of the upper leaf. Treat the cutting with a rooting compound and place the cuttings in a sand and perlite medium, cover lightly, water, and keep moist. For division: Divide well-established clumps in the fall or spring. Separate the rosettes or basal offshoots from the mother plant, replant these divisions, and water immediately. For seeding: Collect stalks by cutting below the capsules, then place stalks upside down in a paper bag. Leave the bag opened so capsules are exposed to the air for a few days. Shake the bag to release the seeds. Seeds need light to germinate, so place them on the surface of a prepared seed bed in late fall so that the seed overwinters and germinates naturally in spring.

Remedy Form: Not recommended for internal use, though *Lobelia inflata* is sometimes prescribed by homeopathic practitioners. Externally, plant parts can be crushed and applied as a poultice, compress, or wash for muscle pain, rheumatoid arthritis, bruises, sprains, insect bites, poison ivy, and ringworm.

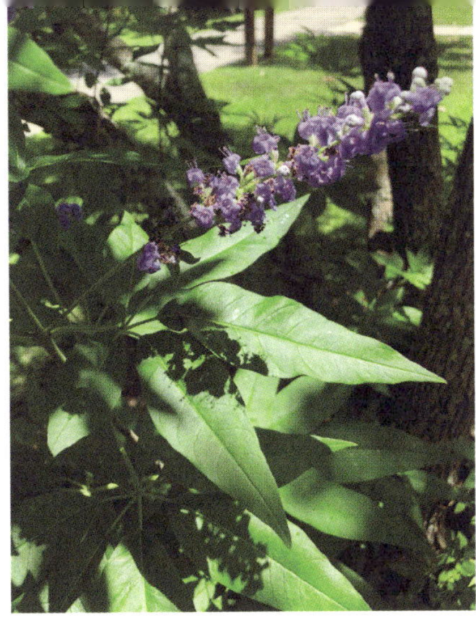

CHASTE TREE & THE MONKS

WINTER

Chaste tree
(*Vitex agnus-castus*)

In early December, I am out to watch the sunrise over the bayou. It's a surprisingly cold morning. Temperatures hover around freezing, ice has formed over a few puddles, and the sidewalk is slippery. Despite the cold, it's a beautiful day. A thin fog is rising up from the canal, and egrets wade in shallow water, foraging for breakfast. Along the boardwalk, some goldenrod is still lush and bright in a protected spot, and though beautyberry has started to seed, some of its twigs still bear the bright magenta fruits like those I harvested months ago. I take a few photos of the sunrise and then suddenly spot an herb I've been researching lately—chaste tree! Although it has already started to scatter dried gray seeds along the ground, a few slender twigs still bear pretty lavender flowers despite the cold.

Chaste tree was one of the first plants I learned about in herb school. It was reported to be especially useful for women's reproductive health and was recommended for menstrual irregularity, breast pain, and mood fluctuations. When I began to practice as an herbalist, I recommended the herb to women who experienced premenstrual symptoms, or who had irregular cycles and were hoping to get pregnant, and often noted good success. Then, when I was going through menopause, I found it useful for symptoms associated with that change of life. And the herb has often been used by midwives and herbalists to help prevent miscarriage. While there are still many questions about exactly how the herb works, there is enough evidence of its efficacy to maintain its status as an important herb of commerce.

The plant's common name was supposedly based on its use by medieval monks living in cloisters who were trying to suppress libido and stay chaste.

Over the years, I've gained so much appreciation for those same monks who, it turned out, preserved many medicinal plants in their gardens and kept track of the lore concerning their use. In the last few decades, that information has been key to pharmaceutical researchers and the medical community as they explore the potential for healing plants both as home remedies and as future medicines for a wide variety of health conditions.

Apparently, the focus of the monastic life is to grow ever more deeply into the interior spiritual reality, and to deepen one's commitment to the mystery that underlies all of life. One of the most important supports of that quest was having solitude and silence to ward off the pressures of the world. In many monasteries, each monk would have his own room, or cell, and also his own small garden in which he could spend hours meditating in nature. Often, the monks offered remedies to members of the surrounding community who were ill, and the monastic gardens were especially vital as they provided food that would otherwise only be found in noisy, distant cities.

And it turns out that monastics might be women as well as men. St. Hildegard of Bingen (1098–1179) was a mystic, scholar, composer, herbalist, and scientist. She was well known for her devotion to nature as a healing tool, and her treatises explored the use of medicinal plants for various physical and emotional maladies. She recorded the effects of over two hundred herbs and plants and their medicinal actions in the human body, and she was recognized not only by the pope but by medical practitioners throughout her region. She was one of only four women to be named a "doctor of the Catholic Church," and her writings were acknowledged to have special authority. Hildegard's theology affirmed that both women and men express the "imago Dei," or image of God, and she declared that each sex has equal dignity before God.

Even though Hildegard was dedicated to a deep spiritual life, it turns out that she was pretty feisty! She confronted those in power and refused to settle into her "lowly" role as a woman. She spoke up for those members of the Earth community—human and nonhuman alike—who were disadvantaged and vulnerable, and was an advocate for those at risk.

So, too, have other monks spoken out for social justice through the centuries. Thomas Merton (1915–1968), a well-known Catholic monk, spoke out against war and oppression and focused on social justice issues, including the civil rights movement and proliferation of nuclear arms. Despite being a Trappist monk living in the Abbey of Gethsemani in Kentucky, he was also a writer, a mystic, a quiet pacifist, and a student of comparative religion. He encouraged interfaith understanding and pioneered dialogue with prominent Asian spiritual figures, including the Dalai Lama and the Vietnamese monk Thich Nhat Hanh. Decades after his death, he is still recognized for his contribution to interfaith dialogue and social justice.

And while I'm pretty sure Merton didn't have time to think about the chaste tree, it was definitely one of Hildegard's recommended herbs for menstrual irregularities.

Which leads me back to the chaste tree in front of me. In my recent research on this herb, it is recommended that the fruit be gathered while it is still partially green and attached to the tree. I'll not be using today's find for a harvest, since most of the berries are on the ground. But my cousin Jara has several chaste trees, and I can check to see how far along hers have gotten in their fruiting stage. If the berries are still attached to the stems, I'll make a harvest to tincture up and experiment to see what results I get.

Which leads me back to the monks, and to their importance in the history of healing plants. I'm so grateful for those quiet people, dedicated to a deep interior life, who have throughout the ages tended to the things that make us whole: stillness, time "away," medicinal herbs, and deep concern for all forms of life that help shore up our health. Even now, we continue to benefit from their quiet, dedicated lives. We can learn more about the chaste tree, and plant and encourage it on our own home ground

And maybe, in some curious way, as we continue to explore and share and use herbal lore and healing plants, we are co-participating in that journey as well. May it be so.

Other Names: *Vitex agnus-castus,* monk's pepper, wild pepper, Indian spice, Abraham's balm, hemp tree, sage tree, wild lavender, common chaste tree, true chaste tree, tree of chastity, chaste lamb tree.

Parts Used: Fruit/berry, seeds, leaves, bark.

Medicinal Properties: Anaphrodisiac/aphrodisiac (regulates libido), antibacterial, anticancer, anti-inflammatory, antifungal, antioxidant, diaphoretic, diuretic, febrifuge, galactagogue, infertility remedy, ophthalmic, sedative, stomachic.

Uses: Internal—Reproductive system support for women, regulating heavy periods, restoring hormonal balance, infertility, premenstrual tension, menopause. Has also been used by men for prostatitis, benign prostatic hyperplasia (BPH), and swollen testes. External—Repels mosquitoes, flies, ticks, fleas, and head lice.

Risks: Should be avoided by pregnant or nursing women, and by those taking dopamine-related medications or Parkinson's disease medications, birth-control pills, hormone-replacement therapy, or with a hormone-sensitive condition such as breast cancer. Should not be used by children.

Description: *Vitex* is a large, deciduous flowering shrub with aromatic, compound, palmate, grayish-green leaves. Leaves have five to seven lance-shaped leaflets that are up to 6 inches long. Flowers are tiny, fragrant, lavender to pale violet and occur in loose panicles up to 12 inches long in mid- to late summer.

Habitat: Pastures, roadsides, fence rows, stream valley, waste places.

Distribution: Scattered throughout the state.

Plant Status: Introduced.

Animal Use: Bees, butterflies, and hummingbirds feed on the nectar. Seeds attract several small bird species.

Natural History: Native to Mediterranean region and Asia, plant is naturalized in much of the southeastern United States. The name chaste tree is based on a traditional belief that the plant promotes chastity. Monks in the Middle Ages reportedly used it to decrease sexual desire. Athenian women used the leaves in their beds to keep themselves chaste during the feasts of Ceres.

Designation: Herb of commerce, Cajun traiteur remedy, African American herb, Ayurveda, Unani (Middle East/South Asian/Arabian) medicinal remedy, traditional Chinese medicine, Malaysian healing remedy, European medicine, and used in many Indigenous healing traditions.

Cultivation: Should be planted in full sun for the best blooms but can also do well in partial shade. The trees grow to 10–15 feet in height and can be 15–20 feet wide. Prefers dry, well-drained soil and is very drought-tolerant once established. Avoid organic material as it retains too much moisture. A slow-release, general-purpose fertilizer may be used every year or two to keep shrubs healthy.

Remedy Form: Tea, tincture, paste.

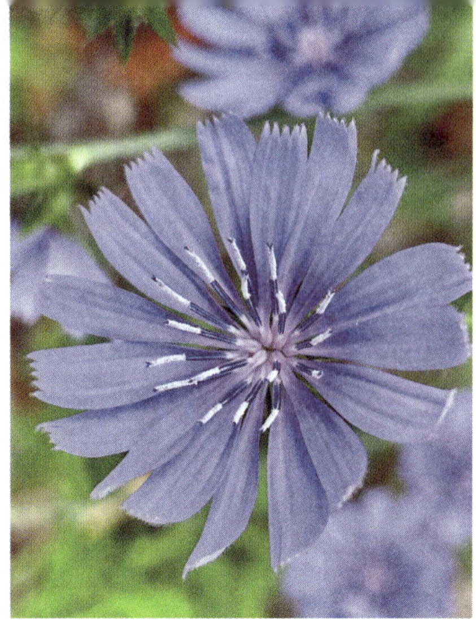

CHICORY & THE CAFÉ DU MONDE

SUMMER

Chicory
[*Cichorium intybus*]

It's an early, gray morning, with heavy dew and hazy sunlight, and Bodi and I are out for our walk before the heat settles in. At sixteen years old, he's more affected by the heat, so we go early these days. He still loves following scent trails along the batture, and he wanders off to see what he can find. While he sniffs around, I spot the usual animal signs. A few fish skeletons, dropped by the eagles nesting nearby, litter the levee trail. Egrets poke through shallow, muddy water, hunting for food. The possum that lives at the edge of the big ditch has worn a path up to the levee and down to the batture woods, and I keep an eye out for her. Occasionally, we'll be out early enough to spot her, but today she's nowhere in sight.

Bodi and I walk over dewy grass to the pond. On the way, I stop to check out the fig trees for the last of the fruit. Bodi isn't impressed with them, but I love the figs and try to get my fill before the birds visit for their daily treat. Today, though, all I find are a few withering, overripe figs with beak holes poked right through them.

Instead of fruit, though, I get a nice surprise. The chicory I seeded at the edge of a neighboring field is finally in bloom. I love the deep-blue flowers that unfurl along tall stems. Apparently, a truly blue blossom is a rare thing in the flower world, and I appreciate them so much that I decided to experiment with seeding chicory here even though this area is more southern than its normal range in the state.

I first heard of chicory when I was a child and my parents would take my sister and me to eat beignets at the Café du Monde in New Orleans. I didn't care much for coffee then, but we couldn't wait for our orders of sweet, powdery treats to arrive while my parents drank café au lait. Inevitably, we would all end up in giggles as we accidentally blew powdered sugar onto ourselves and each other. And we loved sitting in the French Quarter. We never knew what we would see or hear, and that was part of the fun.

As I grew older, I learned to love coffee and to appreciate the chicory root that added depth and flavor to the brew while easing its bitterness. Then, in herb school, I learned about the healing properties of the plant and about how important it could be to gently support various body systems. So many herb books mentioned that chicory supports the liver. But I was kind of confused at first. How the heck would I know if my liver needed support? Was my liver sluggish, even if I felt perfectly fine? Should I be worried?

Since then, I've learned about the liver's many roles in supporting metabolism—it's a vital powerhouse. The organ takes apart nutrients we ingest, converts them into substances that the body can use, then stores these substances and supplies them to cells when they're needed. It also converts toxic compounds into harmless substances or aids in releasing them. And over the years, I've learned how to spot possible signs that might indicate a "stressed" liver. Blood sugar or hormonal imbalances, low energy, headaches, a coated tongue with bad breath, or chronic allergies might be small signs that the liver is taxed. And taking many pharmaceutical medications or being exposed to toxic chemicals in the workplace or at home might impact liver function. I learned that this doesn't mean the liver is damaged, but it might be struggling to deal with the many "insults" of modern life. And I've learned to like the taste of chicory leaves, too.

Last year, on a trip to Italy, a friend and I stopped in a little trattoria near the train station to grab lunch. We were drawn to a grilled panini that featured mushrooms, cheese, and chicory leaves. I knew that chicory had many nutrients and supported digestion, but I wasn't sure how it would taste as an actual meal. Picking it in the wild and chewing a leaf hadn't made it seem very appealing. The herb is pretty intensely bitter, after all, and while I could appreciate small bites of it in a mixed green salad, it was definitely not something I'd want in large amounts. But the sandwich smelled great and looked appealing, so we decided to give it a try. Later, on the train trip, we discovered that when the leaves are cooked, the bitterness disappears but the nutrients are retained, and the sandwich ended up being one of our favorite on-the-go treats.

I like to recommend chicory as a wild or cultivated edible, and as a daily hot beverage. Both root and leaves contain many important nutrients, and one way to access the healing value of the plant is to eat it. Chicory benefits include essential B-complex compounds such as folic acid, pyridoxine, thiamin, and niacin. Vitamins A and C, and minerals like calcium, copper, manganese, iron, and potassium are found in appreciable amounts in various parts of the herb. In addition, the high inulin and fiber content helps to reduce blood sugar and LDL (or "bad") cholesterol levels, and the combination of nutrients boosts carbohydrate, fat, and protein metabolism and encourages healthy gut bacteria. Nutritional content of the herb has also been found to contribute to healthy skin and mucosa, healthy eyesight, and prevention of some malignancies, including lung and oral cancers.

Chicory's many benefits and the beauty of its flowers encouraged me to try growing it near home, and now it seems that my experiment has been a success. I take a couple of snapshots of the chicory blossoms, pluck a few smaller leaves to add to salads, and Bodi and I turn to head home.

Then I get another sweet surprise. There, trucking along the little trail she has laid down across the levee, is the possum! Now I know why I haven't seen her lately—she has at least ten babies holding fast to her back. She doesn't seem to notice us at first and gets pretty close before she glances our way and is startled. She turns to speed-waddle back to the batture woods, forgetting about whatever tasty nibbles she was after. I wonder if maybe she likes the chicory, too—I know that possums eat many kinds of herbs and plants as well as ticks and other harmful insects. So maybe the possum and I have "chicory love" in common. Bodi thinks she's very interesting, but the possum disappears as quickly as she can into the brush, with all the babies still in place. I'm guessing that once we are safely out of her way, the possum mom will come back to feast on chicory leaves, just as I'll be doing later today. Leaving her behind, I steer Bodi toward home and leave the possum—and the chicory—to their important work.

Other Names: *Cichorium intybus,* French endive, succory, blue sailors, coffeeweed, common chicory.

Parts Used: Roots and aerial parts.

Medicinal Properties: Anti-inflammatory, cancer, cholagogue, depurative, digestive stimulant, laxative, diuretic, febrifuge, refrigerant, sedative, nerve tonic, sudorific, tonic, anti-TB; antityphoid. Edible, and a rich source of beta-carotene and other nutrients.

Uses: Internal—Loss of appetite, indigestion, constipation, liver and gall-bladder disorders; hypertension; osteoarthritis; stress. External—Sores, wounds, swelling, inflammation.

Risks: Rare allergic skin reactions. Consuming large quantities of root may cause gas and bloating. Avoid in pregnancy. Avoid if allergic to the Aster/Daisy family of plants (daisies, chrysanthemums, marigolds). In presence of gallstones, consult with a health care practitioner before using. Chicory may lower blood sugar in people with diabetes, so blood sugar should be monitored by those consuming large amounts of this herb. No known drug interactions.

Description: A tall herbaceous plant growing up to 40 feet tall. The stem is tough and grooved, with small hairs. Leaves are stalked, lanceolate, and unlobed. Flower heads are 0.75–1.5 inches wide and range from pale pink or lavender to intense blue. Toward the center of each flower head there are several light-blue stamens with blue anthers. The flower heads bloom during the morning and close up later in the day. The root system is a stout taproot.

Habitat: Roadsides, fields, waste places.

Distribution: Found in several northern parishes, including Bienville, Bossier, Caddo, De Soto, and Madison.

Plant Status: Introduced.

Animal Use: Flowers attract short-tongued bees and other insects. Nectar and pollen are also used. Foliage is eaten by several grasshopper species and beetles. Cattle, sheep, and deer occasionally eat basal leaves.

Natural History: Chicory is native to western Asia, North Africa, and Europe. Its use for healing dates back to ancient Egyptians, who ground up plant parts for medicinal purposes. Chicory grows wild on roadsides in Europe and in Australia, where it has become naturalized. The plant is cultivated extensively in the Netherlands, Belgium, France, and Germany. The use of roots in coffee began on a small scale in Holland, but widespread use can be traced to the Prussian Empire in the eighteenth century, when Frederick the Great restricted imports of coffee, leading to an increased use of chicory as a substitute. In the early nineteenth century, Napoleon Bonaparte blocked the import of foreign goods, and the French turned to brewing chicory for a coffee-like beverage. Over the next few decades, the practice of adding chicory to coffee spread to the French colonies, including parts of modern-day Canada, particularly the Acadian region. Citizens of that region then took this practice to New Orleans, where chicory coffee became a culinary tradition, and the city became the continent's second-largest coffee port by the mid-nineteenth century. Today, coffee and chicory continue to be part of the local flavor of the area.

Designation: Edible, dietary supplement, herb of commerce, Native American remedy. Inulin from the root is used as a sweetener in the food industry.

Cultivation: Chicory likes full sun in a soil with pH of 5.5 or higher. It can be seeded or transplanted in early spring and can tolerate normal winter freezes. The plant requires 1–2 inches of water per week. When harvesting leaves, take no more than one-third of the foliage. Best timing for harvesting the root is late fall or early spring.

Remedy Form: Edible, tea, tincture, food additive.

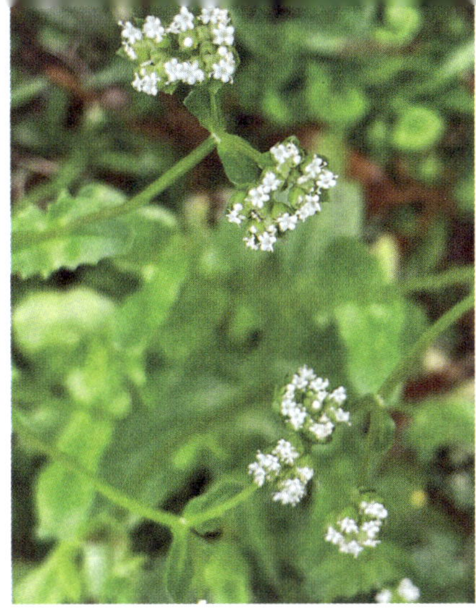

CORN SALAD & THE FORAGERS

SPRING

Corn salad
(*Valerianella radiata*)

It's a lazy Saturday morning, so far. The air is gentle, and blankets of clouds drift overhead. Hazy sun peeks through trees, and the newly hatched sparrows are chatty and busy in their garden world. And it's Easter Saturday—a quiet day. The usual Good Friday crawfish have been eaten, and today's plans are still in the making, but nothing is scheduled yet. For now, I'm savoring the unclaimed time, this morning's trek, and all the growth that's coming up in the yard.

At the back ditch that is half full of yesterday's rain, the usual "yard herbs" are thriving. Wild onions are getting their first little bulblets, the wild *Geranium* is sporting its "crane's bill" seed pods, dandelions are heavy with seed-silk pompoms, and tiny pink *Sherardia* is tucked into the thick clovers. And one of my newly discovered favorite yard edibles is hearty and flowering lately, making me hungry for a *Valerianella* salad.

I had heard of corn salad decades ago and wasn't quite sure what it was. But since coming back to Louisiana and getting more engaged with the foragers in the state, I have my eyes peeled for whatever I can tuck into a meal, and of course, anything I can use for healing. And it turns out that *Valerianella* is actually good for both.

Apparently, the delicate herb is loaded with nutrients, and many of those can help to ward off or correct some health imbalances. When I first discovered the corn salad blooming in the yard, I checked to see if it had any medicinal properties. I was kind of overwhelmed with what I discovered. According to James Duke's ethnobotanical database, *Valerianella* has been scientifically proven to have 220 medicinal compounds, and many of them are easily absorbed and utilized by eating the plant. Research has shown that the little, unassuming corn salad has antifungal, anticancer, antioxidant, antibacterial, antidepressant, antiviral, antibiotic, and many more healing compounds. And the plant can be used for a wide variety of conditions, including anemia, vomiting, abdominal pain, pancreatitis, inflammation, fatigue, diarrhea, and the list goes on.

Some of its healing capacities are attributed to the nutritional compounds found in the plant parts. Numerous vitamins and minerals occur in corn salad, and the plant can be eaten raw or lightly cooked—as a snack or part of a daily meal. Vitamin A, for instance, can help to prevent macular degeneration and can help provide relief against dry eyes. It can also enhance immunity by promoting the function of white blood cells and raising the lymphocyte responses to antigens. It helps prevent or lessen the occurrence of hypertension and supports cardiovascular health. Vitamin C found in the plant can help to lower blood pressure, and can aid in the formation of tendons, skin, blood vessels, and ligaments. It can also assist in healing wounds and reducing the formation of scar tissue. Vitamin B6 helps in the metabolism of vitamins, fats, carbohydrates, and amino acids. It also supports brain development and function and helps to prevent various forms of dementia. And many other nutrients in corn salad help to support optimum health and prevent disease.

From my perspective, some great benefits of the plant are that (a) it grows right at the edges of my lawn, (b) it tastes mild and fresh, and (c) it is free, tasty, easy to use, and is a totally renewable resource.

These days, when so many things seem complicated and require a huge output of energy just to figure out all the important details, corn salad is a treat. And even the animals like it. Many pollinators, including bees, butterflies, wasps, and flies, flock to the *Valerianella,* as do some of the local mammals, including deer.

When I'm trying to learn about the local healing plants, I often come into contact with the wild food folks. They're a fun and resourceful bunch. Several groups and individuals in the state offer educational meetings and classes. My first encounter with Charles Allen in central Louisiana introduced me to many medicinal and edible plants, and follow-up trips to visit him have given me the opportunity to actually eat some of the plants in meals. And while I've never met Johnny Bordelon, he has become a great resource for me and for others by hosting the informative Facebook group "Louisiana Wild Edibles, Foraging & Wild Medicinal Plants & Mushrooms." The site has over seventeen thousand members and offers both beginner and seasoned wild foodies the opportunity to communicate about plant identification, safety, preparation techniques, and other resources. I know that there are other educational foraging clubs in the state and am eager to learn more about them—and about the plants that can help to feed and heal us.

For now, I'm just grateful to have stumbled upon my new favorite wild food, corn salad. I'm looking forward to experimenting with recipes for it, and I'm also curious about preparing it for use as a medicinal—maybe drying some for tea, and also using some for making salves and poultices. For today, though, my little batch of *Valerianella* will go right into a salad. In fact, I've just gotten a call from one of my nearby cousins asking me to an early Easter supper, and I told her I'd bring a veggie dish. I'll shell some peas from the garden, chop up a few wild strawberries and wild onions, and toss it all together with batches of corn salad. Then I'll see if anyone can identify the salad greens. If I know anything about my family, once they've tasted it, I'm pretty sure that the nearby fields will be filled with foragers in search of their own supply, and the gardeners will be plotting ways to grow it in their veggie beds.

Despite the complicated times in which we live, sometimes things are simple. And sometimes, food is the only medicine we need, and it's right under our feet. And that's pretty cool!

Other Names: *Valerianella radiata,* beaked corn salad, woods corn salad, mache, lamb's lettuce, field salad, nut lettuce.

Parts Used: Aerial parts.

Medicinal Properties: Edible, antifungal, anticancer, anti-inflammatory, antioxidant, antibacterial, antidepressant, antiviral, antibiotic, diuretic. Nutritional compounds include vitamins A, B complex, C, E, K, and minerals including calcium, copper, iron, magnesium, manganese, phosphorus, zinc, beta carotene, and fiber. (Roots are known to be sedative and carminative, though are often tiny and hard to obtain.)

Uses: Internal—Anemia; blood sugar imbalances; elevated cholesterol and triglycerides, diarrhea, pancreatitis, gastric outlet obstruction, abdominal pain, nausea, constipation, obesity, ulcers; jaundice; fevers; chronic pain, stress, depression, fatigue. Preventive against osteoporosis and iron-deficiency anemia. External—Alopecia, minor burns or wounds.

Risks: None known.

Description: An annual, square-stemmed plant that grows 4–24 inches tall and has opposing, spoon-shaped leaves. Mature leaves are stemless and clasping. Leaf shape changes as the plant matures. Young plant leaves may be slightly hairy on margins, but hairs disappear when mature. Small, five-petaled flowers are white, and flower clusters have a squarish or rectangular appearance. Each stem forks into two.

Habitat: Moist, low, sandy or clay soils in woods, prairies, meadows, and roadsides.

Distribution: Most of the state, with the exception of a few far southeastern parishes.

Plant Status: Native.

Animal Use: Numerous pollinator species visit the flowers, including bees, butterflies, wasps, and flies. Both deer and bobwhite quail eat the leaves.

Natural History: The plant is mentioned in Gerard's 1633 *Herball, or, Generall Historie of Plantes.* Historically, preparations of the plant have been used externally to treat wounds and internally to treat dysentery and heavy menstruation. Beaked corn salad is named after the sharpened point, or "beak," that is present on the tiny seeds. The name "corn salad" derives from the plant's tendency to grow as a weed in corn or other cereal crop fields.

Designation: Edible, folkloric medicinal plant, Indigenous/Native American food and herb, homeopathic remedy.

Cultivation: Prefers full sun but appreciates some afternoon shade, and can thrive with minimal care. Moderate moisture and good drainage are helpful, and can tolerate a variety of soil types.

Remedy Form: Edible, tea, compress, poultice, salve.

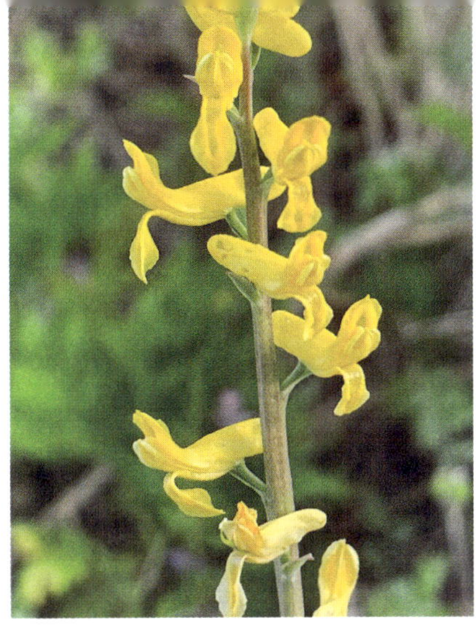

CORYDALIS & THE SNAPPING TURTLES

SPRING

Corydalis
(*Corydalis micrantha*)

I'm out before sunrise this morning and off to see the river. The fading left-over moon hangs over the cane fields, and a glow of first light burns through the batture woods. The air is cool again—only 60 degrees—and a breeze quivers through all the colorful levee wildflowers. Overhead, six little blue herons fly toward their rookery in the marsh, a few pelicans swirl in circles on their way to the diversion canal, and two whistling ducks poke through the shallows of a little pond. I pick flowers to take home for a vase, and head toward the water to see what's changed since last time I visited.

Today the wild fruits are starting to color up. Mulberries on the river-side trees are turning rosy, and the dewberries are larger on their prickly red canes. The purple-flowered vetch is lush and tangles around my legs as I walk, and the horsetail is already taller than I am. But I can't spot the little *Corydalis* that I found a couple of weeks ago. Then, it was bright, delicate, and only about 8 inches tall, though holding its own despite the crowd of its more robust neighbors. All around it, the colorful *Fumaria,* the blooming beggar's ticks, and tangles of prickly cleavers were lush and thriving.

The *Corydalis* is such a beautiful plant—with bright-yellow flowers, an unusual form, and an interesting history. I first got to know *Corydalis* when I was in herb school. On a trek into the New Mexico hills, we spotted a local species there, *Corydalis aurea,* and our teacher introduced us to its uses. He noted that it could be helpful for any kind of tremors, especially for going through the delirium tremens of alcohol withdrawal, or mild Parkinson's disease tremors. He also noted that it could be helpful for anxiety or nervousness. Over the years, I've learned that various species of the plant are employed in healing traditions throughout the world. Emotional disturbances, severe nerve damage, limb tremors, elevated blood pressure, and gastrointestinal spasms are some of the problems that *Corydalis* can reportedly ease. And one species, *Corydalis yanhusuo,* has been used as a painkiller in Chinese medicine for over one thousand years.

Intent on finding the plant now, I push aside the tangled vetch and the beggar's ticks and finally discover what I've been looking for—the *Corydalis!* I try to get closer to it for photos. But stepping over what I think at first is a little mound of sand, I spot a disrupted turtle's nest with many torn, leathery, white eggshells littering the ground. I'm not sure what kind of turtle laid the eggs, but it looks a lot like the snapping turtle nests I see often in Maine summers. Sadly, the condition of the eggshells indicates that the attempt to raise a new generation of turtles in this spot has probably failed. But at least the egg contents have gone to feed another animal for this season, I guess. I know it's not unusual for turtle nests to be preyed upon by other species, but I also have observed how hard the mother labors to dig a nest where she thinks it will be safe and how long her trek back and forth to the nesting site can be sometimes.

The list of turtle egg predators is long. Apparently, foxes, coyotes, raccoons, crows, herons, owls, bullfrogs, fish, and snakes would all be glad to have found this nest. So the eggs provide important food for many of its nonturtle neighbors. And even though the adult turtles have very few predators, they are sometimes attacked by river otters, bears, and coyotes. And humans, of course, either on the lookout for soup protein or for selling to overseas markets.

I know that many folks don't like having the "snappers" around because they can intrude on gardens, and their bite can be pretty tenacious if they're disturbed. But, in fact, they don't normally bite unless threatened, and they can be really great at helping to remove the detritus that can accumulate near ponds or other watery areas. They also help to spread seeds of plants that support fish nurseries and wetland ecosystems.

I have an ambiguous relationship with both *Corydalis* and the turtles. While I love seeing the plant growing in the wild, I also depend on picking small harvests of it to have on hand for some tricky health problems. And though I hope the best for the future of the snapping turtles, my grandmother's turtle soup was one of my favorite childhood foods, and I'm not above ordering turtle soup when I go out to eat.

And so it goes. In order to live, I have to depend upon other lives for my sustenance and support, probably one of the most humbling realities of being human on this lush and fruitful planet.

But maybe I can do something to give back. I can keep an eye out for the turtle nests and do whatever I can to keep them safe, even if it only means carrying an occasional squiggly turtle baby across the road so it will have a chance to live and thrive. And I can figure out how to cultivate and care for *Corydalis* in my own home garden or the neighboring woods, so I can make sure they have a chance to keep on going even when development or weather changes threaten them.

For now, I pat the sandy soil back into place, hoping that there could be a few turtle eggs left intact at the bottom of the nest. And I pick a small handful of the *Corydalis,* thinking I can make a tincture to have on hand. I try to keep some of the roots intact, hoping they will be inclined to sink deep into my garden soil and make a new home there. Then I'll have my own little patch of the herb, and later, if a turtle happens to wander by on her search for a nesting spot, she'll feel right at home.

Other Names: *Corydalis micrantha,* Smallflower fumewort, southern *corydalis,* golden *corydalis,* slender fumewort, slender *corydalis.*

Parts Used: Tuber, root.

Medicinal Properties: Alterative, analgesic/anodyne, antiperiodic, antispasmodic, diuretic, emmenagogue, hypotensive, mild antidepressant, mild sedative.

Uses: Internal—Bronchitis, sore throats; diarrhea, digestive upsets; headache, migraines associated with menstruation, insomnia; irregular or painful menstruation; mild depression, back pain, neuralgia, nerve damage, muscle twitching, sciatica, tremors, traumatic injury; heart disease. Some species of *Corydalis* are used in traditional Chinese medicine for treatment of digestive issues, paralytic stroke, headache, rheumatic arthritis, and sciatica. There is some evidence that it can provide relaxation in the treatment of addictions. External—Compress/poultice for backaches, sores, and minor wounds, and gargle for sore throats.

Risks: Best for short-term use. Avoid during pregnancy and breastfeeding; avoid in the presence of liver disease.

Description: Leaves are up to 3 inches long, and leaflets are deeply divided with lobes further divided into narrow segments, giving them a feathery appearance. Leaf surfaces are hairless, and often have a blue-green or gray-green tint. Multiple stems arise from the base. These are upright to prostate and bear clusters of small, pale-yellow flowers that are approximately 0.3 inch wide and have a curved spur at the back.

Habitat: Fields, roadsides, and moist, sandy soil.

Distribution: Much of the state.

Plant Status: Native.

Animal Use: Seeds have a small, fleshy structure at their base. The seed is taken by ants to their nest, where the fleshy part of the seed is eaten and the remnants are discarded. This process aids in seed dispersal. The plant is pollinated by bees.

Natural History: The genus bears the ancient Greek name of the crested lark, referring to the spur of the flowers. The specific epithet *micrantha,* also from Greek, means "small flower." The subspecific epithet is Latin for "southern." It has been used for medicinal purposes by Indigenous peoples for centuries.

Designation: Indigenous and Native healing remedy, Chinese medicine herb, folkloric herbalism plant remedy.

Cultivation: *Corydalis micrantha* prefers partial shade to full sunlight, and will grow well under trees. It thrives in well-drained, loamy soils with consistent moisture for the plant, though does not like to be waterlogged. It can also grow in sandy soils with added organic matter or heavier clay soils, and is good in a rock garden. *Corydalis* can be propagated through seed or division. Sow seed in early spring, and division should be done in the fall, after the growing season.

Remedy Form: Tea, tincture, compress, poultice, wash.

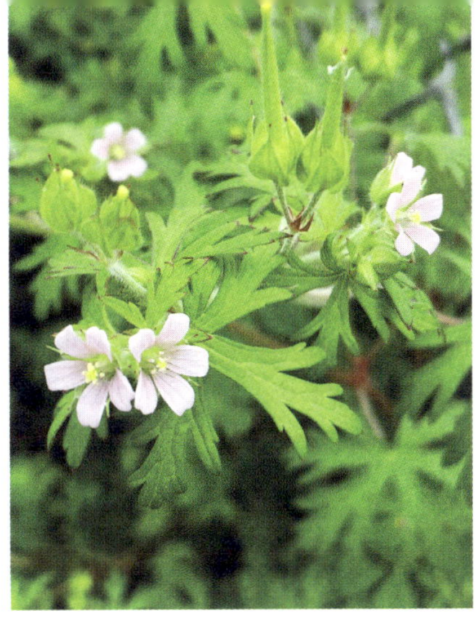

CRANESBILL & THE WILD AMBLING

SPRING

Cranesbill
[*Geranium* sp.]

It's a good and gentle kind of morning, with cooler temperatures after days of heat, sun after clouds, and a quiet, unscheduled day after much busyness. I walk out to the levee just as the sun slips through trees. The sycamore leaves are starting to appear, and dew clings to thready spider webs that stretch from leaf to leaf. Live oak catkins dangle from twigs, and along the wood's edge, wisteria is blooming. At the batture ponds, bullfrogs croak and throb, and a great blue heron stands motionless, keeping an eye out for breakfast. Close by, egrets and stilts and white-crowned night herons line up, looking for their own morning meal.

Today I have time to amble—to stop and peer closely at what's underfoot and near at hand. Black medic and bur clovers tangle into each other. Fleabane is tall, its feathery petals tinged pink, flower heads nodding in the breeze. I taste a few of the herbs. Fleabane's fuzzy leaves have a spicy aftertaste, and spiderwort tastes a bit like grass; betony has downy leaf surfaces but tastes like nothing at all. And the cranesbill, a wild *Geranium* that was recently whacked down by the town mowing crew, is not only rising up out of the shorn levee grass but is sporting pink flowers and sending up spiky seed pods. I feel a new appreciation for its hardiness. Undaunted by most anything, it seems, the cranesbill here is tall and gorgeous.

Lately, I've been wanting to gather this herb to have on hand for several problems. Three species of wild *Geranium* in Louisiana contain a treasure trove of healing properties, and the different species can be used interchangeably. With their high astringency, the cranesbill cousins can help to slow down bleeding and repair wounds externally, and can be used internally for diarrhea and other gastrointestinal upsets, for sore throats and inflamed gums, and to relieve heavy menstrual periods. In herb school we talked about the herb's usefulness for such inflammatory conditions as arthritis, and also about its ability to help remedy swollen and irritated mucous membranes when taken internally. Later this week, I'll be making a spring herbal salve for cuts, bug bites, and minor burns, and cranesbill will be a main ingredient in that preparation.

Remembering so much of its potential for healing, I wade through the knee-high blooming plants and begin my harvest. Pulling up the plants by their roots, I worry a little about yanking this herb out of its native soil, where it does so much to help stabilize the land and prevent erosion. But I'll keep my harvest small. And maybe, once the cranesbill seeds are ripening, I can gather some to plant into a little garden spot at home. Then I can support their growth and harvest them selectively when my supply gets low.

The wild *Geraniums* have a rich history of use not only in herbalism but in the practice of homeopathy and in the flower essence world. It is even appreciated by some for its magical properties. In homeopathy, cranesbill can help in treating bleeding tendencies from different organs of the body and is especially associated with the head and stomach. And rumor has it that a tea of wild geranium flowers is an effective magical remedy to counteract love spells and to attract happiness and prosperity. It was also used in spells for successful pregnancy and childbirth and is said to be spiritually calming and helpful for cleansing the aura. When using flower essences, wild *Geranium* is said to help one reconnect with a sense of self-worth and security. I can't say I've tried *Geranium* for any of these issues, but the herb is certainly helpful for many types of problems, and I'm always uplifted when I see it.

One thing about the wild cranesbill that I've often found confusing is its genus name, *Geranium.* The well-known cultivated garden plant known by that name is actually a member of the genus *Pelargonium* and has many differences from its wild cousin. *Pelargoniums* have big, brightly colored flower clusters and slightly hairy leaves. And their flowers have five petals each, but the top two petals are different in size from the bottom three. In the wild cranesbill, however, all five petals are the same size and shape. And the cranesbills are cold-tolerant, whereas the "garden variety" *Pelargonium* is sensitive to frost. Both types of "geraniums" do have some history of medicinal use, but the wild species known as cranesbill has numerous healing properties, while the garden variety, or *Pelargonium,* is mostly used externally for the astringency of its leaves. It's nice to know that both types have some usefulness, but today it's the cranesbill I'm happy to find.

As the sun rises over the nearby river and mist lifts up from the marsh, I turn to amble home. I so need these gentler days, this unscripted time—not just because I can spot the herbs I want to gather but because in our often-pressured lives it feels so important to just go slowly, to notice and wonder and revel in simple joys. And so I do. Standing on the batture, holding my armload of wild *Geranium,* I come to ground. I settle back into just this—my aging but sturdy body, this lovely, wild tangle of growth, this here and now. And I am grateful, and healed, and home.

Species: Three species of wild *Geranium* occur in the state, and all may be used interchangeably.

Geranium carolinianum

Other Names: Carolina cranesbill, wild *Geranium,* Carolina *Geranium.*

Medicinal Use: Internal—Arthritis, diarrhea, gastrointestinal upsets, stress, and tension; helps promote breast milk production in nursing mothers. External—Gargle for sore throats; cuts, minor burns, insect stings.

Description: A much-branched and sprawling, hairy-stemmed annual or biennial, usually no taller than 12 inches. Leaves are palmately five-parted, with divisions being cleft or lobed again. Pale pink or white flowers with five equal-shaped petals occur in loose terminal clusters. Petals often have dark spots on their bases, and leaves are reddish-green and pinnate, fernlike. Seed pod is long and shaped like a stork's bill; it bursts open when seeds are ripe.

Habitat: Woodland areas, thickets, wet or damp places, swamps, marshes, alluvial forests.

Distribution: Most of the state.

Plant Status: Native.

Animal Use: Visited by insect pollinators and birds. Cattle, sheep, and goats will graze on the plant parts, and seeds are collected by various species of harvester ants and by upland game birds, songbirds, the desert tortoise, and small rodents.

Natural History: Cherokee, Choctaw, Haudenosaunee, Menominee, Meskwaki, and Ojibwa people used the whole plant for various problems, including relief from a sore mouth, as a laxative, as an antiseptic, and as an emetic. It was also included in the diet of several Native American tribes, including the Blackfeet, Shoshone, and Digger Indians.

Cultivation: Prefers full sun to partial shade in poorer soil that is gravelly, sandy, or contains hardpan clay. Plant can become weedy due to reseeding. Use in naturalized areas for the best results.

Geranium dissectum

Other Names: Cutleaf *Geranium.*

Medicinal Uses: Internal—Diarrhea, gastrointestinal upsets, heavy menstruation, internal bleeding. External—Hemorrhoids, sore throats, thrush, vaginal discharges, wounds.

Description: Plant grows to about 2 feet tall and is often prone. The stem is densely covered with short hairs, as is the rest of the plant. The petioled leaves are alternate and deeply, palmately lobed. The main lobes of the lower leaves are also lobed. The lobes of the lower leaves are usually much broader than on the upper leaves. Flowers are deep pink and 0.25 inch wide.

Habitat: Fields, pastures, waste places, and roadsides.

Distribution: Top two-thirds of the state, spotty elsewhere.

Plant Status: Introduced.

Animal Use: Pollinators including native bees, syrphid flies, bumblebees, and honeybees, although the plant can also self-pollinate.

Natural History: Native to Europe and introduced in eastern, southern, and western North America. It is considered a noxious weed in some states.

Cultivation: Needs water during its growth period, especially in the summer when the weather is hot. Control watering in the winter, as excessive watering will make roots rot. Fertilize in spring. Prefers a sunny spot with neutral to slightly acidic soil.

Geranium maculatum

Other Names: Spotted *Geranium*, wild *Geranium*, cranesbill, wild cranesbill, spotted cranesbill, crowfoot, alumroot, alum bloom, storks bill, chocolate flower, old maid's night cap, rockweed, sailor's knot.

Description: A clump-forming herbaceous perennial ground cover growing up to 2 feet tall and 18 inches wide. Flowers are 1.25 inches in diameter, pink to lilac, saucer-shaped, upward-facing, and have five-petal flowers. Leaves are deeply cut, palmately five-lobed, dark green, and up to 6 inches across. Flowers are followed by beaked seed capsules.

Medicinal Uses: Internal—Diarrhea, digestion problems, irritable bowel syndrome (IBS), canker sores, and gum disease. External—Wounds, bleeding sores, hemorrhoids, vaginal discharge, thrush.

Habitat: Dry or moist woods, woodland edges, dappled meadows, and rich or rocky woods.

Distribution: Lincoln, Union, and Vernon Parishes.

Plant Status: Introduced.

Animal Uses: Seeds attract mourning doves, bobwhite quails, and white-tailed deer. This plant is also of special value to native bees and bumblebees.

Natural History: The species name, *maculatum,* means mottled and refers to the dark greenish-brown leaves, which are rather mottled.

Cultivation: Plant it in rich soil with plenty of organic matter in full sun or light shade and provide plenty of moisture for the best growth. Plants flower more prolifically the more sun they receive.

For All Species, Other Names: All species are known informally as cranesbill. See above for individually specific names.

Parts Used: Whole plant.

Medicinal Properties: Astringent, antiseptic, antidiabetic, antidiarrheal, anti-inflammatory, antiviral, diuretic, nervous system support, styptic, tonic, vulnerary.

Uses: Cough, tonsillitis; diarrhea, irritable bowel, hemorrhoids, gastritis; fevers; kidney/bladder conditions; heavy menstrual bleeding, vaginal discharge. In Chinese medicine, cranesbill is used to aid digestion, ease occasional diarrhea, support joint health, and benefit skin health.

Risks: Contraindicated in the presence of dry constipation. Should not be taken if using anticholinergic medication (including some drugs for respiratory, cardiac, gastrointestinal, or some mental health conditions). Check with your health care practitioner.

Animal Use: Seeds—Mourning dove, bobwhite quail. Plant—White-tailed deer. See above for individual species. Caterpillars of nine species of moth are reported to eat the genus *Geranium.*

Natural History: The name *Geranium* is derived from the Greek word *geranos,* which means crane. This refers to the shape of the papery seed capsules that split lengthwise into five long peels and look like a crane or stork.

Designation: Native American/Indigenous remedy, herb of commerce, homeopathic remedy, flower essence remedy, traditional Chinese medicine herb.

Remedy Form: Internal—Tea, tincture, edible. External—Compress, poultice, wash.

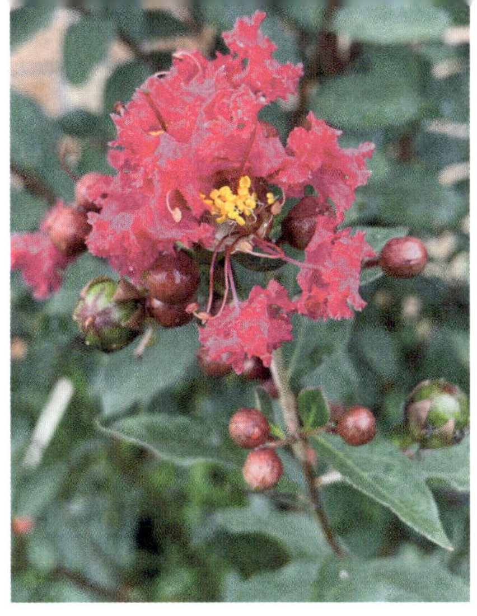

CRAPE MYRTLE & THE MOTHER TREE

SUMMER

Crape myrtle
(*Lagerstroemia indica*)

With another steamy day on its way, Bodi and I trek out to the levee and down to the river before the day gets sweltering. He hates the heat. I guess his little doggy self, bred and born from Maine "doodles," feels most at home somewhere between 20 and 60 degrees. But he's adapted pretty well here, and if we go out before the sun is up, he can come home and settle into the air-conditioned house, then nap for the hottest part of the day.

But I'm okay with the steamy days. Today I'm hoping to do a bit more yard work before giving up and joining Bodi for a nap. One of the yard chores will be to figure out how to help my crape myrtle tree that seems unbothered by heat but is fighting with its neighbors for space.

I'm not sure who planted the crape myrtle in my front yard—but she had made herself at home for years before I arrived. These days, she's overshadowed by the tall, grand magnolia that has become pushy, bushy, tall, and strong. The crape myrtle is persistent, though. She has sprouted long branches up through the *Magnolia*'s thick limbs, and every spring she buds and then blooms with pale-pink flower clusters. Still, I worry about her some—wonder how to help her survive the *Magnolia*'s intrusion and whatever weather changes may come. I want her to keep going because she's beautiful—offers frilly flowers once the air heats up, and a smooth, mottled "skin" of pale and darker-brown barks. And it turns out that she provides some healing benefits as well.

Apparently, crape myrtles have a long history of medicinal uses around the world. James Duke's Phytochemical and Ethnobotanical Databases list more than ninety organic compounds found in crape myrtle that have healing properties. Bark and leaves and flowers and even the roots have been used for pain relief and inflammation, asthma, cancer, flu and colds, viruses and sore throats, heavy bleeding, cuts and scratches, blood sugar regulation, and to protect the liver from damage. The tree was also employed to promote healthy skin and to dissolve kidney stones, decrease cholesterol, prevent heart attacks, and reduce blood pressure. In the Philippines and Japan, leaves are used daily as a tea, and a powder of the roasted fruit is used to brush teeth to make them white and strong. In Ayurveda, the medical system of India, the plant is used to treat diabetes, aid digestion, and promote weight loss.

Although the tree isn't used much by modern Western herbalists, it turns out to be a component of some flower essences, where the blossoms are thought to provide emotional strength, impart courage, and induce calm, a sense of wholeness, the grace to endure change, and greater creativity. It is also reported that witches prefer crape myrtle wood for wands, as it symbolizes strength and stability.

Now that I have learned some of its uses, I want to start experimenting with the plant parts. But normally I recommend that folks use the particular species of a plant as it grows in the wild, and I have no idea whether this tree is close kin to the "original species" of *Lagerstroemia* or is some motley mix of species blended to produce the prettiest bark and the frilliest flowers. And I'm not sure how to find out.

But in doing more reading, I learn that our love for this tree is shared across the globe. I find her name in dozens, even hundreds, of languages—Vietnamese, Bulgarian, and Swedish, Thai and Russian and Malaysian. It's kind of nice to know. But with such a humongous number of places where the tree has grown, it would likely be impossible for me to find an actual "original" species to grow in my own yard.

I think a lot about trees lately, and where they originated, and wonder how they will fare in a changing climate and world. I've been reading a book about trees by forest ecologist Suzanne Simard. In her research on how forests grow, she's come to understand that "trees perceive one another, learn and adapt behaviors, recognize neighbors and remember the past." All of nature, she says, "is an interconnected and sentient community," and at the center of these natural "families" are what she calls the "Mother Trees," who “nurture the forest in the way that families and communities influence human societies.”

Reading that, I’m curious about where the Mother Tree of crape myrtle might have been. Did it occur in the middle of a forest of siblings and cousins? Did it sing in the wind, and hum to all its children? And what about these random crape myrtles in so many yards? Do they communicate, even though they’re separated by distances and roads? Do they miss each other? Are they lonely? Or have they somehow learned to stretch beyond all the human-made structures that chop their world and web into bits? Are there still a few crape myrtle Mother Trees growing in some far-off spot, sending out care and instructions about how to get along in this world? And does my own little tree keep straining to hear and to soak up that love? How much has she changed from her original “family” of trees? And if she’s been genetically tweaked to produce brighter colors and long-lasting blooms, will she still offer healing?

Probably most of my neighbors who love their own crape myrtles haven’t ever thought about nibbling on their trees, or making a tea of leaves and bark, or of crushing the frilly flowers to use as a paste on little cuts, or brushing their teeth with her roasted fruits. In fact, I’m pretty sure they’d think I was rather strange if they knew I was considering that. And I probably won’t do the “toothbrush” thing, after all. But I might someday be working in the garden, get wounded by some prickly tangles, and grab a fistful of crape myrtle flowers to press against the scratch—at least until I can go inside to use an antiseptic wash.

Maybe I can ask my local garden clubs and an LSU agricultural agent my question about the species. Despite all my questions and concerns, though, I’m happy to know that my crape myrtle holds a gentle key to some health issues, and that local birds will be fed by her seeds and the bees will visit her flowers.

For now, I’ll take care of the little “foreign” wanderer who has persisted, through changes and storms and pressure from her neighboring *Magnolia.* I’m sure I won’t ever take the place of what would have been her Mother source—but I can shower her with love, keep an eye out for her health, welcome the wild animals she feeds, and care about her life. I can use some of her freely given parts to shore up my own health. And maybe that will help. Maybe, together, we can make a tiny family, even if I’m not the least bit related to her far-distant Mother Tree. And who knows—maybe, somehow, each year when she buds, far across the oceans other crape myrtle trees will be celebrating as she bursts into bloom.

Other Names: *Lagerstroemia indica* (and some cultivars are a blend of *L. indica* and *L. fauriei*), crapemyrtle, crape myrtle, crepe myrtle, crepeflower, pride of India, queen crape myrtle, queen of flowers, queen of shrubs, queen's flower, cuddle tree, banabá, giant crepe myrtle, Indian crape myrtle.

Parts Used: Bark, leaves, flowers, seeds, roots.

Medicinal Properties: Analgesic, anti-Alzheimer's, anti-asthmatic, anticancer, antiflu, antihemorrhagic, anti-HIV, anti-inflammatory, antioxidant, antiseptic, antiviral, astringent, bronchodilator, hepatoprotective, insulin-sparing.

Uses: Internal—Bark: Fevers, sore throats; cancer (cervix, colon, esophagus, mouth). Flowers: Colds. Leaves: Fluid retention/edema; diabetes; blood pressure irregularities; indigestion. Root: Fevers, sore throats. External—Bark, flowers, and root: Cuts, wounds. In Ayurvedic medicine, dried leaves have been used to help relieve diabetes and to help regulate blood pressure and aid in digestion. A paste of the flowers can be applied to cuts and scratches.

Risks: Avoid in pregnancy and breastfeeding; avoid for two weeks prior to surgery. Possible side effects might include dizziness, headache, and upset stomach. Medications for diabetes and/or high blood pressure may interact with crape myrtle. Regular use may also interfere with the body's ability to utilize some drugs. Check with your health care practitioner for guidance.

Description: Crape myrtle is an upright, wide-spreading, multi-stemmed, deciduous, ornamental shrub or small tree that grows up to 20 feet tall with a spread of 12 feet, and has a moderate growth of about 10 inches per year. The plant has an aggressive and dense root system. Twigs are slender, brown (initially red or green), ridged or angled, and buds are very small. Barks are gray-brown, smooth, and exfoliate to expose shades of brown, reddish brown and green.

Habitat: Gardens, yards, parks. Some have escaped from cultivation to settle in waste places, around parking lots, along highways and rivers, and in some disturbed forests.

Distribution: Many parishes across the state.

Plant Status: Introduced and escaped from cultivation.

Animal Use: A pollen source for honeybees and a number of common native bees at a time of year when resources are scarce. Goldfinches, dark-eyed juncos, house finches, cardinals, and house and white-throated sparrows visit the trees continually from early December through late February. Crape myrtle aphids and their sugary honeydew are food for twenty to thirty species of beneficial insect predators.

Natural History: The genus name honors Magnus von Lagerstroem (1691–1759), a Swedish botanist, director of the Swedish East Indies Company, and friend of Linnaeus. The most common species in the United States is *Lagerstroemia indica.* Although native to China and Korea, the species name (*indica*) indicates that the plant originated on the Indian subcontinent. It was introduced into South Carolina in the late 1700s. *L. fauriei,* native to Japan, is another species found in the United States. Hybrids of the two species generally produce excellent selections.

Designation: Used in folkloric herbal tradition and in healing practices of traditional Chinese medicine.

Cultivation: Prefers sunny locations with well-drained soil and average to medium moisture. It can also tolerate loamy, clay soils with good drainage. Fertilize in early spring and mulch for best weed control. May be susceptible to powdery mildew, aphids, and bark scale. For best growth, tree should not be "topped." The plant needs hot summers in order to flower successfully. Once established, it is drought-hardy, though benefits from occasional deep watering during summer months.

Remedy Form: Internal—tea, tincture. External—poultice, compress, wash.

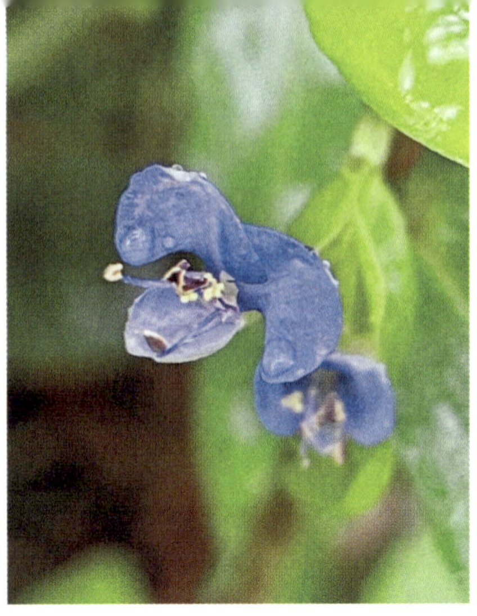

DAYFLOWER & THE GARBAGE

WINTER

Dayflower
(*Commelina* sp.)

This morning I'm in love with the fields. After making it through the droughty summer heat, the land all around has settled into its usual winter green. With a recent rain, a few leftover wildflowers are showing up. Though the usual flashy growth of summer has passed us by, the hardiest plants are still around. I say hello to a few favorites—spiderwort with its lavender-blue blooms; the little, pink-flowered oxalis trying to take over the worn-out yard; the yellow snakeberry flowers just budding up. And one of my favorites—and also one of the most common—the dayflowers.

I love this genus of plants partly because of the beautiful blue petals of most species, but also because dayflower is one of the common, "simple" herbs that is mild in action, helpful for a wide variety of problems, and has been proven safe to use. And it is not limited to just our area but can be found throughout the world. In fact, it's so feisty and persistent that it is often listed as a troublesome weed—appearing in farm fields, city lots, roadsides, and lawns, and growing as far away as Korea, Sweden, Ethiopia, Nepal, Haiti, Ecuador, and Peru. It has found its way into the healing traditions of Indigenous and folk medicine in this country and many others. And it is used for not just physical ailments but for emotional and even spiritual conditions as well. Used in some parts of Latin America for nervous system conditions, it is recommended for calming the spirit and for warding off the evil eye.

In China, some species are used for their antifevers, anti-inflammatory, and diuretic effects. They have also been used in that country for treating sore throats and tonsillitis. Recent pharmacological investigations have revealed that various species of the *Commelina* have cleansing and diuretic properties and can reduce fevers. Used as a gargle to relieve sore throats and tonsillitis, a tea of the dried plant is also used to treat bleeding and diarrhea and can act as an antibacterial. Having read more lately about this plant genus, I'm eager to start a harvest of the small herb so I can test out these claims.

First, though, when I try to take a few photos, I run into a problem. So much garbage litters the road that it's hard to capture the beauty without also capturing the trash. Today's items: crushed soda bottles, an empty beer can, a pile of broken glass, a whole bag (tied up tidily) of leftover food items from the nearest convenience store. At least today there are no poopy diapers.

Every time I see the mess, I try to figure out why it happens. Don't people have garbage cans at home? Or trash bags in their cars? Why would anyone treat their home ground like garbage? Maybe it's just a matter of convenience for all those workers speeding toward their jobs along River Road. Or maybe it's apathy in an area where so many struggle with poverty, in a state that often suffers from neglect and underfunding. Maybe after a while it doesn't seem like anything can change, and people just give up. If you're treated like garbage, maybe that becomes the way you treat yourself, your home, your town. It makes me sad and disheartened. But maybe I can do something to help. I can bring an extra bag with me next time I come, and take a few things home with me, along with whatever herbs I've collected. I can volunteer for the annual trash pickup day in the spring and try to figure out a way to encourage more concern about how the town looks.

For now, I pick up a few bits of trash that aren't too yucky and stuff them in a big pocket. As I turn onto the road home, I find a skeleton from a roadkill and pick up a few bits of jawbones with complicated teeth, putting that in my other pocket so I can look it up to identify its source. I like to know what's in my neighborhood—not just the people and the plants but the animal neighbors as well.

As I head on home, I'm pretty sure my little tidying chores today won't make a bit of difference, but at least I'll have cleared a spot where the dayflowers can flourish, and I'll feel safe harvesting a batch later this week. And maybe, somehow, making my little notes every day—these love letters of appreciation—might help folks to know that the beauty matters, the lushness matters, the healing and the herbs and the caring all matter. And so does where we live. For a while, I guess I'll just continue to pick herbs and pick up trash as part of my morning ritual, a couple of small things I can do to help promote the plants and to cherish the land where I live.

Species: Several *Commelina* species in the state have been proven to have a history of use for healing. These include:

Commelina caroliniana

Other Names: Carolina dayflower.

Medicinal Uses: Internal—Diarrhea, gastrointestinal tract disturbances, hemorrhoids; colds, coughs, flu, fevers, laryngitis, sore throats, pharyngitis, respiratory tract infections, otitis media; mumps; arthritis; urinary tract infections, edema. External—Swelling, eye irritation, conjunctivitis, nose bleeds, insect bites.

Description: An annual herb with a spreading growth habit and will readily root at the nodes when in contact with the soil. Hairless leaves are lance to lance-elliptic shaped, and measure 0.275–4 inches in width and 1–4 inches in length, with rough margins. Stems may rest on the ground or may rise at tips to climb. Flower has three blue petals, with two larger upper petals and one smaller bottom petal that turns white toward the center of the blossom.

Habitat: Fields, yards, waste places, along roadsides or railroads, or occasionally in forests. Also found in crops, especially those involving heavy irrigation such as rice, sugarcane, and corn.

Distribution: Scattered across the state in undisturbed areas.

Plant Status: Native.

Commelina communis

Other Names: Asiatic dayflower, common dayflower.

Medicinal Uses: Internal—Bleeding; fevers, flu, influenza, sore throats, tonsillitis; diabetes; diarrhea, enteritis, obesity; urinary tract infection. External—Poultice/compress for boils, cuts, abscesses, and insect bites.

Description: A weedy, sprawling plant that can be erect at 3 feet high or spread across the ground for up to 10 feet. Flowers are blue, with two relatively large blue petals and one much smaller white petal. Blossom is 1 inch wide and appears singly on a 2-inch stalk from midsummer to early fall. Each flower blooms in the morning and lasts for a single day. Root system is fibrous and the plant can root and form new plants easily.

Habitat: Low, moist woods, riverbanks, thickets, shaded gardens, and waste places. Grows best in partial shade or full sun.

Distribution: Spotty throughout the state, more concentrated in northern and southern parishes.

Plant Status: Introduced.

Commelina difusa

Other Names: Climbing dayflower, spreading dayflower.

Medicinal Uses: Internal—Diarrhea, gastrointestinal tract disturbances, hemorrhoids; colds, coughs, fevers, flu, laryngitis, sore throats, pharyngitis, respiratory tract infections, otitis media; mumps; arthritis; urinary tract infections, edema. External—Swelling, eye irritation, conjunctivitis, nose bleeds, insect bites.

Description: Can be distinguished from its species cousins by the fact that the three petals are blue, the leaves are narrowly elliptical, the spathe is elongated and open, the seeds are shallowly reticulated, and there are no stolons. Spreads diffusely, creeping along the ground, branching heavily and rooting at the nodes, and may be up to 3 feet long. Stems may have small hairs. Leaves are variable, from lance-shape to ovoid, and are up to 1 inch in width and up to 4.7 inches in length. Flowers are blue (or occasionally lavender) with three petals. Two upper petals measure up to 0.2 inch and lower petal is smaller.

Habitat: Open swamps, marshes, forests, thickets, riverbanks, and humid, open places.

Distribution: Scattered across the state, mainly in disturbed areas.

Plant Status: Native.

Commelina erecta

Other Names: Whitemouth dayflower, erect dayflower, widow's tears, day flower, white-mouth dayflower, hierba del pollo.

Medicinal Uses: Internal—Diabetes; diarrhea; hypertension; infertility; influenza, viruses; rheumatism. External—Skin infections, rashes, sores, and bleeding.

Description: Flowers are terminal and have two large, ear-like petals that are purplish-blue and a much smaller white petal that appears below the others. Leaves are linear to lance-shaped, sessile and clasping. They are alternately arranged. Stems are soft and jointed. Fruits are inconspicuous capsules.

Habitat: Sandy or clay soils in pinelands, open woodlands, dry woods, grasslands, limestone slopes, and stream banks throughout Louisiana and Texas. Can be weedy in fields and gardens.

Distribution: Spotty throughout the state, more concentrated in northern and western parishes.

Plant Status: Native.

Commelina virginica

Other Names: Virginia dayflower.

Medicinal Uses: Mild anxiety and spasms; fevers; urinary tract infections, fluid retention.

Description: May grow up to 2 feet tall. Leaves are arranged in a spiral, with the sheaths having red hairs on the edges, and are up to 5 inches long and 1.5 inches wide. They are elliptic-lanceolate with sheaths up to 1 inch long. Stems at base of leaf sheaths are slightly enlarged. Leaf sheaths wrap tightly around the stem. Flowers are small, open at daybreak, and quickly wilt and fall off. Flowers have two upper petals and a slightly smaller lower petal. Petals are light blue and slightly ruffled with a narrow, stalk-like base.

Habitat: Low, moist woods in Louisiana and East Texas, especially swamps, river and stream banks, ditches, and bottomlands.

Distribution: Most parishes—heavily concentrated in top two-thirds of the state.

Plant Status: Native.

For All Species, Parts Used: Whole plant.

Medicinal Properties: Various species have been proven to be antibacterial, anti-inflammatory, antipyretic, antispasmodic, antitussive, astringent, demulcent, depurative, detoxifying, diuretic, emmenagogue, expectorant, febrifuge, hemostatic, laxative, nervine, refrigerant, styptic, and tonic.

Uses: Internal—Diarrhea, gastrointestinal tract disturbances, hemorrhoids; colds, coughs, flu, laryngitis, sore throats, pharyngitis, respiratory tract infections, otitis media; mumps; arthritis; fevers; urinary tract infections, edema. External—Burns, swelling, eye irritation, conjunctivitis, nosebleeds, insect bites, skin irritations, wounds. Many species are used as a wild edible.

Risks: Numerous studies of *Commelina* species report low risk of using the plants. Check with a health care practitioner if pregnant or nursing.

Animal Use: Eaten by pigs, ducks, chickens, and fish. Plant and seeds eaten in the wild by mourning dove, bobwhite quail, redwing blackbird, and cardinal (seed) and white-tailed deer (plant). Blooms attract a variety of pollinators, especially bees and sylphid flies. Foliage is sometimes consumed by gopher tortoises.

Natural History: The genus was named by Linnaeus after three Dutch botanists in the Commelin family, Johann (1629–1698), Kasper (1667–1731), and a third who died young. Linnaeus felt the flowers represented the three botanists, with each flower having two showy petals and a third inconspicuous petal, referring to the two accomplished botanists and the third who died before accomplishing anything of great botanical significance. The species name *communis* refers to the fact that the plants "grow in colonies."

Designation: Traditional Chinese medicine, folk medicine remedy in many countries across the globe, Indigenous healing traditions.

Cultivation: The *Commelina* are not particularly picky about growing conditions but are sometimes considered weedy plants, so it is best to check with your local agricultural agents about the plant's growth in your area. One way to control weedy plants is to harvest and use them for healing and wild foods (in safe areas).

Remedy Form: Edible, tea, tincture, compress, poultice.

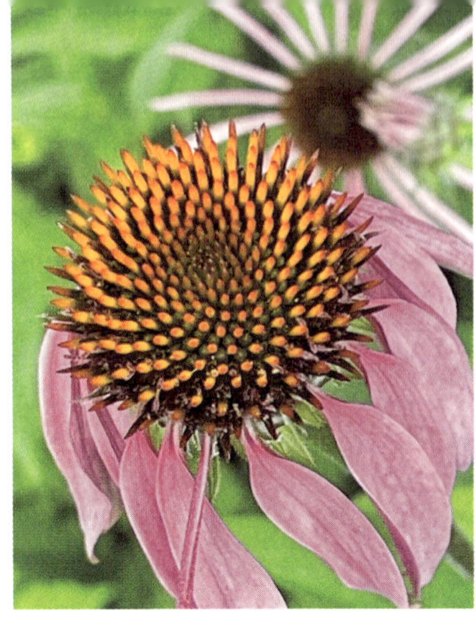

ECHINACEA & CANCER ALLEY

SUMMER

Echinacea
(*Echinacea purpurea*)

On a late-summer morning, I sit at the kitchen window and watch birds flit in and out of the tattered garden. Finally, after a dry and fiery summer, the air is a little cooler—only up to 90 degrees predicted for later today. But there's still no rain in sight, and everything is struggling. The usual visitors to the yard—coons and possums and bunnies—come early and are gone by sunup. And the birds that come for seed depend on the birdbath and other low dishes I keep filled with water in the yard. But, fortunately, most of the flower beds are doing okay. They are still lush with blooms, and some of my favorites—the coneflowers—are right at home with arid soil and the big heat.

Even before I went to herb school, I knew about *Echinacea* and its usefulness for supporting the immune system. Over the last four decades, much research has been carried out on the herb internationally, and several species have been documented to have over six hundred medicinal compounds. In many states, *Echinacea* species grow wild but are sometimes threatened by overharvesting. Gardeners love the plant, too, and it is easily grown in home flower beds, producing great summer blooms and attracting many pollinators.

For many years now, I've counted on *Echinacea* for health as well as garden beauty. Most often, I utilize it at the early outset of a cold that seems to be going around, or a flu, or just a vague sense of feeling not quite right. It's often the first thing I reach for when I start to feel unwell. It's a great herb to have on hand.

But sometimes threats to health are more subtle or complicated than cold symptoms. Other factors like diet, stress levels, exercise, and social support systems can impact our wellness. There are also times when the very lands and waters and air around us can be the source of illness. We live in complicated times. No matter where we reside, or how much we do to take care of our bodies, we are constantly bombarded with threats to our health.

And Louisiana has more than its share of challenges. Poor air quality, questionable water safety, conflicting priorities, and weak governmental commitments afflict not only our health but also our very safety. Communities that occur within what is known as "Cancer Alley"—an eighty-five-mile stretch along the banks of the Mississippi River between New Orleans and Baton Rouge—are home not only to state residents but also the sites of over two hundred fossil fuel and petrochemical operations. In recent decades, it has become obvious that citizens living in these areas have much higher cancer rates than do other residents of the state, or of the nation.

There is much information available on this, and, in fact, some parts of Louisiana have been informally dubbed a "sacrifice zone"—where it is just accepted that residents will be exposed to more toxins from petrochemical plants. A recent report from ProPublica, a nonprofit investigative news group that takes on important issues, noted that those living in Louisiana's Cancer Alley are sometimes exposed to forty-seven times the level of risk deemed acceptable by the Environmental Protection Agency. Residents in these areas have begun to demand remediation and protection, and there is some hope that things will move in a healthier direction, but not without much effort on their parts, and not without lots of support. For now, the struggle continues.

I guess we all know these things in a vague way—we read and hear about the challenges everywhere. But after a while all that information becomes white noise in the background of our lives. So often, we feel that there is not much we can do, so we do the best we can. And we know that can never be enough, so we just kind of give up.

My older daughter, who lives in Maine, has visited me here several times in the last few years. She loves Louisiana—has childhood memories of visits to grandparents and trips down the bayous, alligator swamp tours, meeting her hundreds of cousins, the joie de vivre of Louisiana folks. And even though she is nowhere near retirement age, she once thought this would be where she landed after her work years ended. But lately, she's found herself adrift. Reading all about the state's struggles with environmental issues, and disturbing information about Cancer Alley, she's changing her mind. She's done her research, and she's found that many state-level governmental policies still seem to lean toward favoring the desires of big oil and chemical companies over the needs of citizens. So she's given up on the idea of coming "home." She still loves to visit, but she says she just can't make a decision that would put her health, and life, at risk. And I understand.

I guess living in Louisiana may always mean living with risks as ever-present storms, corporate greed, and political waffling keep us all on shaky ground.

So what do we do? My daughter has made her decision to not settle here. But some people just can't leave. My own family, with seven generations who lived and thrived here, will now have to decide what the future holds, and where it lies. But my ninety-year-old cousins can't be uprooted. Where would they go, when their ancestors lie in the soft, damp ground all around them?

Despite the gloomy outlook, some good things are happening. People are rising up, in gentle ways and sometimes in feisty rebellion, to speak and act against the unhealthy, unconscious, and often-deliberate ignorance that allows whole areas in the state to become sacrifice zones.

As for me and my future, in light of the huge challenges and health threats that plague the state, I figure anything that can support my own immunity and healing capacity seems like a great idea, which leads me back to the coneflowers. There are three species of *Echinacea* that grow wild in the state, and I'm happy to be growing them in my own garden. I love using my own homegrown plants for healing, and I'm happy to be hosting so many pollinators that love the plants, too.

One good thing about using *Echinacea* is that there is much research throughout the years on the efficacy and safety of the herb. And while the plant is often recommended for the early, acute stage of an illness, it is also possible to take it preventively. *Echinacea pallida,* in particular, can be helpful for that.

And in terms of the health of the land, there are some bright, hopeful spots. Lately, I'm hearing about groups of folks committed to native plants and their many benefits. They are working tirelessly to restore some areas—including their own yards and grounds—to the way the land was before mono-cropping and pollutants and sacrifice zones were the norm.

Down the bayous, where the lands that people lived on are sinking rapidly and residents are scattering and sad, people are thinking creatively of ways to stay connected and to share memories, loves, and fears both in person and digitally. Important groups like the Bayou Cultural Collaborative work hard to connect those "interested in the intersection of traditional culture, the arts, and science in the face of Louisiana's land loss and the impact of migrations upon our culture in the coming years."

And I'll continue to be here, for a while at least, and to find herbal and other ways to shore up my health. In that effort, *Echinacea* just might become a regular support—small doses, taken over a shorter period of time, could become one of the ways I head into the future.

This place is so at-risk that it tears at my heart. But maybe, if we work together, we can move in the direction of positive changes. In the meantime, thank God for the beauty. Thank God for communities, and hope, and feisty folks who will not go down easily. And thank God for the healing plants. Amen.

Species: Reportedly, three species of *Echinacea* grow wild in the state, and all species have been documented to contain many medicinally active properties and are often used interchangeably. These include:

Echinacea pallida

Other Names: Pale *Echinacea,* pale coneflower, purple coneflower, pale purple coneflower.

Medicinal Uses: Best for short-term use and acute conditions. Internal—Acute respiratory distress syndrome (ARDS), common cold, cough, bronchitis, fevers, inflammation of the mouth and pharynx; arthritis, rheumatism; infections; urinary tract infections. External—Insect bites and stings, minor burns and wounds. Used in Ayurvedic medicine for balance and support of the body's defenses. Used in more Westernized/integrated Chinese medicine.

Description: The plant grows 2–4 feet tall, stems are stout, flower heads have lavender (and occasionally white) rays that droop from a large, spiny, cone-shaped center. Ray flowers vary in length and width. Leaves are coarsely haired, narrowly lance-shaped, and attach to the plant near the base. *E. pallida* is the only species in the genus to have white pollen.

Habitat: Prairies, woodlands, roadsides, dry, open, rocky sites.

Distribution: Almost two dozen parishes in the western to central half of the state.

Plant Status: Native.

Echinacea purpurea

Other Names: Purple coneflower, eastern purple coneflower, snakeroot, Kansas snakeroot, narrow-leaved purple coneflower, scurvy root, Indian head, comb flower, black Susan, hedgehog.

Medicinal Uses: Prevention against and treatment of upper and lower respiratory system illnesses, coughs and colds, bronchitis, upper respiratory infections, ear infections, flu, gingivitis, canker sores; vaginitis, yeast infections; wound infections; inflammation; certain cancers, and prevention of metastasis.

Description: An herbaceous perennial that may grow up to 4 feet tall and 10–12 inches wide. Leaves are mostly alternate (though sometimes opposing), 3–6 inches long, 1–3 inches wide. Surface is somewhat rough, shape is lance-like, broader at the base, tapering to a point. Leaves are stalked, becoming smaller and stalkless as they ascend the stem, and have serrated edges and three or five distinct veins along the length. Cone-shaped, flowering heads are most often purple in the wild.

Habitat: Rocky prairie in open wooded regions and road banks.

Distribution: Spotty across top half of the state. Found in eleven parishes in central and extreme upper-left corner of the state. Widely cultivated.

Plant Status: Native.

Echinacea sanguinea

Other Names: Sanguine purple coneflower.

Medicinal Uses: Colds, flu, respiratory infections; inflammation; insect bites. Anticancer for breast, cervix, colon, liver, lung, skin, stomach, and anti-metastatic for stomach. Research has proven this species to have even stronger anti-inflammatory effects than other *Echinacea* species.

Description: Stiff, upright, slender stems may be 1.5–3 feet tall. Each stem bears a single flowerhead that is composed of ten to twenty ray flowers that are often drooping and range from pale pink to purple. Disc flowers occur in a central, cone-shaped area that is purplish brown on the outside and greenish in the center. Leaves are rough, 4–9.5 inches long, and are arranged alternately at base of stem. Seed heads are rounded and have yellow pollen.

Habitat: Prairies, open sandy fields, and pine and hardwood forests.

Distribution: Documented in Caddo Parish, may be found in nearby parishes as well.

Plant Status: Native, though plant habitats have experienced loss and degradation due to prairie conversion, woodland logging, and other factors.

For All Species, Parts Used: Whole Plant.

Medicinal Properties: Adaptogen, alterative, antibacterial, anticancer (for breast, cervix, colon, liver, lung, skin, stomach, and anti-metastatic for stomach), antidepressant, anti-inflammatory, antioxidant, anti-osteoporosis, antiseptic, antiviral, anxiolytic, depurative, diaphoretic, digestive, immunomodulary, larvicidal, sialagogue.

Uses: Internal—Arthritis, rheumatism; treatment for and prevention of Acute Respiratory Distress Syndrome (ARDS), colds, coughs, bronchitis, fevers, flu, upper and lower respiratory infections, sore throat, inflammation of mouth and pharynx, ear infections; gingivitis, canker sores; vaginitis, yeast infections; urinary tract infections. External—Insect bites, wounds.

Risks: Echinacea species may cause chemotherapy to be less effective. Use under the guidance of health care practitioners if suffering with autoimmune conditions. While research on the usefulness of *Echinacea* in the treatment of viral infections that provoke excessive cytokine production, such as SARS Co-V-2/COVID-19 is ongoing, there is no conclusive evidence of its safety and effectiveness, and it is best to follow the recommendations of a family physician for prevention and treatment of this condition.

Animal Use: Coneflowers attract a variety of animals and pollinators, including insects, butterflies, and birds. Specific animals that are drawn to coneflowers include bumblebees, long-horn beetles, soldier beetles, monarchs, swallowtails, goldfinches, hummingbirds, and blue jays. Cattle, deer, rabbits, and woodchucks may browse on the plants.

Natural History: *Echinacea* use is reported to have originated with North American Indigenous Indians around the eighteenth century. Traditional healers employed various parts of the plants to relieve snakebites, wounds, burns, and insect bites externally, and for pain, coughs, throat infections, digestive infections, and rheumatic conditions internally. White settlers began to use *Echinacea,* and the first pharmaceutical preparation, known as Meyers Blood Purifier, became popular around 1880 for rheumatism, neuralgia, and rattlesnake bites. In 1939, commercial cultivation was undertaken in Germany, followed by cultivation in Switzerland around 1950. Since then, the genus has undergone extensive research and is currently one of the most widely used medicinal plants worldwide.

Designation: An important herb of commerce, folkloric herbal remedy, Native American medicinal herb, and European healing plant. Also used in Ayurvedic and traditional Chinese medicine.

Cultivation: *Echinacea* species are generally low-maintenance and can tolerate a range of soils from sandy to clay as long as there is good drainage. They prefer full sun to light shade in hotter climates. Propagation may be carried out by seed, division, basal cuttings, or root outings. Dividing every few years will keep them healthy. Avoid overwatering after initial planting because *Echinacea* prefers drier conditions once established. Plants often do not flower well in first year.

Remedy Form: Internal—Tea, tincture. External—Compress, poultice, wash.

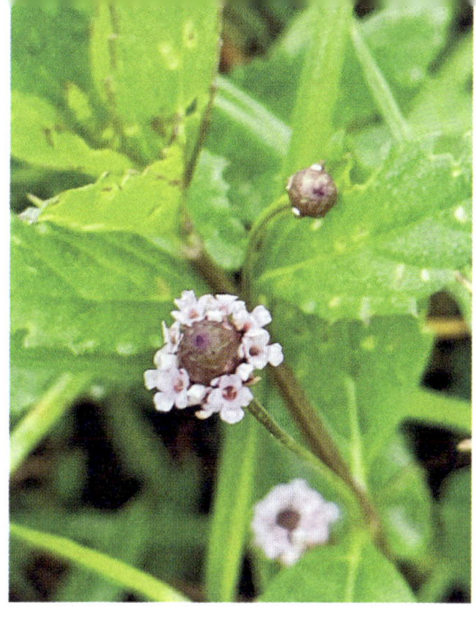

FROGFRUIT & THE NATIVE PLANTS

FALL

Frogfruit
(*Phyla* sp.)

Bodi and I take a short walk this morning in a blessing of light rain. We're so happy to have a reprieve after much heat and drought this summer that we don't mind getting a little wet.

It's a quiet start to the day. We walk down to the riverbank, where lately the water is so low that there are worries about how the cities and towns that line the bank will deal with the water shortage, or how the boat traffic will manage. Despite the worries, though, some things are pretty dependable. Our ragged garden is still producing tomatoes, and the winter squash is ripening, so I'll be lugging them in pretty soon. And the last of the bright trumpet creeper flowers hang onto the vine, even though some long, ridged seed pods are starting to form. It won't be long before the plant starts its winter rest.

Along the levee, there are still some green patches of grass and other low growth—and I spot one of my favorite native herbs. Frogfruit is getting near the end of its own blooming season but is still looking pretty healthy despite the weather challenges. The little lavender and white flowers are still nodding on stalks, and even though other wildflowers have been daunted by the heat, this plant is abundant and beautiful.

I'd never seen frogfruit before coming back to Louisiana. It wasn't one of the attention-grabbing flowers I first stumbled upon when I returned here. Some of the obvious "stars" were the showy *Magnolias,* the *Echinacea,* the mamou. But after a while, I started noticing the smaller plants, and eventually my eyes settled on the small flowers of frogfruit, so I did some research on them. And as is so often the case, they were interesting, intriguing, and medicinal.

I began to learn some of its healing properties. And researching *Phyla nodiflora* (and its cousins) made me curious about other native plants that grow in the area, and about the fairly recent movement toward landscaping with the plants that are at home here. I began to imagine a future where our landscapes and gardens could be allowed to include those "volunteer" plants that are right under our feet. In addition to beauty, often they also contain some important nutrients, and many have healing properties.

As an herbalist, I had never paid much attention to how a plant arrived at the spot where it was growing—I was more interested in what could be done with it once I found it. Of course, I was careful about plant populations, harvesting with awareness of whether an herb might be at risk where it was growing. But I basically just appreciated the plants for what they could offer. As it turns out, though, I had been unintentionally harvesting native plants for decades. And when I found myself writing an herb journal about Louisiana wild medicinal plants, I found that I had included a preponderance of natives in the book.

I've learned that one of the great things about native plants is that they're not finicky. No matter the weather, these plants can handle it. They've adapted over time to whatever the soils and skies and nearby creatures offer up, and they're right at home. They often provide food and nectar to local animals and are an integral part of how various species survive. It also turns out that many native plants contain natural chemical compounds that help them to thrive and reproduce. And other chemicals in the plants, known in the herbal world as secondary metabolites, offer a host of healing properties to those of us interested in using them.

My research on frogfruit revealed that the plant has many biochemical activities that make it useful for a range of problems including bronchitis, asthma, colds, coughs, and other respiratory ailments, and for fevers. It's also been used in numerous other parts of the world for constipation, fluid retention, menstrual irregularities, and pain. In Ayurvedic medicine, the herb has been employed internally for blood disorders, wounds, diarrhea, joint pain, indigestion, respiratory ailments, and kidney or gallbladder stones. Externally, a poultice of the herb has been helpful for boils, acne, wounds, and hemorrhoids.

And if that were not enough, it turns out that *Phyla nodiflora* is an easy and adaptable native herb to include in home gardens. It has a long bloom period and is a host plant to many butterflies and other pollinators. And its seeds provide food for many birds, especially waterfowl. And it's not hard to grow! Clippings of the plant can be easily rooted in a garden, where they can be used for a ground cover, a walkway, or even an herbal lawn. The more I read about the use of native plants in our home gardens, the more impressed I am with their possible contribution to a more sustainable future for the state. As Louisiana Native Plant Society past president Tammany Baumgarten noted in a recent article, "Intentionally putting native plants back into our ecosystems has become increasingly . . . important, because we are starting to see biodiversity losses, (and) less of the birds and insects and all of these things that use Louisiana's native plants."

With all of that in mind, I decide to start experimenting with frogfruit right now. Bodi waits patiently while I bend down to snip off a handful of the herb to dry for tea. Now that I know more about its benefits—both for healing, and for the landscape and wildlife—I'm eager to have it on hand. I want to try some for colds, coughs, fevers, and pain. In fact, I might decide to come back later to dig up a small patch of the herb to plant in my garden. Then I'd have it close at hand whenever the need arises, and I'd be supporting the local animals that coexist with me on my few acres.

Bodi and I turn around and walk slowly toward home. I'm savoring the new harvest and appreciating the time to notice what's growing all around us. And we are both happy. I love these small, simple moments of life—walking with my aging dog, checking on the fruits of my garden work, and appreciating the native plants that can handle most any weather and still thrive.

Sometimes I think that the most modest and unassuming things are the most healing and powerful. Maybe learning to identify and use the little frogfruit and the other "common," unfinicky native plants can act—for all of us—as a reminder of the unconditional generosity that underlies all of life. Working with native plants, we may find small ways to move forward into a more balanced world. Maybe, in some way we can't yet understand, in these simple tasks, we are inextricably linked with, and co-participating in, the future of Healing, and a verdant life on Earth. May it be so.

Other Names: *Phyla nodiflora,* fog fruit, turkey tangle, sawtooth frogfruit, Mat Lippia, Mat Frass, capeweed, Texas frogfruit, creeping charlie, matgrass, hierba de la vargen maria.

Parts Used: Whole plant.

Medicinal Properties: Anodyne, antibacterial (against E. coli, pseudomonas, staphylococcus, etc.), anticonvulsant, antidiabetic, antifungal, antioxidant, antiparasitic, antitumor, anxiolytic, diuretic, emmenagogue, hepatoprotective, antilithic, antitumor, anti-inflammatory, antihypertensive, antimelanogenesis, antityrosinase, refrigerant, renoprotective.

Uses: Internal—Bronchitis, asthma, colds, coughs, and other respiratory ailments; constipation; fevers; fluid retention; menstrual irregularities; pain. Used in Ayurvedic medicine for blood disorders, wounds, burning sensation, boils, diarrhea, joint pain, indigestion, asthma, bronchitis, hemorrhoids, and kidney/gallbladder stones. External—Boils, acne, hemorrhoids.

Risks: Avoid during pregnancy and nursing or seek out guidance from a health care practitioner.

Description: A long-lived, low-growing, mat-forming perennial with prostrate hairy stems that grow to about 18 inches long and can root at the nodes, often forming large colonies. Growth height is 3–6 inches. Leaves are opposing with a few large teeth toward the tip, and the leaf is widest above the middle. In flowers, white to pinkish petals surround a purple center. Flower head is about 0.25 inch wide, and flower stalk is erect and about 1.25 inches long.

Habitat: Damp lawns, beaches, hammocks, disturbed sites, marshes, wet pinelands, and glades. Somewhat salt-tolerant. Likes sandy soil and limestone outcrops.

Distribution: Occurs in most of the state's southern parishes, and sporadic in other areas.

Plant Status: Native.

Animal Use: An acceptable forage for cattle. Seeds are eaten by waterfowl. Attracts numerous insect pollinators and serves as the larval host and/or nectar source for numerous butterfly species.

Natural History: Reportedly, the plant was initially called "fog fruit." In ancient times, fog would sometimes hang over the recently hayed fields, and the new low-growing plants would look as if they were sown by the fog. The general name "fog fruit" was given to the low-growing *Phyla nodiflora.* Over time, the common name transitioned from "fog fruit" to "frogfruit" and included four different species (*Phyla nodiflora, P. lanceolata, P. cuneifolia,* and *P. stoechadifolia,* and occasionally *P. intermedia,* an apparent hybrid of the species). All of them look pretty similar, and all of them are native to the United States.

Designation: Indigenous/Native medicinal remedy in many cultures, Ayurvedic healing herb, Chinese medicine herbal tea used for the treatment of inflammation, menstrual disorders, and infectious diseases, and for inflammation and liver and kidney failure in Taiwan and China.

Cultivation: Best cultivated by transplanting. Collect sections with several nodes and rootlets attached, and plant in a shallow container until well established; then transplant into new soil. Water regularly until established. Can be trimmed back in the winter if it gets too dense. Prefers full sun to partial shade and is able to survive a wide range of conditions and soil types, tolerating both drought and flooding. The plant is a good alternative to grass turf and can tolerate some foot traffic. It can be mowed once after it flowers. (If mowed during flowering, it will take years to flower again.)

Remedy Form: Internal—Tea, tincture. External—Compress, poultice, wash.

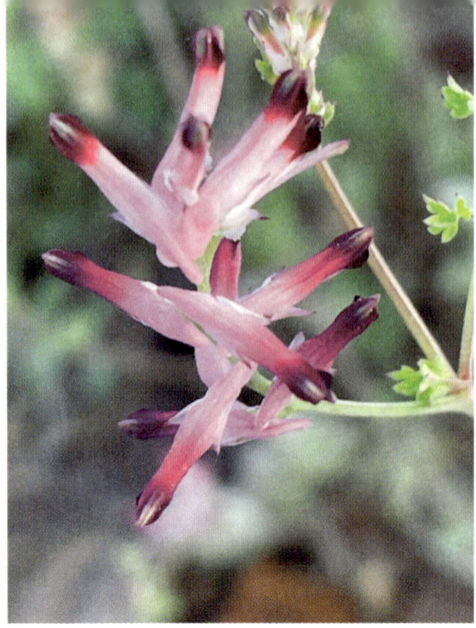

FUMITORY & WHAT WE LEAVE BEHIND

WINTER

Fumitory
(*Fumaria muralis*)

I walk out early this morning, down to the river while Bodi sleeps. Very dark clouds crowd the sky, and the usual storm crows are out, flying and noisy. At the bayou fleet trail, wind-blown sand has packed down, the dunes are tall, and high grasses and fading goldenrod lean into the path.

And the river is busy. Even on this day when storms are coming, and the sky has just started to pale, tugboats shift into place behind barges and push out into the river. An eagle sails from treetops, and a small flock of pelicans hangs over the ships. A fish flips up and out of the water, plunges back in, over and over—silvery in the first promise of sun.

Alongside the riverbank, debris from the latest hurricane is tangled in low growth and small trees. The waterlogged sand is littered with trash—a red plastic hardhat, hospital masks, many empty soda bottles and caps, brushes, bits of colored plates, old tubes of industrial lubricant—either dumped from busy tugboats or scooped up by stormy winds and tossed ashore. I gather up whatever I'm not afraid to touch and stack it into piles to pick up later and haul away. While I work, killdeer slip along the curve of damp sand, poking about for breakfast.

I think about "stuff"—how much we humans seem to accumulate and how much we leave behind as we make our way through the natural world. So many things travel along this river. Apparently, commercial use of the Mississippi waterway is continuing to grow. Sometimes, I see huge ships traveling, and other times there are lines and lines of barges, all loaded down with freight. Petroleum, coal, iron, steel, chemicals, sand, and crushed rock are common freight. And, apparently, about 60 percent of all U.S. grain exports are shipped by barge to ports in New Orleans and south Louisiana. As one of the most important riverways in the country, and one of the major river systems in the world, the Mississippi helps to provide supplies that are vital to our lives. But along with that growth comes trash! A recent study on the amount of waste found in the river noted that at least 75 percent of the trash is plastic. Other common items include cigarette butts, which contain several pollutants and take up to ten years to decompose. Plastic bags, food wrappers, tin and aluminum cups, grocery bags, bits of foam, masks—all join the "leftovers" from our daily lives. Given the increase in violent storms and the unpredictability of water levels lately, I guess it makes sense that some of the debris would end up sloshing along the river's edges at one point or another. But seeing it makes me sad, and I worry about negative effects on the riverside wildlife.

Soon, though, I get tired of thinking about trash and take the path away from the river and around the constantly changing sand-pit ponds. Here, it's another world. Animal tracks intersect, tall horsetail crowds the edges of the trail, a few mulberry trees anchor the dunes, and a beautiful little creeping plant draws my attention. It is tiny and low-growing, with unusual, deep-pink flowers whose tips are tinged with dark red. Even the leaves are pretty—deeply cut and frilly. I check my phone app and discover that, once again, what's underfoot is medicine. It seems that I've stumbled upon what I've heard called "fumitory of the wall," because of its habit of climbing up nearby structures.

Although I've never seen the plant before, I vaguely remember that it has been traditionally used in Europe and other countries for a few health issues. Externally, the crushed plant is recommended as an application to small wounds or scratches and can be especially helpful for the irritations caused by eczema, psoriasis, or acne. I know that the plant has also been used internally for such problems as gallbladder and liver issues and for digestive upsets. But I also know that this herb is a member of the poppy family, and there are some cautions about internal use. I'm eager to get home and look up more about the plant. And I'm excited that even now, when so much of the surrounding land is frost-beaten and brown, in this tucked-away spot, fumitory is lush and thriving. I haven't seen *Fumaria* in many Louisiana areas, but now that I know it has made itself at home here, I'll be on the lookout for it in other spots. Apparently, the herb knows how to take up residence wherever it lands, and it is thought to be a weed in some parts of the country. And after this morning's visit to the trashy riverside, I wonder if maybe its seeds were first brought in on some of those same ships that contribute to the riverside litter.

Next time I'm able to leave Bodi snoozing late into the morning, I'll slip past the busy river, the bustling ships, and the piles of trash, and visit the tucked-away *Fumaria* stand again. I'll bring a bag and some plant shears and clip off enough to dry for tea and an herbal wash and try that on myself. I'll probably tincture some fumitory, too, for future use. I'd like to know more about its usefulness for bowel issues like irritable bowel syndrome, since I know a couple of folks who struggle with those conditions. I'll be happy, then, to have something to check out besides the trash.

And I'll try to be careful about what I leave behind—hopefully only footprints in the dusty river sand.

Other Names: *Fumaria muralis,* common fumitory, earth smoke, climbing fumitory, Allegheny vine, fumitory of the wall.

Parts Used: Whole plant.

Medicinal Properties: Analgesic, anthelmintic, antidyspeptic, anti-inflammatory, antirheumatic, antispasmodic, aperient, cholagogue, diaphoretic, diuretic, hypotensive, laxative, and mildly tonic. Research has proven that some chemical compounds in the plant have antitumor, antimicrobial, and anti-inflammatory properties. Also considered edible and used as a culinary herb in some countries to provide a slightly bitter taste.

Uses: Internal—Dyspepsia, flatulence, gallbladder and liver problems, nausea; fevers, influenza, respiratory infections. External—Acne, eczema, psoriasis, scabies.

Risks: Internal use should be limited to one week. Excess doses may cause sedative effects. Avoid during pregnancy and lactation. Reported side effects of internal use include gastrointestinal complaints and flushing.

Description: A delicate vining plant with stems that are initially erect but become sprawling and/or climbing, are weak and hairless and much branched. Individual stems grow up to 39 inches. Flowers appear in spikes of twelve to fifteen. The flower cluster is shorter than the stalk.

The slender, tubular flowers are pink with a dark-red tip. Leaves begin as single, are up to 0.6 inch wide, and then become compound and lobed. Mature leaves are three times deeply lobed with three or more leaflets and form a rosette. One-seeded fruit is round or oval, and smooth to slightly wrinkled.

Habitat: Found in moist, disturbed areas, particularly along streams and waterways. It prefers to grow in open, bare patches and is often found in pastures, roadsides, gardens, and footpaths.

Distribution: Identified in several areas around Baton Rouge and New Orleans, possibly spreading in lower parts of the state.

Plant Status: Introduced.

Animal Use: Provides food and habitat for a variety of insects, including bees, butterflies, and moths.

Natural History: In 1753, Linnaeus established the genus *Fumaria* in his *Species Plantarum.* He derived the name from the Latin *fumus terrae,* "smoke of the earth," referring to the smoke-like smell of some species or to the appearance of smoke rising from the ground. The species name *muralis* is from Latin and means growing on the walls.

Designation: Used as a European phytotherapy remedy, and in Turkish folk medicine as a blood purifier and an anti-allergic agent. Species of *Fumaria* are used in Ayurveda, Siddha, and Unani healing systems. In some European folklore, the plant was believed to have magical properties and was used in love spells and was also hung over doorways to ward off illness and bad luck and to protect the home and its inhabitants from harm.

Cultivation: Can be propagated from seed or transplanted from cuttings. Prefers full sun, moderate to low water, and can tolerate poor soil. While considered a weed in some areas, it is a valuable component of many ecosystems and can be attractive as an interesting groundcover.

Remedy Form: Internal—Capsules, tea, tincture, powder. External—Compress, poultice, wash.

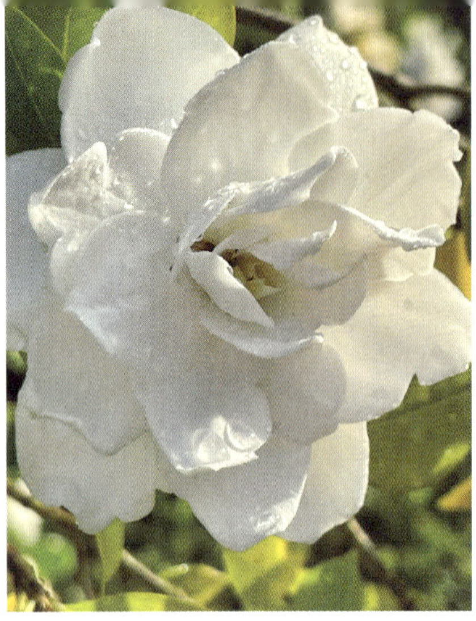

GARDENIA & BODI & THE MOON

FALL

Gardenia
(*Gardenia jasminoides*)

At 12:45 a.m., in the middle of another moonlit night, I am up with Bodi and out in the back field. Poop trip number three, so far. We tramp over the unmown lawn that is wet and tangled and stand under Orion and the waning gibbous moon. I brought a flashlight but don't need it. Bodi navigates more with his nose lately, anyway, and he is curious about what nighttime wild wanderers might have passed through the yard. I am wearing my old winter pajamas that are tattered around the cuffs, and my fuzzy slippers have grown sodden with dew in just the little trek from the house. But the neighbors are asleep, dreaming, I imagine, of their busy lives, and no one cares what I look like—which is a good thing.

The woods glow slightly in the moonlight, tawny with the colors of late fall. And even though I am task-driven, and keep urging Bodi to poop, he thinks it's a fine time to sniff the nighttime scent trails in the dark.

And I have to admit, I am loving my own favorite scents. Late-blooming gardenias have weathered drought and relentless heat and still offer a few more small but fragrant flowers. Their lovely perfume has called to me for my whole life. Growing up in Louisiana, gardenias were ever-present. My mom had a handmade ceramic dish she called the "gardenia bowl." Flat, with slightly upcurved sides, the bowl was just deep enough for the short stems of the picked flowers to rest on the bottom so they could drink up water but not sink down. As a child, I just wanted to stick those fragrant petals right up my nostrils, they smelled so delicious. Little did I know then that I could actually have eaten the petals or made a tea from the flowers. It took me decades of practicing as an herbalist before I realized that the oriental shrub *Gardenia jasminoides* had a number of medicinal properties and was a mainstay in tradition Chinese medicine for various ailments.

So far, I've never used the plant for healing and am eager to try. But one thing stops me. According to my research, the most useful part of the *Gardenia* plant is the fruit. What? Since when has *Gardenia* had a fruit? I try to imagine how I could have missed a fruit after picking and loving the flowers for so many decades—but maybe I have a clue. I remember that when I deadhead a gardenia flower, the small bit of blossom just above the stem does seem to be slightly bulbous as it yellows and gets ready to fall. But would that count as a fruit? Guess I'll have to do more research on this, but I will certainly be happy to try those lovely white petals as a tea and am eager to use the crushed leaves and bark as an external application for cuts or small sores.

I recently bought a very tiny and insanely expensive bottle of *Gardenia* essential oil. I had heard it was good for the skin, and after struggling with a few precancerous sunspots, I think my skin could use some help. I've also heard that it can be useful for insomnia as well. According to the National Institutes of Health, it has melatonin-like activity, can reduce "digital stress," and can help reverse signs of aging—all of which I could certainly use. I'm not sure exactly what digital stress is, but having spent quite a few hours in what I call "cyber-hell," I'm pretty sure I'm afflicted with it. Certainly, a little dab of *Gardenia* oil couldn't hurt. And it's fun to know how many healing properties *Gardenia* has. In folkloric herbalism and in Chinese medicine, the herb is used to treat inflammation, headache, edema, fevers, hepatic disorders, and hypertension. Apparently, the herb is also useful for anxiety and depression and has a spiritual effect of bringing great joy. Remembering all of its potential uses for healing, I pick a pocketful of the sweet flowers that are left on the bush. I'll figure out what to do with them when we get back to the house.

Meanwhile, Bodi continues to follow scent trails through the cold, dewy grass, and I follow him. By now, our feet are wet and cold. We'll be ready for bed soon. But so far, we are feral-wild and glorious under this moon.

The rural, small-town silence wraps around us, and we can hear ourselves breathe. And then the chorus begins. From the levee and from the tallest trees, the owls start up—two different kinds, tonight—the barred owl's "who cooks for you," deep and thrumming, and then another call, a long, wheezy hoot. I stand still for a moment, trying to remember which owl this is. And then the coyotes begin, their songs and the owls' weaving together and echoing in the night. The sounds and the damp, cold darkness hang over us, over the yard, over this luminous land. And Bodi and I stand still for a while, happy in our half-wild home. Here we are, this old pooch and I, doing what we have done for so many years—walking in the night, slipping back into our ancient, half-remembered selves, when we were wild. We breathe and listen and watch and wait.

After a bit, we both give up—head back into the warmth and light our normal, everyday selves have gotten used to. But we are thrilled, once again, by that moon that called us out. And by the scents of healing flowers, and of whatever wild critters passed us by in the dark. We won't have many more nights like this, I guess, since I am seventy-six and he is sixteen. But for now, we are chilled and damp and so alive. And so alive.

Other Names: *Gardenia jasminoides,* cape jasmine.

Parts Used: Flowers, fruits, leaves, bark.

Medicinal Properties: Whole plant—Alterative, antiseptic, antispasmodic, antiperiodic, cathartic, anthelmintic, antiseptic. Leaves and fruit—Antibacterial, antifebrile, demulcent, cholagogue, diuretic, and edible.

Uses: Internal—Anxiety, agitation, depression, pain; bladder infection; bleeding; cancer, immune system support; constipation, gallbladder disease, high cholesterol, liver disorders, swelling of the pancreas; diabetes; fevers; high blood pressure; insomnia; flu; menopausal symptoms; rheumatoid arthritis. It is also used as an antioxidant and to reduce swelling. External—Bleeding, wound healing, sprains, and muscle soreness.

Risks: Avoid if taking stimulant laxatives such as bisacodyl (Correctol, Dulcolax), cascara, castor oil (Purge), and senna (Senokot).

Description: *Gardenia* is a shrub that ranges 1–10 feet tall in the wild, with cylindrical to flat branches that are first covered with hairs that fall early, leaving the branch smooth. Leaves occur in opposite pairs or rarely in groups of three along the branches and have either short or absent petioles. Leaves are 1.2–9.8 inches long and up to 3 inches wide and can be oblong-lanceolate, obovate, oblanceolate, or elliptic in shape. Upper surface is smooth and shiny, or slightly hairy along the primary veins, while the undersurface is sparsely hairy to smooth. Each leaf has eight to fifteen pairs of secondary veins. Flowers are solitary and terminal, arising from the ends of the stems. White flowers have a matte texture and gradually become creamy yellow in color. They can be up to 4 inches in diameter and are loosely funnel-shaped. Flowers are strongly fragrant and are followed by small oval fruits.

Habitat: Grows in woods and along streams in tropical and subtropical regions. Often cultivated.

Distribution: Widely cultivated in hardiness zones 8–11.

Plant Status: Introduced.

Animal Use: Attracts bees and butterflies. (All known species of *Gardenias* are poisonous to dogs, cats, and horses.)

Natural History: The genus was named by Carl Linnaeus and John Ellis after Alexander Garden (1730–1791), a Scottish-born American naturalist. The plant originated along the stream banks of southern China and Japan and is native to tropical and subtropical regions of Africa, Asia, Madagascar, Pacific Islands, and Australia. Tradesmen brought them to South Africa and Europe in the eighteenth century, though they struggled to thrive in the harsh English cold weather. Around 1752, Garden himself became the first-known person to grow gardenia flowers in North America successfully.

Designation: Traditional Chinese medicine herb, folkloric herbal remedy, Indigenous healing herb.

Cultivation: *Gardenias* are best planted in the fall. They need moist, well-drained soil that is high in organic matter. Optimal soil pH is acidic, 4.5–6.0. *Gardenias* can grow in full sun to partial shade. The more sun they get, the more they will flower. An ideal location would get morning sun (four hours or more) with afternoon shading to protect the plants from the intense heat of the summer sun. Fertilize *Gardenias* using a fertilizer formulated for acid-loving plants with a ratio of 2:1:1.

Remedy Form: Internal—Tea, tincture, edible. (Flowers can be eaten raw, boiled, pickled, or preserved in honey.) External—compress, poultice.

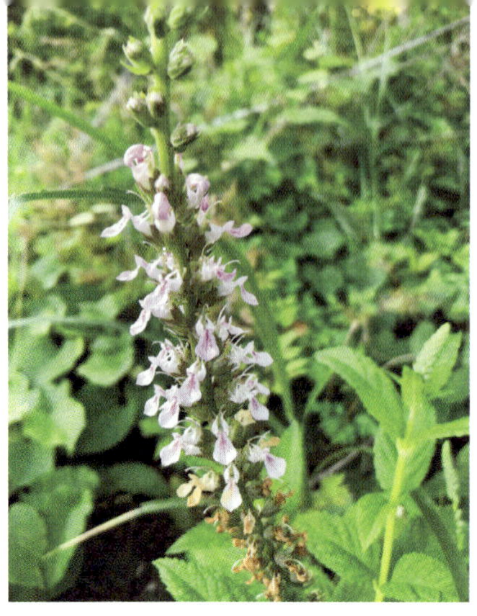

GERMANDER & THE BEAVERS

SPRING

Germander
(*Teucrium canadense*)

On a warm spring afternoon, my cousin Jara and I trek over the levee and around to the river's sandy edge looking for blackberries. Earlier this spring, there were so many blackberry flowers that the batture looked like it was covered in snow. Today, the canes that bore flowers earlier are loaded with berries just starting to ripen, so we're here to see what we can harvest. We stop and taste a few. The fruit turns out to be very juicy, but not quite ripe, so we will give them a week or so before we return to harvest.

In the meantime, it's a beautiful spot. From where we stand, we can see the Mississippi and hear it lap against the shore. I wonder if maybe this is part of the reason the fruit is so abundant here. When the river is high, it probably washes in and deposits its nutrients on this soil, and the berries and other plants thrive.

We look around to see what else is growing, and spot something large and lush and healthy-looking that we can't identify. Though there are no flowers yet, the plant is already about two feet tall, with sturdy stems, kind of wrinkly, dark-green leaves, and what looks like the beginnings of a flower spike. I mention to Jara that a couple of years ago, when I was at another area of the batture, I found germander in flower, lush with pale-pink blooms. We take a photo of the plant leaves in front of us, check our phone apps, and find that that's exactly what we've discovered!

I've heard that germander is a useful medicinal herb that can be helpful for regulating blood sugar, lowering cholesterol, fighting infections, and even relieving some cancer symptoms. But I also remember that, in recent years, it has been used as an adulterant for the look-alike herb skullcap, and that numerous research studies found the herb to cause liver toxicity. Increased regulation in the herbal trade has managed to control the substitution of *Teucrium* for *Scutellaria,* but in that process a number of countries have banned the use of *Germander* in any herbal products. It's kind of hard to give up on a healing plant that could have some important uses, but much more vital to help prevent any harm the herb may cause.

Suddenly, we hear someone coming up behind us on an ATV. We move aside, and the driver stops to chat. He turns out to be someone Jara knows. He loves to drive back into this wilder spot, he says. As a child, he and his brother played for hours at a time on the sand dunes and in the woods at the river's edge. Now he comes often just to be away from the busyness of life and to spend time in nature.

Recently, he came here early and spotted a couple of beavers working away at a newly dredged canal. They were building a dam. The next day the town crew tore down the dam so water from the river could move freely. But now it appears that during the night, the beavers completely rebuilt their dam! They're terrific engineers, the man says. He loves watching them. And they're pretty docile. He can sit right next to them, and they don't seem bothered at all. And they're known to be an important keystone species wherever they live, so it's nice to have them here.

But even though we all love watching the beavers work, they have a mixed reputation. They often antagonize landowners by "redesigning" the landscape around them, and are felt to be a pest species. But beaver activity can lead to increased water storage on the land over time and can support the reintroduction of various species of insects, birds, amphibians, mammals, and fish in an area. Prevention of future wildfires, wetland stabilization, and the renaturalization of heavily degraded environments are some of the biggest benefits that occur wherever beavers settle.

The three of us chat about this woodsy area, and the beavers and berries, and how important places like this can be—not just for local residents but for so much wildlife as well. And no matter who "wins" the water right-of-way contest between the town crew and the critters, we are always thrilled to see the beavers work and will come back soon to keep track of how they're doing.

It occurs to me that our two finds of the day—the germander and the beavers—are great examples of the complexity of things. Germander has so many helpful healing qualities but has recently been found to have very harmful effects on the liver. And the beavers do such important work in preserving wetlands and mitigating brushfire threats over time, but they can also make immediate impacts on the land that can cause economic and land management hardships for some.

Now that I know some of the complex effects of having beavers around us, I'll try to learn more about living neck and neck with them on our home ground. And having learned more about the pretty serious potential side effects of using germander internally, I'll stick to employing it only for external use. From what I've read, it can be a pretty good insect repellant. Having spent hours harvesting blackberries on a number of steamy mornings in the past, I could certainly use some help with that. And I'll feel pretty confident that crushing up a handful of *Teucrium* leaves and flowers and rubbing them over my arms and neck will be a safe use of them and may discourage the mosquitoes from thinking of me as breakfast.

Jara and I turn and head on back, sampling a few blackberries as we walk. But we'll be eager to return in a week or so to make our ripe berry harvests and to see the germander in bloom. And maybe, if we're lucky, we'll get another glimpse of the beaver dam and its wild inhabitants.

Other Names: *Teucrium canadense,* American germander, wood sage, hairy germander, Canada germander.

Parts Used: Aerial parts.

Medicinal Properties: Antiseptic, diaphoretic, diuretic, emmenagogue. Various species of *Teucrium* have also been found to have antipyretic, antioxidant, antibacterial, antifungal, anticancer, cholesterol-lowering, hypoglycemic, antimalarial, spasmolytic, and anti-inflammatory properties.

Uses: Internal—Historically used for gallbladder conditions, digestive upsets, diarrhea, weight loss; diabetes; fevers; gout; hypercholesterolemia. External—Insect repellent, mouthwash for halitosis.

Risks: Liver toxicity has been documented in numerous cases with long-term use.

Description: A sturdy perennial plant that forms clumps up to 3 feet tall. Upright, squarish stems are hollow, hairy, with opposing leaves and topped by a terminal spike of purplish-pink flowers. Leaves are ovate or lanceolate, deeply veined and coarsely toothed, up to 5 inches long and 2.5 inches wide. Terminal flowers occur in a raceme that is up to 8 inches long and contains numerous whitish or pale-lavender lipped flowers with large, shelflike lower lips. Flowers have no scent. Fruits contain yellowish-brown seeds.

Habitat: Grows in water and/or mud along streams, canals, lakes, marshes, wet grassy swales, low, moist woodlands, and meadows.

Distribution: Most of the state.

Plant Status: Native.

Animal Use: Flowers attract insect pollinators including bumblebees, honeybees, digger bees, cuckoo bees, and megachilid bees, and are also visited by flies and butterflies and occasionally by hummingbird moths and hummingbirds. Leaves are bitter and are unattractive to deer and other mammals.

Natural History: The genus was reportedly named in honor of the first king of Troy (Teucer), who, according to the Roman historiographer Pliny, was the first one to employ the plant for medical purposes. The species name *canadense* refers to the original species being first observed in Canada.

Designation: Native American remedy, traditional herbal medicine in northern Africa, the Middle East, and southern Europe.

Cultivation: Prefers moist, fertile, well-drained soils in full sun. Tolerates partial shade. Propagate through seeds, cuttings (taken in spring or summer, just below where leaf attaches to stem), or division. Germination of seeds improved when buried in the ground over winter.

Remedy Form: Avoid internal use. Externally, may be applied as compress, poultice, or wash for insect bites and minor wounds. May be crushed and rubbed on skin to keep biting insects away. Leaves may be made as a tea that can be gargled for sore throat (but should not be swallowed).

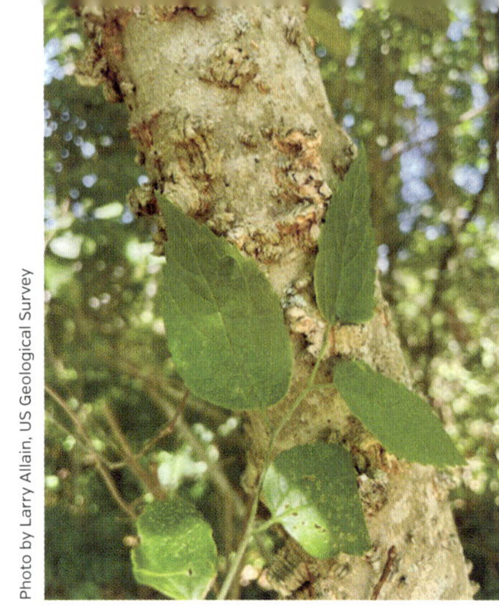
Photo by Larry Allain, US Geological Survey

HACKBERRY & THE COW PASTURE

LATE SPRING

Hackberry
(*Celtis laevigata*)

Today my cousins Nanette and Dede and I get ready to pick blackberries in the back cow pasture. It's high season for the fruit, with the air steamy, hot, and buggy. No one's been out to the pasture for a while, but Nanette warns that we'll need to be prepared. There are lots of prickly bushes to get through on our way to the fruit, and the hackberry trees have made a volunteer fence we'll have to climb around. The cows who graze there won't bother us, she says, but the bull definitely will if he isn't hiding back in the woods.

We pack up things that we'll need and toss them into the bed of the old truck—bags for the fruit, hats, bug spray, water bottles. Nanette hands me a baseball bat and a machete. I figure the bat could be used to fed off the bull, but I try to imagine what I'm supposed to do with the machete. Maybe swipe at the bull if it charges at me? No, Nanette says, the machete is for chopping our way through the thick vines as we try to find the fruit.

We drive over the old railroad track, jump out to open the creaky, rusted gate, and then walk back, back, back through history. I try to imagine how many cousins in this big motley family have trekked back here, eager for fruit.

We make our way through the hackberry fence, and I wonder if these scrubby volunteer trees have any medicinal uses. So often the plants that show up in neglected places have been used by Native peoples or early settlers for their healing properties. I make a mental note to check on this once we're back home.

We come to an old shed and start to make our way through the brambles to get berries. The cows are curious, but so far, we haven't spotted the bull. We all hope he hasn't spotted us! We laugh and chat as we pick, and

I wonder again how many of our people worked at this same bit of land, gathering free food to make up into something tasty they could share. It's such a good tradition, the family working together to eat from the land.

The berries are sweet, though not as abundant as we had hoped, so we have to work harder to get much fruit. After a while, as we're just getting tired of picking, we see the bull slipping around the edge of the cow crowd, and we decide it's time to leave. We don't have much of a harvest, having helped ourselves to the fruit as we worked. But we have purple mouths and hands and have had much fun working together, so it's been a good morning.

At home, I pop my cup of berries into a bowl to rinse them off, thinking I'll make muffins with them later. Then I grab an herb guide so I can check out the hackberry trees. Apparently, there are two species of this tree that have been used for healing, though only one species is found throughout Louisiana. On reading, I'm surprised at how many medicinal recommendations I find for hackberry.

According to ethnobotanist Daniel Moerman, the Houmas Indians used hackberry bark to make a tea for sore throats and a decoction to treat venereal disease. The Iroquois used hackberry to regulate a woman's menstrual cycles. And a dozen or more tribes used the tree as a source of food. The Kiowa pounded hackberries into a paste and baked that over an open fire. The Comanche would beat the fruits to a pulp, then mix the pulp with fat, roll the mixture into balls, and roast them over a fire. The Apache, Chiricahua, and Mescalero ate hackberries fresh and also made them into jelly and dried cakes. The Dakota used dried fruits to season meat. The Meskwaki made porridge out of the ground berries, and the Pawnee pounded the berries into a powder and mixed it with fat and parched corn.

So, despite the general thinking around here that hackberry is a kind of "weed tree," in other parts of the world it is held in high regard. Scientists in Egypt have found that hackberry leaves contain significant antioxidants, and the plant parts are used in many areas as a helpful medicine for diseases of aging and for cancer prevention. It is also used for diarrhea and dysentery, and an extract of the bark has been used in the treatment of jaundice and for sore throats.

Related species of the tree have been proven to have antimicrobial and antifungal activities, and the leaves have proven to be active against *Candida albicans* and other pathogenic yeast infections. The tree also has some ecological importance in dry areas, where it is used as a shade tree in urban environments because of its drought tolerance and size.

Hackberry has a rich history of magical uses as well. Apparently, hackberry is the Druidic birth tree for those born February 9–18 and August 14–23. Traits of those who were born under the sign of hackberry include impulsiveness, optimism, intelligence, and heightened ability for deductive reasoning. Some famous people born under this sign include Galileo, Darwin, and Goethe. The tree supposedly bestows nobility, pride, and dedication.

It also turns out that hackberry was used as the fuel source for the altar fire at peyote ceremonies. At the beginning of each of the four stages of the ritual, the altar fire was fed with hackberry wood. In addition, the flowers of this valuable tree are visited by pollinators including honeybees and butterflies, and apparently the fruit is preferred by many bird species and wild animals.

With the tree so thick in the cow pasture, and so abundant in the state, I probably won't be planting it on my own land any time soon. But now that I know about its many uses for healing, I'll have a good excuse to return to the cow pasture where I can harvest some bark and leaves from the trees. And I'll have one more excuse to visit that land my grandparents walked, and loved, for so many years.

Other Names: *Celtis laevigata,* sugarberry, sugar hackberry, hackberry, Texas sugarberry, palo blanco, American hackberry, Mississippi hackberry, nettletree, northern hackberry, sugarberry, beaverwood.

Parts Used: Bark, berries.

Medicinal Properties: Astringent, anodyne, antioxidant, cytotoxic, emmenagogue, nutritional.

Uses: Fruit—Edible; abnormal menstrual flow; colic, peptic ulcers, diarrhea and dysentery; pain relief. Bark—Sore throats; regulating menstrual cycles and reducing heavy menstrual flow. Bark and leaves—Peptic ulcer disease, diarrhea, and dysentery.

Risks: Should not be taken in pregnancy. Hackberry pollen may be an allergen for sensitive individuals. No drug interactions known.

Description: The tree has a broad, rounded, and open crown of spreading or slightly drooping branches. Grows 60–70 feet tall and equally as broad.

Leaves have asymmetrical bases and partially toothed margins. Smooth, pale bark is marked with cork-like, lighter patches. Fruit matures to reddish purple.

Habitat: Rich bottomlands, stream banks, floodplains, alluvial woods, sandy loam, thickets.

Distribution: Most of the state.

Plant Status: Native.

Animal Use: Fruit—Wild turkey, ring-necked pheasant, quail, grouse, lesser prairie chicken, cedar waxwing, robins, and other bird species and mammal species. Deer eat berries and will browse leaves once their preferred browse species are gone. The tree provides good cover for species such as mule deer, white-tailed deer, upland game birds, small nongame birds, and small mammals. Many species of songbirds, including mockingbirds and robins, eat the fruit and use the tree for nesting habitat. It is a larval and nectar host for two butterflies: hackberry emperor (*Asterocampa celtis*) and American snout (*Libytheana carineta*).

Natural History: The Acadian French name for hackberry is *bois connu,* or "known tree." The fruit of all hackberries is edible and palatable. The Houma Tribe used hackberry bark for sore throats and crushed shells for venereal diseases. Iroquois used decoctions of the fruit to regulate menstrual cycles.

Cultivation: Hackberry trees like a sunny location but will tolerate partial shade. They prefer a slightly moist, organic soil, but can handle clay, compacted soil, alkaline soil, and drought. Account for large size of mature tree when spacing. Dig a hole as deep and at least twice as wide as the root ball. Set the tree in gently and upright. Fill the hole half full with soil and add plenty of water. Allow water to drain before filling the hole with the remaining soil. Firm the soil lightly to remove any air pockets. Water the tree every week the first season after planting, especially during dry conditions, until the roots become established.

Designation: Native/Indigenous medicinal plant.

Remedy Form: Edible, tea, tincture.

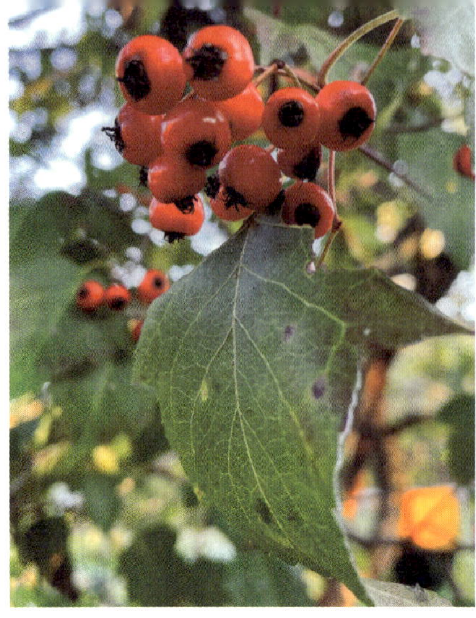

HAWTHORN & BODI'S RAINBOW BRIDGE

WINTER

Hawthorn
[*Crataegus* sp.]

This morning, I start walking on the levee before the sun comes up. It's a cool day, and layers of cloud whisk by overhead. And it's quiet—the birds are not so chatty, maybe because of the chill. I'm out to see what might be coming up on the batture, when suddenly my phone rings. It's a call from the veterinarian's office letting me know that Bodi's ashes are on their way home. They should arrive today.

Back in Hahnville this winter, I am solo—without Bodi. And though he is with me in spirit, I am missing him since he's moved on. Lately, every walk I take is someplace I've been with him. Now, as I trek into the little tangle of woods that edge the river, I step over the newly unfolding violets, over prickly dewberry vines, past butterweed and chickweed and wild geranium. If Bodi were with me, we'd be trucking along together, both of our faces aimed down at the ground. He'd be crashing through the tangles on some scent trail or other, and I'd be checking for new growth. Once we got home, I'd be picking leaves and petals out of his curly hair. And we'd both be excited and happy after our early walk.

But now he's gone. And I'm so sad. I know he's okay, wherever he is—he was happy to his last breath, that funny guy. After more than a year of his increasing physical frailties, though, I am exhausted, swamped with love, and shaken with loss. And now, waiting for his remains. I'm not sure what I'll do with them, but it will be good to have him back. I haven't been able yet to pack up all his stuff and tuck it away, so lately I've been arranging little piles of his favorite things and decorating each pile with photos of him.

In the spring, when I find hawthorn in flower, I'll gather some petals and add them to the altars and also save some to use for tea.

In herb school, hawthorn was our go-to remedy for cardiovascular support and the prevention of heart disease. It seemed like a perfect, safe remedy for someone with a family history of heart disease and could also help to lower blood pressure while strengthening cardiac muscle tissue. With my family's history of heart issues, I was happy to hear about it, and as I entered my later years, I began to include the herb in my regular health-support regimen. But recently, I learned that the hawthorn is not only helpful for cardiac conditions but could also be used for those wounds of the heart that are emotional or even spiritual in nature. Now I'll get to find out how well that works.

I guess I'm lucky to live in a place that has so many species of *Crataegus* growing in the wild. While the "official" hawthorn species of the herbal world (*C. oxycantha* and *C. monogyna*) don't grow wild in Louisiana, many others occur in the state and have been found to have the same complex of healing compounds that make this plant a star of the herbal healing world. Apparently, eight hawthorn species can be found in Louisiana, and I'm eager to track them down. I'd love to make a hawthorn tincture of flowers, leaves, and fruit to use in these hard months without Mr. B.

The herb has a very long history of use for various heart-related health conditions including hypertension, arrhythmias, the cardiovascular changes of aging, mild congestive heart failure, recovery from heart attack, and coronary artery disease. And, apparently, so many *Crataegus* species are recognized for their usefulness that they are known collectively as "hawthorn." One thing I love about this herb is its gentle action and relative safety. While there are some cautions, hawthorn is really one of the safest herbs to take for physical health problems.

And it's nice to know that the herb can help to relieve even some emotional challenges as well. I have my own particular pain of losing a beloved companion, but lately all of us carry burdens as we try to figure out how to live in a challenged world. Climate changes, social unrest, political gridlocks, increased financial pressures all make for challenging times. Maybe hawthorn will be one of the ways we make our way forward. Maybe some of its qualities—gentleness, abundance, nourishment, inspiration—will help us to find a way forward that is kind, supportive, and healing.

All in all, it's pretty amazing, really, how much the heart can hold—great loss, great relief, and so much love, and even the tiny troubles that losing a pet can bring. Lately, at the very same time that my body feels so adrift in the newfound emptiness of the house, it also feels a much-needed release. I don't know how all these things can be true—can stand in the same exact place without canceling each other out—but life, and emotions, are complex.

I do know that even though the last couple of years have been hard, Bodi made me a better person. I wish I could say that I deserved him, but I don't know that. I do know that he opened my heart and climbed right in. He made me laugh out loud even when I was trying to be grumpy. He taught me about resilience, about keeping things in perspective, and about being in pain but still being happy enough to play. He taught me about love, and forgiveness, and letting things go. So I'll keep on keeping on—missing B, trying to adjust to my new single life, and sipping hawthorn tea to ease the grief left in the wake of such sweet love. That might be just what I need.

Species: Eight species of *Crataegus* can be found in the state, and all are native. Most species have been proven to produce healing effects, and preparations of various species can be used interchangeably. The Cajun name *cenellier* is used to refer to any members of the genus *Crataegus* that have red berries.

Crataegus brachyacantha

Other Names: Blueberry hawthorn.

Description: Tree height is 40–50 feet. Leaves are ovate, 1–2 inches long, and dark, glossy green. Flowers are small, cup-shaped with five petals, and are tinged orange in the fall. Fruit is dark blue, 0.3–0.5 inch across. Tree has short, recurved thorns that are up to 1 inch long.

Habitat: Borders of streams in rich, calcareous soils.

Distribution: Concentrated in more northern parishes and a few central areas.

Plant Status: Native.

Crataegus crus-galli

Other Names: Cockspur hawthorn, bush hawthorn, aubépine ergot-de-coq, cockspur thorn, Newcastle hawthorn, Newcastle thorn.

Description: Often seen as a dense, low-branched, broadly rounded tree 25–35 feet tall with horizontal branches and armed with numerous large thorns 1.5–3 inches long. Lower branches often sweep near to the ground. May also occur as a tall, flat-topped shrub.

Habitat: Pastures and stream banks.

Distribution: Northern parishes, top half of the state

Plant Status: Native.

Crataegus marshallii

Other Names: Parsley hawthorn.

Description: Seen as a small native tree growing up to 20 feet. Leaves are simple, alternate, grow 0.75 to 2 inches long on slender stalks. Serrate margins resemble parsley leaves. Flowers white to pink with red anthers. Fruit is a small red pome that ripens in fall and may overwinter. Thorns are unbranched.

Habitat: Alluvial woods, swamp forests, sandy woods, hillsides, fencerows, pastures.

Distribution: Concentrated in top two-thirds of the state.

Plant Status: Native.

Crataegus opaca

Other Names: Riverflat hawthorn, western mayhaw, apple haw, mayhaw.

Description: A small tree or large shrub, 12–36 feet in height. Tall, narrow trunk has a rounded crown and spiny branches. Leaves are oval and dark green. Clusters of pink or white flowers become cranberry red, and fruits are relatively large, juicy, and edible. Thorns are 0.5–1.5 inches long.

Habitat: Seasonally wet depressions, borders of swamps.

Distribution: Northern and a few central parishes.

Plant Status: Native.

Crataegus spathulata

Other Names: Littlehip hawthorn, pasture haw.

Description: Large shrub or small evergreen tree with broad crown, slender branches, and large thorns. Grows 8–20 feet tall. White flowers later produce bright-red, edible fruit. Dark-green toothed leaves are spoon-shaped (spathulate).

Habitat: Sandy or sandy clay woods, fencerows, pastures, stream banks, low woods, moist and fertile soil.

Distribution: Top half of the state, a couple of central parishes.

Plant Status: Native.

Crataegus triflora

Other Names: Three-flower hawthorn.

Description: A multistemmed shrub, up to 20 feet tall. White flowers are large and occur in small clusters, typically with three blooms but may have up to seven. Leaves are up to 2.8 inches long, oval, with toothed margins. Leaf surfaces are slightly hairy. Fruits are red with orange flesh and contain five seeds.

Habitat: Hardwood forests on rocky, limestone slopes.

Distribution: Only in Caldwell Parish.

Plant Status: Native.

Crataegus uniflora

Other Names: Dwarf hawthorn, one-flowered hawthorn.

Description: An upright, small shrub growing up to 12 feet tall with a slender trunk. Silver bark is lined with numerous branches that bear large thorns. Leaves are shiny, dark green, downy, and whitish on the underside with rounded, serrated edges. Single white flower and greenish to dark-red fruit distinguish it from other species.

Habitat: Dry sandy and rocky uplands in open woods, forest borders, thickets, and old fields.

Distribution: Bienville, Caddo, Vernon, and Winn Parishes.

Plant Status: Native.

Crataegus viridis

Other Names: Green hawthorn, southern thorn.

Description: Grows up to 25 feet. Clusters of white flowers produce bright-red, persistent fruit in the fall. Bark of older trunks may exfoliate to expose an orangish-brown inner bark. Thorns are minimal. Leaves are dark green, simple, alternate, and 1–2 inches long, changing to red/gold in fall. Flowers are 0.75 inch in diameter with five white petals and grow in 2-inch clusters. The fruit is less than 0.5 inch in diameter, round, fleshy, abundant, orange to red, and persists in winter.

Habitat: Open woodlands, meadows, prairie, plains, pastures, savannas, alluvial woods, and swamp forests

Distribution: Heavily concentrated in northern parishes and also found in a number of southern parishes.

Plant Status: Native.

For All Species, Parts Used: Flowers, leaves, fruits.

Medicinal Properties: Cardiovascular tonic, cardioprotective, anticoagulant, anti-HIV, antihyperglycemic, anti-ischemic, antioxidant, antispasmodic, astringent, diuretic, carminative, gastroprotective, hepatoprotective, hypotensive, neuroprotective, sedative, anti-Alzheimer, vasodilator. Research has documented its ability to protect heart tissues, promote coronary circulation, repair coronary arteries, and relieve cardiac hypoxemia. Hawthorn has both immediate and long-term benefits, and the whole plant preparations have proven to be more effective than those made from isolated constituents of the herb.

Uses: Cardiovascular tonic, atherosclerosis, chronic heart disease, hypertension, degenerative conditions of the cardiovascular system, mild congestive heart failure, coronary artery disease, recovery from heart attack, gradual age-related loss of cardiac function, palpitations, tachycardia; blood sugar irregularities; anxiety, insomnia, cerebral insufficiency. Hawthorn is especially indicated in the treatment of weakened heart combined with high blood pressure. Prolonged use is necessary for it to be effective.

Risks: Generally recognized as safe. High dosages can cause mild symptoms including dizziness, lightheadedness, nausea, or sedation. More severe symptoms may include cardiac arrhythmia and low blood pressure, but these are very rare. Avoid if taking Digoxin or beta-blockers, or anticoagulants/antiplatelet drugs (or use under supervision of a health care practitioner for medication dosage adjustment). Avoid if taking medications for male sexual dysfunction (including Phosphodiesterase-5 inhibitors).

Description: There may be as many as one thousand species of hawthorn worldwide. Most occur as a shrub or medium-sized tree and can range from 10–50 feet in height. Bark is brown-gray, knotted, and fissured, and twigs are slender and brown. Branches have thorny twigs and clusters of small, cup-shaped white or pinkish flowers that bloom in spring. Fruits occur in autumn and are generally red or orange, though a couple have blue or greenish coloration. Dark-green leaves have serrated and sometimes lobed margins. Thorns are 1–3 inches long.

Animal Use: Hawthorns support a variety of bees, butterflies, flies, and songbirds and are a host plant for over twenty-five species of moths.

Natural History: *Crataegus* is a derivative of the Greek word *kratos,* meaning "strength," referring either to the hardness of the woody bark or to the strengthening of the cardiovascular system. The Old English name "hawe" referred to the space encircled by a hedge (which was often hawthorn or *Crataegus*).

Designation: Major herb of commerce, Indigenous traditional remedy, African American herbal remedy, Chinese medicine (some species), Iranian medicinal herb, homeopathic remedy.

Cultivation: In general, hawthorns are adaptable and can tolerate sun to partial shade and average to wet conditions and are not picky about soil type or pH. Cultivation may be done from seeds, cuttings, or layering.

Remedy Form: Edible, tea, tincture, syrup, paste.

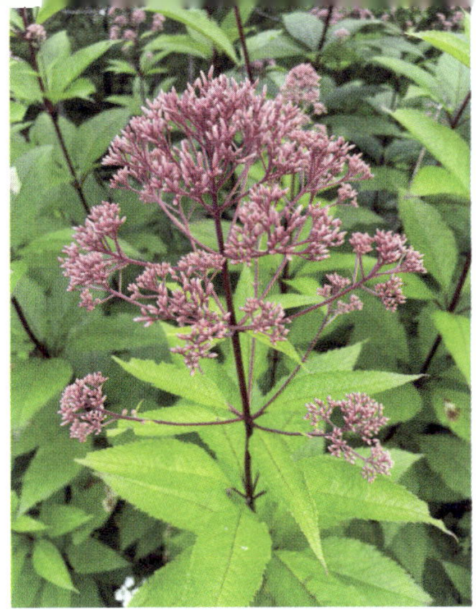

JOE PYE & THE HUMMINGBIRDS

SUMMER

Joe Pye weed
(*Eutrochium* sp.)

It's a buggy morning. Mosquitoes, gnats, and deer flies dive-bomb Bodi and me as we walk. And today, Bodi is pokier than usual, which, for a sixteen-year-old pooch, is pretty slow. And I'm encumbered, with one hand lugging a bag full of just-picked cucumbers to give to my neighbor for pickle making and the other hand holding Bodi's leash. This leaves me no hand to swat at the bugs, which makes me pretty grumpy. But B is doing fine. A little wobbly this morning, he is still curious, nosing at scent trails left by whatever critters passed by in the night. Eventually, I drop off the cukes, swat at a few bugs, nudge Bodi toward home, and start to enjoy myself.

After days of rain, the sky is finally blue, the rain-saturated garden is abuzz with bees, and hummingbirds are air-dancing over the Joe Pye flowers. This late in their migration season, the birds are headed back down south and are always happy to find a source of nectar. And the Joe Pyes are nothing if not stunning. I try to take close-up photos of the blooms and birds, but the plants are so tall that the blossoms tower over my head. Despite their unphotographable heights, though, I'm happy to see the Joe Pye, and for more reasons than one.

When I first started studying herbal healing, I tried to identify the plants around me so I could learn their possible medicinal properties. Some of the plants were tiny, or kind of bland-looking, or hidden by lush foliage. But the Joe Pye was a delight. Not exactly shy once it started to sprout up, it was easy to identify. Enthralled with its beauty, I tucked a few seedlings into my home garden and researched its history.

As far as I could discover, this member of the *Eutrochiums* (formerly known as *Eupatoriums*) were named after a real person—a Mohican chief, Joseph Shauquethqueat, who lived in Massachusetts and New York in the eighteenth and early nineteenth centuries. During a typhoid epidemic, he was reported to have used a wild plant growing in the nearby woods to alleviate the illness. Since his remedy gave so much relief, the plant was given his nickname, Joe Pye. Native Americans and early settlers continued to use the plant for various problems, including rheumatism and gout, fevers, diarrhea, lung ailments, and especially bladder and kidney issues.

In herb school, we called the plant "gravel root" because of its ability to help dissolve small kidney stones. Several members of the *Eupatorium/Eutrochium* genus were known for their usefulness as diuretics and antilithic plants that could relieve these conditions.

As I began to practice as an herbalist, I recommended the herb for various kinds of urinary tract ailments, and for a few other problems. I'd heard that Joe Pye was best used along with other herbs, so it was often added to formulas for fevers and arthritis. I was happy to hear that the leaves, stems, and flowers could be used in addition to the root. At that point, I wasn't looking forward to digging up the plant that produced such gorgeous blooms. But over time, the plant spread and sometimes needed a bit of taming. Then I was happy to uproot some of the herb and add the roots to my stash of Joe Pye for future use.

Three species of *Eutrochium* are commonly known as Joe Pye, and all of these have been found to have diuretic, antilithic, and anti-inflammatory properties. Two of those species—*Eutrochium fistulosum* (hollow Joe Pye) and *Eutrochium purpureum* (sweet-scented Joe Pye)—are native to Louisiana, and a third species, *Eutrochium maculatum* (purple Joe Pye), can be readily cultivated in the state. All make beautiful, tall backdrops to a home garden and invite numerous pollinators. And all of the Joe Pyes produce blooms over a longish period of time and are attractive for both their color and nectar. This makes them a great food source for the hummingbirds. In spring, these tiny birds come for the bright beebalms, the cardinal flowers, and other colorful blooms. But in late summer, when they're on their way back farther south and will have another long trek across the Gulf of Mexico to their wintering grounds, they're on the lookout for home gardens and for feeders where they can rest and fatten up before they go.

My neighbors and I love hosting the birds, so I've researched some details about their lives. Apparently, Louisiana is the first landfall the birds make after their very long spring flight. And the birds are amazing! During migration, a hummingbird's heart beats over 1,200 times a minute, and its wings flap up to eighty times a second. In preparation for the long flight, hummingbirds will typically gain 25–40 percent of their body weight before they set out. And they fly alone, often on the same path they have flown earlier in their life. Young hummingbirds have to navigate the trek without parental guidance. The tiny travelers can travel as much as twenty-three miles in one day, though during migration across the Gulf, they may cover up to five hundred miles at a time.

Knowing how hard the hummers work to get here, my neighbors and I keep an eye out for their arrivals every year. Many folks put up feeders, and some of us make sure to include favored hummingbird plants in the garden. Once the birds have arrived, they are said to visit one thousand to two thousand flowers a day to maintain health and strength.

According to the LSU AgCenter's website, the ruby-throated hummingbird is the only species that mates and raises chicks in the state, but up to fourteen species of hummingbirds have been spotted here. In summer, flowering gardens or woodland edges offer places to hide and nest. The birds also depend on household nectar feeders.

Now that I know more about the hummingbirds in Louisiana, I am even more eager to increase the numbers of my pollinator plants. And knowing how helpful the various species of Joe Pye can be for some common health conditions, I'll make sure to build up my stand of them in the coming years.

For now, it turns out that what started as a grumpy day has turned out to be pretty fine. Bodi is down for a nap, the tall Joe Pye flowers nod in a small breeze, and the hummingbirds are still dive-bombing into purple blossoms. What could be lovelier?

Species: Two species of Joe Pye weed are native to the state, and another species can be readily cultivated in the garden. All have a history of medicinal use.

Eutrochium fistulosum

Other Names: Trumpetweed, queen of the meadow, hollow Joe Pye weed.

Medicinal Use: Used alone or along with other *Eutrochium* species for bladder and kidney complaints, fevers, and other inflammations.

Description: An erect, clump-forming perennial growing 4–7 feet tall, with coarsely serrated, lance-shaped, dark-green leaves that are up to 12 inches long and occur in whorls of four to seven (frequently six) on sturdy, upright to arching, green, hollow, purple-spotted stems. Large, rounded flower clusters, up to 12 inches across, are composed of hundreds of dainty, pinkish-mauve flowers that are produced mid- to late summer and into fall.

Habitat: Alluvial woods, meadows, bogs, marshes, and stream banks.

Distribution: Spotty in top half of the state (reported in nineteen parishes), mostly in northern and central parishes.

Cultivation: Sow seeds in the fall and plant thickly, as germination is usually low. Propagation is also possible by cuttings taken in late spring, or by division. The plant prefers damp, moist to wet, rich soils, but it will also grow in gravelly or sandy soils if they get sufficient moisture. Prefers full sun to partial shade and neutral to slightly acid soils. Plants should be cut back to the ground in late winter.

Plant Status: Native.

Eutrochium maculatum

Other Names: Spotted Joe Pye weed, queen of the meadow.

Medicinal Use: Fevers, colds; kidney and liver complaints; rheumatism.

Description: *E. maculatum* is a 4–7 feet tall, clump-forming perennial with branched, purple-speckled stems clad with serrate, lance-shaped, medium-green leaves that grow up to 8 inches long and typically appear in whorls of three to six. Tiny, light- to deep-purple flowers in compound inflorescences.

Habitat: Prefers full sun to partial shade, and moist-wet soil.

Distribution: Does not occur in the wild in Louisiana but can be cultivated.

Cultivation: Grow in average, medium to wet soils in full sun or light, afternoon shade. Prefers moist, fertile, humus soils and does not like to dry out. Cut plants to the ground in late winter.

Plant Status: Cultivated.

Eutrochium purpureum

Other Names: Sweet-scented Joe Pye weed, purple-node Joe Pye.

Medicinal Uses: Cystitis, incontinence, kidney/bladder inflammations and infections, small kidney stones (gravel); gout, rheumatism.

Description: An erect, clump-forming perennial growing 4–8 feet tall. Leaves are coarsely serrated, lance-shaped, dark green, up to 12 inches long, and grow in whorls of three to four on sturdy green stems with purplish leaf nodes. Tiny, vanilla-scented, dull pinkish-mauve flowers occur in large, terminal, domed, compound inflorescences. Each flower cluster typically has five to seven florets. Seed heads persist into winter.

Habitat: Moist prairies, wood edges, thickets, open wooded areas, drying sites, and wooded slopes.

Distribution: Only in Caldwell Parish, though can be cultivated in other areas.

Cultivation: Grows well in average, medium-moisture soils, in full sun to partial shade. Prefers moist, fertile, humus soils. Tolerant of clay soils. Cut plants to the ground in late winter. Best propagated by stem cuttings. This species generally grows well in open woodland areas.

Plant Status: Native.

For All Species: Parts Used: Whole plant, though roots and flowering tops are most often used.

Medicinal Properties: Antilithic, anti-inflammatory, astringent, antiseptic, diaphoretic, diuretic.

Uses: Historically used for arthritis, gout, rheumatism; asthma; chills, fevers; cystitis, incontinence, kidney stones.

Risks: Best for short-term use; consult with a health care practitioner if pregnant or breastfeeding.

Description: The Joe Pye *Eutrochium* are all tall, erect herbs with leaves arranged in whorls along the stems. The species may hybridize widely in nature, sometimes making identification a challenge.

Animal Use: Butterflies, native bees, skippers, moths, and flies pollinate flowers. Caterpillars of several moths feed on the foliage. Various species of *Eutrochium* are visited by insect pollinators, which in turn attract insectivorous birds. Seeds are eaten by seed-eating birds like the American goldfinch, mallards, ruffed grouse, wild turkeys, and swamp sparrows. Foliage may be browsed by deer, rabbits, and livestock.

Natural History: Long known as being in the genus *Eupatorium,* these species have been placed into the genus *Eutrochium.* A tea from the roots or flowers was used by the early settlers to break fevers. The former genus name, *Eupatorium,* is attributed to an ancient Asian ruler named Mithridates Eupator. Reportedly, the ruler discovered a *Eupatorium* that was an antidote to poison, and he drank nonlethal doses of it to keep himself from being poisoned by his enemies as his father had been. He was eventually captured by his enemies and tried to poison himself but had so much antidote in his system that he did not die. Supposedly, he then asked a friend to stab him instead. The genus name *Eutrochium* is derived from the Greek words *eu,* meaning "well," and *troche,* meaning "wheel-like," referring to the whorled leaves. Used by many Native American tribes including Abenaki and Cherokee.

Designation: Herb of commerce, Native American herbal remedy, folkloric herbal preparation, Cajun healing plant, Ayurvedic herb for kidney and gallstones.

Remedy Form: Internal—Tea, tincture. External—Compress, poultice, wash.

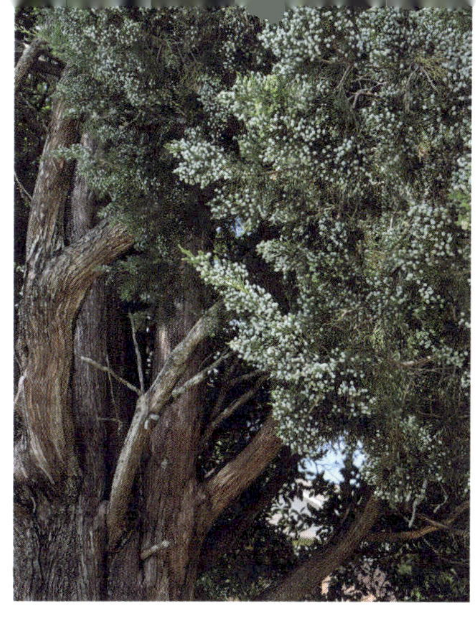

JUNIPER & THE GIN TRAIL

SPRING

Juniper
(*Juniperus virginiana*)

After days, even weeks, of rain, the sun is finally out. We are all so dizzily happy! The neighbors race out to check their marshy gardens, try to mow saturated lawns, worry about nearby trees whose roots could pull up from the watery soil. And even though the sun makes the air steamy, which makes us all hotter, it's such a welcome break from so many gray days. Even Bodi is happy! He isn't a big fan of hot sun, but today he's eager to walk along the roadside without getting sopping wet. As we amble along, Bodi sniffs for animal trails, and I inhale deeply as sun hits the prickly leaves of the surrounding juniper trees. Their scent reminds me that it's about time to make a harvest of one of my favorite herbs.

In my early years of practicing as an herbalist, I relied on juniper as a trusted remedy for bladder infections, joint pain, and chest congestion. I loved harvesting the herb. The fragrance seemed to take me into a deep sense of restfulness. I remember hearing that the aromatic properties of all species of juniper have spiritual properties as well and have been used by many cultures to ward off negative influences. Many Indigenous tribes tossed the berries onto hot rocks in sweat lodges or dried the berries and made them into incense. These days, an aromatherapy oil of juniper is thought to be an aid for meditation and other spiritual practices and to provide a sense of calm, relaxation, and emotional balance. No matter what it is used for, though, juniper definitely reminds me of healing—and also of gin.

Much to the consternation of my Louisiana family and friends, I'm not much of a drinker. Several years ago, when I told a cousin that I was making plans to visit Italy, she said, "Oh, what a waste! You're going to Italy and you don't even drink!" Of course, as an adolescent, I did the usual sampling of whatever alcohol was kept in my parents' cupboard, followed by the usual teen experimentation in my first year of college. But basically, (a) I didn't like the way alcohol tasted, and (b) I hated the way I felt after drinking it. One episode of imbibing some strange cocktail combination had me sitting on the dirty bathroom floor of a dingy bar hoping not to throw up. Eventually I wondered, what was the point?

But I have to say that the one flavored alcoholic beverage I could sort of tolerate was gin. Even before I was an herbalist and understood the healing uses of juniper, I thought the taste of gin was sort of interesting. Since then, I've learned more about its origins and have discovered that it was originally utilized for its medicinal properties.

Apparently, the long, winding trail of gin's history began with eleventh-century Benedictine monks in Salerno, Italy, whose monastery was surrounded by rolling hills and many juniper trees. It was not uncommon for monks to be involved in maintaining medicinal herb gardens and to act as local healers for the small, often-isolated villages in which they lived. And they also routinely produced alcoholic beverages, including wine and beer. These were felt to provide a nutritious beverage, as well as to lift the spirits, and were generally safer to drink than the local water, which could contain dangerous bacteria. Often, these alcoholic beverages were flavored with local herbs and plants, including juniper berries.

It wasn't long before various European apothecaries were offering juniper-based tonics for coughs and colds, pains and cramps. Centuries later, gin was partnered with another useful herbal drink—tonic water. In the 1800s, the antimalarial properties of quinine from local *Cinchona* tree bark were sought out by British soldiers stationed in India. They began drinking tonic water made from *Cinchona* to prevent and combat the disease, but due to the bitter taste of the bark, gin was added to make the tonic taste more tolerable. Soon, a twist of lemon or lime was added for flavor, but even then, healing was involved. It turned out that the citrus could help to combat scurvy that afflicted sailors on long voyages.

In modern times, juniper is an important herb of commerce and is utilized for a variety of health problems, including urinary tract complaints, chest congestion, and inflammation. It is also an important plant in aromatherapy. The essential oil and the fragrance are reputed to be analgesic and anti-inflammatory, to aid in the elimination of toxins, and to help with arthritis and neuritis. It is also known to support lymphatic circulation and drainage.

As the juniper continues to release its perfume on this warm morning, I hope that the sun will stick around for a while. I'm looking forward to another trek out to the junipers with Bodi in the next few days, and I'll be bringing a bag to pick some of the fruit and leaves. I'll be using my harvest to make a new batch of tincture and to dry for tea. I might even try a recipe I've found recently for a "botanical gin" that includes a few spices along with juniper berries. Soon, the whole house will be perfumed with that powerful and restful scent—and I'll have another batch of the herb on hand to share with neighbors and friends. As Bodi and I head on back to the house, we're both grateful for sun, and I'm grateful for this lush and fruitful place, and for the monks who began the long and winding journey of the gin trail.

Other Names: *Juniperus virginiana,* pencil wood, juniper bush, pencil cedar, Virginia juniper, red cedar, red savin, Carolina cedar, red juniper.

Parts Used: Bark, root bark, fruit, leaves.

Medicinal Properties: Leaves—Antibacterial, anthelmintic, antimalarial, anti-inflammatory, antiseptic, diaphoretic, diuretic, rubefacient, stimulant, tonic. Fruit—Anthelmintic, diaphoretic, diuretic, emmenagogue and mildly antiseptic.

Uses: Internal—Bladder infections, fluid retention; asthma, bronchitis, coughs, colds; hypertension; joint pain; weakness following a long illness. External—Acne, canker sores, rashes, hair loss, eczema, fungal skin infections, hemorrhoids, rheumatism, insect repellant, warts. In aromatherapy, juniper is used to produce a grounding and calming effect, to help balance emotions, and to support mental health.

Risks: Should not be taken in large amounts. Essential oil should not be ingested. Avoid if pregnant or breastfeeding, or in the presence of kidney disease. Avoid if taking sedative medications.

Description: A small- to medium-sized native evergreen tree that grows up to 70 feet tall. Plants are dioecious with separate male and female trees. Male cones are small, terminal, solitary, and oblong-ovoid. Female cones are aromatic, fleshy, berrylike, globular, 0.25–0.4 inch in diameter, and turn dark blue to purplish. Bark is light reddish-brown, separating into large, fibrous strips. Two kinds of leaves can be found on the same tree. The more common kind is dark green, minute, scalelike and clasping the stem in four ranks so that the stem appears square. The other kind, usually appearing on vigorous young shoots, is awl-shaped, sharp-pointed, spreading, and whitened. Young trees bear only this kind of leaf, making them look different from older trees.

Habitat: Found in dry hillsides to swamps, sandy and rocky soils, commonly in old fields, along fencerows, and on the edge of forests.

Distribution: Much of the state, except for extreme southeast parishes.

Plant Status: Native.

Animal Use: Fruit—Eaten by cedar waxwing, northern bobwhite, ring-necked pheasant, ruffed grouse, sharp-tailed grouse, wild turkey, American robin, starling, mourning dove, northern mockingbird, willow flycatcher, purple finch, common crow, northern flicker, myrtle warbler, downy woodpecker, evening grosbeak, pine grosbeak, hermit thrush, fox sparrow, yellow-bellied sapsucker, eastern bluebird, kingbird. Also eaten by mammals including rabbits, foxes, skunks, opossum, and coyote. Many mites, worms, and beetles will feed on different parts of the tree.

Natural History: Reportedly, the city of Baton Rouge (meaning "Red Stick") is named after the eastern red cedar because the Indians were carrying a pole made from the tree. Numerous Native American tribes and other Indigenous or cultural groups have utilized various parts of the plant for healing. These include Rappahannock, Dakota, Omaha, Pawnee, Ponca, Comanche, Cree, Chickasaw, Chippewa, Dakota, Ojibwa, Delaware, and Fox tribes. In African American home-health practices, juniper was used internally for rheumatic pain, urinary tract inflammations, and blood sugar control, and externally for snakebite and wounds. In Appalachia, tree parts were boiled and inhaled for bronchitis, and in New Mexico, a boiled mixture of bark and water was used for skin rashes.

Designation: Herb of commerce, Native American remedy, African American home remedy, folkloric herbalism plant.

Cultivation: The tree can be propagated by seed or by grafting, layering, or from cuttings. Cuttings may be rooted outdoors during the winter by taking tip cuttings. Germination is improved by warm moist stratification followed by cold/moist stratification.

Remedy Form: Internal—Tea, tincture, edible. External—Compress, poultice, oil/rub.

BOTANICAL GIN
(MAKES ONE 750 ML BOTTLE OF GIN)

- 8 tablespoons juniper berries
- 3/4 teaspoon coriander, whole
- 1/4 teaspoon ground allspice
- 1/4 teaspoon fennel seeds
- 3 green cardamon pods
- 3 black peppercorns
- 1 bay leaf
- 1 sprig fresh or 1 teaspoon dried rosemary
- 1/4 teaspoon citrus zest or 1 citrus slice
- 1/4 teaspoon lavender
- 750 ml vodka

1. Put the herbs in a glass jar. Add vodka, cap tightly, and let sit one month or more in a cool, dark place. Then strain the liquid into a glass bottle.

(https://campustrees.umn.edu/eastern-red-cedar)

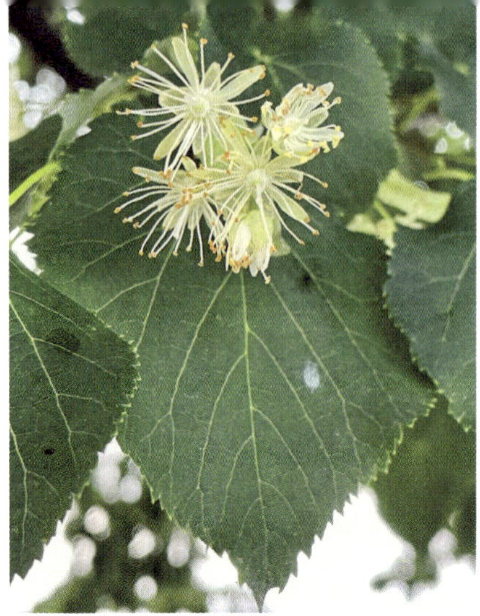

LINDEN & CONSERVATION BIOLOGICAL CONTROL

SUMMER

Linden
(*Tilia americana*)

It's a cooler-than-usual July morning, and I'm out before dawn. The air is gentle and sweet with summer perfumes, and the linden trees are blooming. Their drooping clusters of buds have finally opened, and the flowery fragrance drifts over the pond. The leaves are glossy and lush, and the ivory flowers are already hosting nectar-loving bees, so the trees literally hum, which means it's a perfect time to harvest from the tree.

My first encounter with linden trees occurred decades ago. Living in an old farmhouse that was situated on top of gently rolling hills and surrounded by rambling fields, I loved my country place. And I got to know its inhabitants. Coyotes would hide out beneath the weathered pear trees and gobble up fruit in late summer. Deer would nestle down into the long field grasses, then rise up to wander into the woods at dawn. And so many herbs grew wild. I kept track of them all. They were kin, in a way, so much a part of my small, half-wild world.

The animals often flocked around an old linden tree that grew in the middle of a field. I'm not sure how the tree got there, but the bees busily worked its flowers, and the larger animals rested in its shade on any hot day and fed on its various parts. Seeds were cherished by chipmunks, mice, squirrels, and some birds. Deer would nibble on the bark in fall and winter, and many woodpeckers and other birds made their homes in cavities that were created when old limbs broke off in a storm. But it's that fragrance I remember most, so now it's nice to have a linden close to home again and to see it in bloom.

I've known for years about the healing properties of *Tilia* species and have looked forward to gathering enough plant material to have a ready stash of it on hand. Long employed in European countries for its healing properties, linden is often called "lime blossom" there and is felt to be helpful for various illnesses, including tension and anxiety, upper respiratory complaints and coughs, fevers, and for helping to alleviate high blood pressure. It's also held in much regard worldwide as a central part of many community ceremonies and rituals. Linden is often planted along town roads and streets and has been a highly symbolic and holy tree to many cultures throughout the world.

And it turns out that *Tilia* has benefits additional to its medicinal uses. Apparently, linden species are excellent candidates for a method of environmental management called "conservation biological control." Lately, I'm trying to understand what that means. So far, here's what I know: In recent years, it has become common knowledge that toxic, wide-spectrum chemicals often used to control insect damage in agricultural crops can have negative effects on the land and its natural inhabitants. The chemicals do, indeed, destroy the destructive bugs on farm crops and in home gardens, but they also kill off the local helpful bees, butterflies, birds, and even small mammals that normally feast on the pests that cause much damage to crops. And the negative impacts last months and even years into the future. Unlike toxic chemicals with their negative environmental effects, plant species like *Tilia* actually encourage the balance and health of the land where they stand by hosting so many helpful species of wildlife that normally prey on those harmful bugs.

I don't exactly understand how all this works—in a way, it seems like it's just about leaving nature on its own to find the balance it needs and tolerating a few garden bugs instead of spraying the heck out of everything. It's a lot to think about, and much of the information seems to be above my knowledge level. But I'm glad to know that the linden can help provide an alternative to the heavy use of pesticides, and I'm also happy to have it on hand to count on for my own health

And I'm happy to know that this linden tree will not only be appreciated by me and used in the future for my healing but will also support a whole host of beneficial insects and wildlife that can help to keep a balance between harmful and helpful natural lives in the area. Today, this linden tree offers me beauty, a lovely fragrance, and healing for the future. I decide to pick some flowers to use for tea and tincture. Being careful not to bother the bees, I poke fingers into the delicate blossom clusters and pull, over and over, until my pockets are filled with the blooms. Then I amble on home, with their lovely fragrance wafting all around me.

At home, I grab my plant snips, trim the sweet-scented flowers into bits, and begin packing the blossoms into a bowl. It takes a while, but soon I have enough linden flowers to fill a glass jar for tincture and enough left over to use for a fresh linden blossom tea. While I boil water, I decide to taste the flowers to see if they are as sweet as the scent. But, at least in this one tasting, that's not true. I chew a few blossoms and find that the taste is not objectionable at all—more like a mild spring green from the garden. But the interesting thing is that the flowers turn out to be mucilaginous. A slightly slimy mouthfeel is noticeable immediately and then lingers. I swallow a bit and wait to see if there's an aftertaste. Minutes later, I'm left with just the slightest slippery taste and a mild, vegetably flavor. I'll have to do some online searching to see if the wild food folks in the state mention using linden for food or tea and see what they might have noticed. But it's nice to know what to expect from the flowers.

Waiting for my tea to steep, I do a little search on *Tilia* and find that the slippery quality of the flowers is not so surprising. It turns out to be part of the Malvaceae family—a group of plants that includes marshmallow, hibiscus, and other mucilaginous plants—all of which have a number of soothing and healing properties.

With so many medicinal properties, and so much potential for helping to relieve some of the challenges facing our planet as we stumble into the future, it seems that *Tilia* will continue to be a blessing and gift to us in many ways. In this quiet moment, I'm grateful for the scent that wafts up from the flowers, for the bees that hover just outside the window screens, and for the balance the lindens offer as we search for a wiser way to live on this remarkable planet.

Other Names: *Tilia americana,* basswood, American basswood, American linden, lime tree, bee tree.

Parts Used: Flowers, leaves, bark, sap.

Medicinal Properties: Analgesic, anticonvulsant, antispasmodic, demulcent, diaphoretic, diuretic, edible, ophthalmic, sedative, vermifuge.

Uses: Internal—Anxiety, grief, stress; colds, fevers, chest infections; hypertension; migraine headaches; heart burn, indigestion. External—Minor burns, muscle aches, sunburn, wounds.

Risks: Avoid excessive amounts and long-term use. Avoid if taking lithium or in the presence of heart disease. Avoid if you have many allergies, or use only under guidance of a health care practitioner. Frequent consumption of the tea made from the flowers may cause heart damage.

Description: *Tilia americana* is among the largest deciduous trees of eastern and central North America and can live up to two hundred years. Bark is gray and furrowed with flat ridges. Leaves are alternate, unevenly heart-shaped, and blades are 2–5 inches wide, thick and slightly leathery, with shallowly toothed margins. Flowers are yellowish-white, 0.3–0.5 inch broad, fragrant and nectar-bearing, in drooping clusters of six to twenty flowers dangling on a stalk that diverges from near the center of an oblong, leaflike, and strongly veined bract 2–4 inches long. Fruits are mostly rounded, hard, and dry.

Habitat: Upland, deciduous woods, and north and east slopes of mesic ravines.

Distribution: Top two-thirds of the state, a few parishes in bottom third.

Plant Status: Native.

Animal Use: Provides abundant nectar that will attract birds, native bees, and honeybees. Seeds are eaten by chipmunks, mice, squirrels, and songbirds. Rabbits, deer, and voles eat the bark, and leaves are eaten by various caterpillars. The canopy shelters various species, and cavities in trees are used by wood ducks, pileated woodpeckers, other birds, and small mammals for nesting. *Tilia* may serve as a larval host plant for eastern tiger swallowtail, red-spotted purple, and mourning cloak butterflies, and sixty-six species of insects from twenty-nine families were identified as pollinators of *Tilia* flowers.

Natural History: *Tilia americana* is a species of tree in the family Malvaceae and is native to eastern North America. *Tilia* is also a highly symbolic and holy tree to many cultures throughout the world. In the Germanic pre-Christian mythology, local communities held dances and celebrations under a linden tree and carried out their legal meetings there. In the Slavic Orthodox religious tradition, linden was the preferred wood for panels used for making icon paintings. The most notable street in Berlin, Germany, is called Unter den Linden, named after the trees lining the avenue and leading from the center of Berlin to the country residence of the Prussian kings. In northern China, where there was no Bodhi tree like those felt to be sacred in Buddhism, *Tilia* (with some similarities to the Bodhi tree) was planted in temples instead. Linden also played an important role in Greek literature, with Homer, Horace, Virgil, and Pliny all mentioning the linden tree and its benefits. And in Sweden, where the lime tree is named "Lind," the one hundred most common surnames in 2015 included seventeen Lindbergs (Lime-hill), twenty-one Lindströms (Lime-stream), twenty-two Lindqvists (Lime-twig), twenty-three Lindgrens (Lime-branch), and ninety-nine Lindholms (Lime-island).

Designation: Herb of commerce, Native American medicinal remedy, European healing plant, homeopathic remedy, flower essence preparation.

Cultivation: May be propagated by seeding, cuttings, layering, or grafting. The tree prefers moist, well-drained, loamy soils, and full to partial sun. It tends to be moderately drought-, salt-, pollution-, urban-, and heat-tolerant. It will require plenty of room to grow and needs pruning to develop a strong structure. Dig the planting hole twice as wide and to the same depth as the root ball. Place in hole and backfill, gently firming down. Mulch around base with organic mulch like bark chips, woodchips, or pea straw, keeping it away from the trunk. Water regularly until well established.

Remedy Form: Tea, tincture. Some species of *Tilia* are used in homeopathic remedies.

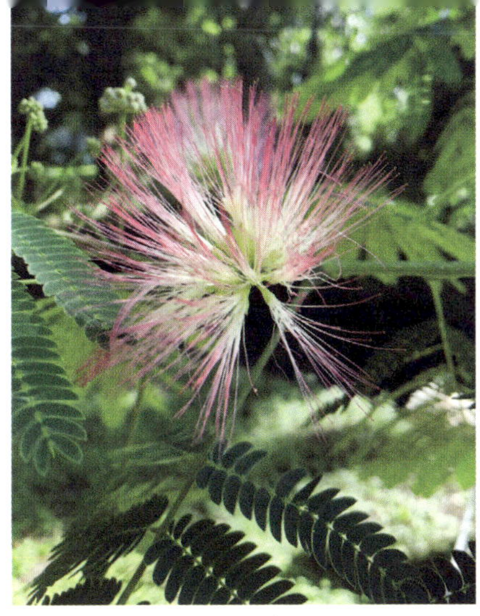

MIMOSA TREE & WALKING BODI HOME

EARLY SPRING

Mimosa tree
(*Albizia julibrissen*)

In late February, the days are finally heading toward warmth. After last week's blustery winds and cool temperatures, this morning is warmer already, with a promise of sixties by midday. Today I'm out alone for my morning walk. My little labradoodle, Bodi, now almost sixteen years old, has had some health struggles lately, and I've decided not to disturb him when he's sound asleep. He probably needs all the rest he can get as he navigates his senior years. With two recent knee surgeries and increasing food sensitivities, it's not uncommon for us to be up several times a night for a potty visit to the backyard. I don't mind too much, though. I get up grumbling, but once I step out under the sky, I'm rewarded with the stars and constellations overhead—and the late-night quiet along the usually busy road. Still, it's a challenging time for both of us.

With Bodi's "rainbow bridge" approaching, I'm getting prepared for the grief I know I'll experience when he moves on. Years ago, when my favorite aunt passed away, grief became my whole world. I didn't exactly feel depressed, but I was definitely in another realm—still more with her than I was present in my everyday life. I wouldn't have given that time up, though. As hard as it was, I found beauty in it, too. It was an opportunity to listen to my own inner process and needs and to spend time celebrating the relationship with my aunt that lingered even though she was gone. Fortunately, in the decade since her death, the medical community and the general public have begun to understand the deep challenges and meaningful gifts of the grief process.

With all that in mind, lately I'm getting prepared for Bodi's last walk. I recently happened upon an article on the many medicinal plants that can help relieve feelings of loss, and I've started to work on a little "grief apothecary" to have on hand. This morning, I'm out to check on the mimosa tree in my neighbor's yard. In the last few days, she's been doing some pruning of the smaller branches, and I'm pretty sure she'll let me make a harvest of the bark before the logs dry out. Last summer, I gathered lots of the pink, fluffy flowers to dry for tea, and now I'm hoping to round out my mimosa supply with enough bark to make a tincture.

As a child, I spent as much time outdoors as possible. Nature was a sanctuary for me—a place where I could quiet down, be at peace, and ponder the mysteries of the world and my place in it. And my favorite way to do that pondering was by climbing trees. Sitting above the ground and all its busyness, I'd rest and observe and imagine and have a little time for myself. And the easiest tree to climb in our yard was the mimosa. Smooth-barked, with comfortable and safe crotches where I could wedge myself securely, it was a perfect perch. What I didn't know then was that the mimosa trees were good for more than beauty or hiding out from the busy world. Once I started learning about medicinal properties of plants, I discovered some surprising information about this tree.

I found that the mimosa has a history of use in the healing traditions of many cultures. In traditional Chinese medicine, a remedy from the tree is known as the "Collective Happiness Bark" and is felt to "nourish the heart and calm the spirit." Reportedly, it can help to relieve worry, anxiety, confusion, and depression. According to Chinese medical philosophy, a vital connection exists between the mind and the health of the heart. In Western medicine, we now know that mental anxiety can lead to heart palpitations and high blood pressure, so something that could gently relieve stress would be helpful.

In addition to helping ease grief, *Albizia* flowers and bark are recommended for supporting general mental health, relieving anxiety, promoting restorative sleep, and calming irritability. In scientific studies, *Albizia* has been proven to enhance neurotransmitter secretion and regulation, and the flowers have been used for mild amnesia associated with insomnia. A tea of the leaves and bark can also relieve muscle aches after rigorous exercise. In addition, traditional Mayan healers used the bark and flowers externally for skin wounds and traumatic injuries. And modern research has proven that the crushed or powdered bark contains important steroid compounds that act as a helpful anesthetic, reducing pain for up to three hours. It also aids in regenerating skin.

By the time I get home, Bodi is stirring and ready for a short walk. I give him a few bites of cooked turkey and rice and then head outdoors again. Bodi can visit the mimosa tree with me this time and sniff for animal trails around its base. Even though he's slowing down, he's still curious and snarky, still has a bit of appetite, and is happy to be outside—all a few good signs that he's not heading for the rainbow bridge just yet. But I'm glad to build up my stock of *Albizia* to have on hand when Bodi's leaving time is near. And I know the mimosa tree will continue to be a haven for me—offering beauty, solace, a place to perch safely above the ragged worries and challenges of life, and a source of healing for those wounds of the heart that are part and parcel of living in this world.

Other Names: *Albizia julibrissin,* silktree, powderpuff tree, silk tree, tree of happiness.

Parts Used: Flowers, bark, leaves, gum.

Medicinal Properties: Flower heads are anticonvulsant, antitumor, anti-inflammatory, carminative, digestive, sedative, and tonic. Bark is anodyne, anthelmintic, astringent, carminative, coagulant, digestive, diuretic, oxytocic, sedative, stimulant, tonic, vermifuge, and vulnerary. Gummy extract from the plant is highly astringent and vulnerary.

Uses: Internal—Flowers: Anxiety, depression, grief, insomnia, irritability, poor memory. Bark: Insomnia, irritability, pain, muscle soreness, depression, anxiety. May also speed up healing in fractures. External—Abscesses, boils, burns, and minor wounds.

Risks: May cause mood swings in those with bipolar disorder.

Description: A small, flat-topped tree with branches spreading wide, and up to 40 feet tall. Bark is smooth and blotched with gray. Fernlike leaves are alternate, deciduous, 8–15 inches long, and bipinnately even compound. The leaflets are dull green, asymmetrical, and about 0.5 inch long. Leaves close up at night. The pink (rarely white) flowers occur in headlike clusters and bloom from May to August. The fruit is a flattened legume, 5–8 inches long and up to 1 inch wide, and contains five to sixteen seeds. Seeds are toxic to dogs and livestock.

Habitat: Old fields, fencerows, gardens. Often cultivated as an ornamental that escaped.

Distribution: Many parishes (though not much in south and central areas).

Plant Status: Introduced from Asia and naturalized in southern states.

Animal Use: Seeds may be eaten by birds and squirrels; flowers attract several species of bees, hummingbirds, and butterflies.

Natural History: The mimosa tree is a native of Iran, Japan, and southern Korea, and was introduced to Europe and North America in the mid-eighteenth century. It may have been introduced to the United States by French botanist Andre Michaux in 1787, when he grew seeds brought from Persia to his nursery in Charleston, South Carolina.

Designation: Traditional Chinese medicine remedy, African American medicinal plant, Indigenous traditional herb, Iranian traditional medicine, Mayan healing remedy.

Cultivation: Best done from seed, and the tree will seed readily on-site.

Remedy Form: Tea, tincture, oxymel, powder, syrup.

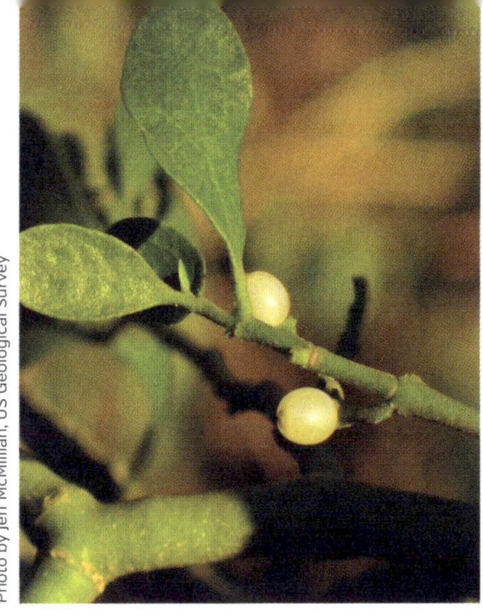

Photo by Jeff McMillian, US Geological Survey

MISTLETOE & DADDY'S GUNS

SPRING

Mistletoe
(*Phoradendron* sp.)

I grew up with guns. My dad had a shotgun and a rifle and was off hunting as often as he could get away. It wasn't unusual to see him cleaning his gun at the kitchen table when he was getting ready to go out with the guys. And the table was host to his catch once he returned. In fact, one of the ways I learned to love nature was by looking closely at what my dad brought home. I watched him pluck ducks and skin squirrels and scale fish, so before the bounty ever hit the dinner table, I'd have learned a lot about the animals. At some point, after seeing a Disney movie, I realized that my dad would probably have shot Bambi's father if he could have, and that was the end of being comfortable with eating wildlife for me! But guns, at least when I was a kid, were tools—just one of the ways we got some of our food.

Louisiana people are inextricably linked to the land and water and air. Even now, even if folks aren't the least bit likely to go hunting or fishing or trapping, just about everyone who lives here knows when the oysters will be cold and salty, the crawfish will be large, and the crabs will be fat. They know when the cane trucks will be lumbering along the back roads, and the alligators and snakes will be coming out of their hidden homes and sliding along the swampy ground. It's hard to escape nature here—it has seeped into our skin from the day we were born and become our home.

Over the past decades, my time away from the state and my basically peace-centered temperament have shifted my ideas of the possible scary results of having guns around. But I did go hunting a few times with my dad. It was a nice way for me to be outdoors and to have him for myself for a while. On one trip, we walked into a grassy field to stand under old trees, and my dad taught me how to spot mistletoe. He was eager to get some to take home for our Christmas tree, so he just lifted his rifle and shot down a large, rounded clump of it. It was too hard to get it otherwise, he said. And that's how he and his brothers had gotten the plant down when they were boys.

My own knowledge about mistletoe was a bit different than his. As an herbalist, I had heard about the uses of the plant, especially for seizure disorders and other neurological conditions. But I knew that there were many questions about its safety, and so I hadn't tried using it yet. At one point, I was living in a tiny rural town in Virginia and had a neighbor who saw me out harvesting herbs one day. She asked what I was doing, and when I replied that I was studying medicinal plants, she asked me about a health concern. She had a seizure disorder, she said, and didn't want to take any medications for her condition. She'd prefer to use foods and plants to stop the seizures. It posed a bit of a quandary for me. While I appreciated her desire to take care of her health using natural remedies, I also knew that seizure disorders are complex and can vary greatly from person to person, both in terms of what triggers them and what medications can help. I recommended some other, milder herbs that might help support the nervous system, and told her she would probably fare better if she tried to work out an approach under the direction of her family doctor.

To this day, even though I love seeing the great round balls of *Phoradendron* high in the trees, I've never harvested it. Given the potential side effects of mistletoe, I'm not too likely to use it internally for healing. And despite my dad's comfort with hunting, I have no intention of buying a gun. But I have a respect for both traditions—for the hunting activities that make up such a big part of what it means to live the Cajun lifestyle, intimately connected with the land, and for the use of mistletoe not just for stolen holiday kisses but for its healing properties as well. I guess keeping both these traditions alive makes me feel a little less sad about some of the ways of life that are threatened in the state. And I'll continue to keep an eye on current herbal research. The U.S. National Institutes of Health recently reported that various species of *Phoradendron* showed much promise in the future development of pharmaceutical drugs for seizures and other nervous system conditions—offering us one more step in the direction of bridging conventional and holistic health.

Other Names: *Phoradendron serotinum* and *Phoradendron leucarpum* are two species often called American mistletoe or Christmas mistletoe.

Parts Used: Leaves, flowers, seeds.

Medicinal Properties: Antiproliferative, antioxidant, anti-inflammatory, antimicrobial.

Uses: Mistletoe has been widely used in Europe and is regarded as among the most widely employed natural therapies for cancer. In addition, it has many uses in traditional Chinese medicine as well as in healing systems of Indigenous groups in Australia and Latin America. Navajo healers in the past used the mistletoe occurring in juniper trees to create a soothing lotion for bug bites, to cure warts, and to ease stomach pain.

Risks: Nausea, vomiting, diarrhea, decreased heart rate, hallucinations, and heart problems may occur. It is best to avoid taking the plant internally.

Description: The *Phoradendron* are hemiparasitic, living in the branches of trees. Leaves are leathery and thick, and opposing, simple, and ovate. Flowers occur as short, jointed spikes. Berries are white, 0.12–0.24 inch in size, and are pulpy and sticky. Shrub or ball can grow to 3 by 3 feet.

Habitat: May occur on branches of deciduous trees exposed to sun, including apple, oak, maple, elm, pine, and poplar.

Distribution: All of northern half of the state, much of southern half.

Plant Status: Native.

Animal Use: Fruits are covered with a sticky substance that is eaten by birds. They spread the seeds through their droppings and by wiping their beaks on branches, where a new plant may become established. The most important birds for effective dispersal include the cedar waxwing, euphonias, silky-flycatchers, bluebirds, and thrushes. Mistletoe also provides essential food, cover, and nesting sites for an amazing number of animals including birds, butterflies, and insects.

Natural History: Ancient cultures valued mistletoe as a sacred, mystical plant, and it was placed in cradles to protect infants from being stolen by fairies. It was also once considered a symbol of peace. The ancient Celtic Druids collected mistletoe for their ceremonies just after the winter solstice, which is near December 25. Mistletoe was considered sacred to them and was believed to have great powers. They cut down the mistletoe with a golden sickle and adorned their homes with the foliage to bring joy while protecting the family from bad spirits. These rituals were later frowned upon by those practicing Christianity, and this custom has faded away.

Designation: Indigenous and folkloric herbal remedy. Sometimes employed in European phytotherapy practice.

Cultivation: Done by birds.

Remedy Form: Not recommended for internal use until more pharmacological studies have been done. External—Poultice for boils and insect bites.

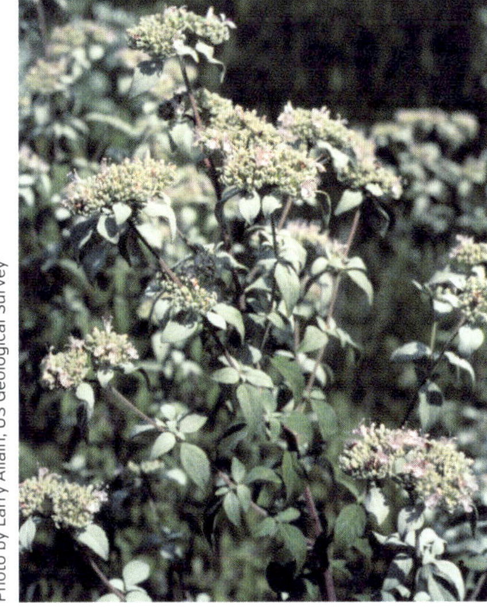

Photo by Larry Allain, US Geological Survey

MOUNTAIN MINT & THE RAIN

SUMMER

Mountain mint
(*Pycnanthemum* sp.)

It's been an odd summer so far—first, with no rain at all for what seemed like weeks. And then, lately, at least one big, sloppy deluge a day, if not more. Every morning, before the sun rises, all the neighbors are out as early as possible to check the waterlogged gardens, mow raggedy lawns, and run errands before cloudbursts start up again.

I've tried to prepare folks from away for Louisiana rains when they visit. "No matter how hard you think it rains where you live," I say, "there's no comparison. If the sky darkens and the winds pick up, you will definitely not make it home before it pours! And you cannot do without a longish raincoat, because within ten seconds you will be soaked to the skin. And forget about umbrellas—inside out and totally useless once the gusts pick up. And if you think that a couple of inches of rain is a lot, ha! Try fourteen inches overnight! Imagine your huge garbage bin, your heavy potted plants, your loaded wheelbarrow, or any patio furniture just floating away. That is Louisiana rain."

Nope, rain is no stranger here. According to recent records, the average annual rainfall for southern Louisiana can be up to seventy inches, and for central and northern areas, around fifty inches. And apparently it has been increasing over the past few years, with more flood events, especially during storms. But I remember childhood rainstorms when streets were pretty frequently underwater, and folks from down the bayous would just get in their cars and drive to (relatively) higher ground, knock on someone's door, and ask to be let in to wait out the flood. At our house, we'd fill the bathtub with water and freeze lots of ice cubes, my mom would cook up plenty of food that could be eaten at room temperature, and my dad would board up windows. Just as we did then, we still know how to get ready. But even without hurricanes or gusty storms, high water is a given.

With all that in mind, this morning I'm out for a quick trek to the levee trail before the daily deluge starts. At the beginning of my walk, the sky is gorgeous—the coming sun glows through huge clouds and paints everything orange and pink. The usual little blue herons and egrets are out early, too, hunting in the marsh. Much wild petunia is flowering in the fields and along the sidewalk, and honeybees are sipping nectar from the newly blooming grass flowers. By the time I get home at 6:00 a.m., the air is already hot and steamy, and mosquito hawks and monarch butterflies are busy in the messy garden. *Gaura* blossoms bob on long stems, waving in the first of today's breezes. And the mountain mint is tall, its flowers full and just beginning to set seed.

Before I visited Charles Allen's bed-and-breakfast in Pitkin, I'd never heard of mountain mint. I was quite familiar with the mints of the northeastern states. *Mentha arvensis* grows there like a weed, and I love picking new leaves and nibbling on them as I walk in early summer. And I am really familiar with the cultivated mints—spearmint continues to take over my flower bed every year and hangs in bundles to dry every fall. And peppermint is a regular there, too. But the mountain mints were a curiosity—and not even an official *Mentha* family member! In a recent class I attended at Allen's Acres, a small group of us wandered all around the feral gardens that are a mix of wild and lightly cultivated growth. Charles explained the many edible and healing properties of the plants and then gifted us with samples. I took home a couple of species of the native mints to encourage in my own garden.

Curious about their history of healing, I recently read up on *Pycnanthemum* species and found they have as many, if not more, medicinal properties than members of what we regularly think of as mints. Three species grow wild in Louisiana, and each of them is rich in important chemical compounds that promote healing. Many mountain mints have had an important place in Native American healing traditions. Apparently, the Choctaw used a hot tea made from the leaves of *Pycnanthemum albescens,* or white mountain mint, as a diaphoretic for colds and fevers. Cherokee tribal healers used another species to relieve headaches and to break a fevers, and the Lakota took an infusion of the leaves for coughs. And several species of the herb were used by the Chippewa for food or to season meats and soups. Leaves, buds, and flowers were also used to help settle indigestion, relieve menstrual irregularities, and reduce the symptoms of coughs or colds. In recent years, scientific studies have documented antibiotic properties in the essential oils of various *Pycnanthemum* species. And USDA ethnobotanist James Duke noted numerous uses worldwide for the three species of mountain mint found in Louisiana. The healing benefits documented include analgesic, anthelmintic, antiacne, antiallergic, antiasthmatic, antibacterial, antibronchitis, anticancer, anticonvulsant, antiflu, antifatigue, antirheumatic, antiseptic, antispasmodic, antistaph, antistrep, antitumor, antitussive, antiviral, antiyeast, hypotensive, immunomodulary, refrigerant, and sedative. Good grief! Who knew?

For all those reasons, I was excited to start experimenting with the mountain mints. Last week, during a few bright days, I tried my first sample of the plant. And I have to say, I wasn't wild about the taste. I picked a midsize leaf and chewed it for a while. I noticed its astringency right away. Then came the strong minty flavor that was similar to the *Mentha,* but a little different. Even though I wasn't thrilled with the taste, I'd heard that the tea can be very soothing, so I was willing to give it a try. I gathered several bundles of the plant and hung them to dry. Now that they're dried and stored, I'm eager to try the plant again. Maybe it will taste a little milder as an iced beverage. After I do a few chores, I'll try mountain mint tea with a little lemon and some of my neighbor's honey for a touch of sweetness and see what I think.

Now the clouds that were glorious early in my walk are rumbling with thunder. They press down over the levee and break open to drench the fields and gardens. Again. But I'm pretty sure there won't be as much accumulation as a week ago, when fourteen inches of rainfall registered on my patio at one point! And despite the tiresome, everyday rain, there's something I love about it. It's another excuse to nap, to curl up with a good book, and to do more herb work later. Today, it will be making up teabags from the mountain mint I harvested recently and stored in glass jars. And I'll be paying attention to any effects I might notice as I sample my first cup of iced mountain mint tea.

Species: Three species of *Pycnanthemum* can be found in Louisiana and may be used interchangeably. These include:

Pycnanthemum albescens

Other Names: White mountain mint.

Medicinal Uses: Colds, fevers, headaches.

Description: Grows about 1–4 feet tall. Leaves are 1.5 inches long and 0.5 inch wide (nearest the middle). The terminal one-half to two-thirds of each margin has six to eight widely spaced, shallow teeth. Upper surfaces of lower leaves are dull olive-green; lower surfaces are greenish-gray. Upper leaves and flower bracts are whitened with a dense, thin coating of grayish-white hair. The white coloration slowly spreads over these leaves, creating the silvery bracts.

Habitat: Low open woods, along streams, savannas, thickets, and dry, rocky hillsides.

Distribution: Western half of the state, also some central and eastern parishes.

Plant Status: Native.

Pycnanthemum muticum

Other Names: Muticous mountain mint, short-toothed mountain mint, clustered mountain mint, blue mountain mint.

Medicinal Uses: Allergies, asthma, bronchitis, chest infections, cough; acne; antitumor (including breast, colon, pancreas, prostate, stomach); fatigue, sedative, mild tranquilizer; immune system support, staph and strep infections.

Description: The plant bears oval, toothed leaves on strong, square, pubescent stems that branch frequently in the top part of plant. Leaves occur on short petioles along the stems and are opposing and aromatic. In summer, plants are topped by dense, rounded clusters of tiny white-lavender tubular flowers. Leaves surrounding the flower clusters are highlighted with silver.

Habitat: Dry open woods, bogs, savannas, low meadows, low woods.

Distribution: Found in approximately two dozen western and central parishes in the state.

Plant Status: Native.

Pycnanthemum tenuifolium

Other Names: Slender-leaved mountain mint, narrowleaf mountain mint, common horsemint, Virginia thyme.

Medicinal Uses: Allergies, bronchitis, chest congestion and infections, viruses; Alzheimer's disease; anticancer (breast, cervix, colon, pancreas, prostate, stomach); ulcers, yeast infections.

Description: Stems are wiry and green and branch 2–3 feet tall. Stems are square and leaves are narrow, opposite, and simple, measuring up to 2 inches long and less than 0.25 inch wide. Flowers are white and occur in dense, half-round heads. Foliage has a very faint mint fragrance.

Habitat: Grassy, moist, open woods, bogs, savannas, old fields, meadows, marshes, upland woods, dry soil in prairies, pastures, and roadsides.

Distribution: Western half of the state, and some central parishes.

Plant Status: Native.

For All Species, Parts Used: Aerial parts, essential oil.

Medicinal Properties: Analgesic, anesthetic, anthelmintic, antiacne, antiallergenic, antiasthmatic, antibacterial, antibronchitis, anticancer, anticholinesterase, anticonvulsant, antifatigue, antiflu, antihistamine, anti-inflammatory, antilaryngitis, antilithtic, antimetastatic, antioxidant, antirheumatic, antistaph, antistrep, antitumor (against breast, colon, pancreas, prostate, and stomach malignancies), immunomodulary, sedative, vulnerary.

Uses: Internal—Allergies, chills, colds, coughs, fevers, flu, general exhaustion, immune system regulation and support; colic, indigestion; inflammation, pain; menstrual disorders; sinus headaches; stress, anxiety. External—Minor burns, gargle for mouth sores, insect repellent, wash/poultice for wounds.

Risks: Avoid in the presence of gastroesophageal reflux disease (GERD). Limit intake during pregnancy. Do not ingest essential oil.

Description: *P. muticum* is shorter (about 3 feet), has a stronger smell, and has very short or no petiole, while *P. albescens* is taller (5 feet), has a weaker smell and petioles.

Animal Use: All Louisiana species are important pollinator plants and attract numerous bees, butterflies, flies, and birds.

Natural History: Genus name comes from the Greek word *pyknos,* which means "dense," and *anthos,* which means "flower" (indicating its densely packed flowers). Species indicators include *P. albescens* (meaning whitened or grayed), *P. muticum* (meaning short-toothed or blunt), and *P. tenuifolium* (meaning slender-leaved).

Designation: Native American healing remedy, Cajun traiteur remedy, folkloric herbal medicine.

Cultivation: May be grown from seed, root, or stem cuttings, or division. If growing from seed, directly sow into the garden in early spring. Scatter or press seed lightly, but do not bury, as it requires light to germinate. Transplant outdoors once all danger of frost has passed. The *Pycnanthemum* prefer moderate moisture, need a mixture of sun and shade, are not picky about soil, and appreciate some heat/sun protection in hot weather.

Remedy Form: Internal—Edible, teas, tinctures. External—Compress, poultice, wash.

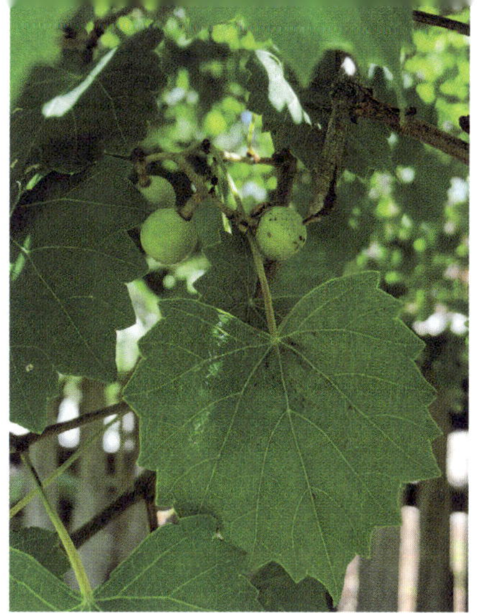

MUSCADINE GRAPES & THE WILD TURKEY

LATE SUMMER

Muscadine grape
(*Vitis rotundifolia*)

All morning long, my neighbor and I keep watch over a wild turkey that has settled into our yards. Crippled by some mishap that has damaged its right leg, it can only hobble, and pretty badly at that. It takes a few hops, then falls to the heat-weathered ground. It will spread out one big wing and peck at fallen seed from the spent sunflowers. It seems to like the fallen grapes from the wild vines beyond the garden, too. Despite its injury, the turkey seems pretty peaceful. We guess that it might be grateful for fruit and seeds, for sun and the mild wind, maybe even for the nearby humans who are keeping watch. But we worry about it. Both of us have seen coyotes around the edges of the neighborhood, and though the turkey is pretty large, we're sure that a group of coyotes could make short work of our injured visitor. Marcia and I text back and forth, each of us trying for a while to get close and see if we can capture it somehow. Kind of unlikely, of course—and what would we do if we could catch it, after all? But the turkey is wily and cautious, hobbling away from us again and again.

We keep texting one another about what to do. She puts in a call to a local wildlife rehab group and then brings bird seed over while I gather some grapes. We think that maybe if we make a trail of the food into my garage, the turkey will follow. Then we could close the door and keep it safe for a while. As we discuss our rescue plan, the bird rehab guy shows up, steps toward the turkey, and it flaps its big wings and flies across a little pond. Back and forth they go, the rehabber and the turkey, until finally we all give up. It can fly, after all, and forage for food. It just can't run or walk.

A few hours later, Marcia and I are still worrying about the turkey, wondering how it's doing. We text about how ridiculous this is, in a way. After all, we both eat turkey often, and it is a feature of some holiday meals. We've probably eaten some of this turkey's relatives! But although that meat has been at the center of our tables, this wounded turkey is now at the center of our hearts. Being close to something makes a difference, I guess. We have watched its struggles, and its resilience, and the way it adapted to its new, unfortunate life. We both talk about how beautiful it was, even with its naked, wrinkly head.

I start to clean up the turkey food mess in the yard and then pop a few ripe muscadine grapes into my own mouth. And I think about healing, and food, and the muscadines that have settled so happily into the little thicket beside my house. I love grapes. In fact, I eat them every day. This time of year, I can gather them in the wild and have them with my morning tea. During other seasons, I buy the fruit at local grocery stores. And the grapes aren't just tasty; they're good medicine as well.

I'm always so excited when the wild grapes start to ripen—I love the sweet, juicy flavor. And even though I buy seedless grapes when the wild ones aren't available, I don't mind the seeds much when I'm picking my own fruit right off the vine. Standing near the edge of the batture pond, I reach as high as I can and fill my pockets. I figure the songbirds can have the highest grapes, and the turkeys and small mammals can have the low fruit, and I can pick from the middle without disturbing the vines.

Much research the past few decades has proven that grapes and their leaves and seeds have many healing properties, and the fruit can be a great addition to daily diets. Many species of *Vitis* provide antioxidant and anti-inflammatory compounds. And it turns out that the muscadine grapes contain more resveratrol than most fruits. A food with this compound can protect against many chronic diseases, including cardiovascular diseases, liver diseases, obesity, diabetes, Alzheimer's disease, and Parkinson's disease. They have also been indicated for preventing recurrence of several kinds of cancer.

For the greatest nutritional benefit, experts recommend that we eat the skins and seeds as well as the pulp and juice. Apparently, research has proven that the seeds can be used for diabetes complications such as nerve and eye problems, improving wound healing, preventing tooth decay, preventing cancer, preventing age-related macular degeneration, and alleviating poor night vision, liver disorders, and hay fevers.

And the vines are easy to grow in home gardens, as they have a natural resistance to diseases and pests that thrive in hot and damp climates. It turns out that grapes offer important nutrition to wild turkeys, and I wonder if the fruit offers some kind of healing for them as well. I imagine they could use whatever help they can get.

Populations of wild turkeys in Louisiana have diminished over the years, so I'm glad that at least our neighborhood turkey can take advantage of the foraged grapes. And for all I know, maybe turkeys have heart troubles, too, and maybe the muscadines can help today's turkey in more ways that I can imagine. In any case, I'm happy to know that wherever the injured turkey has landed, it will at least have food—grapes and seeds—and the shelter of the woods.

For a while, my neighbor and I will continue to keep watch for our disabled visitor. And I'll keep including grapes in my daily diet. I might even consider growing some myself. I know that the LSU AgCenter has recommendations and support for those interested in growing muscadines. If I have my own vines, I can continue to support my health with native grapes, and I'll have some on hand if another wounded turkey ends up in my yard. A pretty good deal for us all.

Species: Several grape species make their home in Louisiana. While many of the species probably have similar medicinal properties, most have yet to be evaluated for healing potential. The species with documented or historical medicinal uses include:

Vitis aestivalis

Other Names: Pigeon grape, summer grape.

Medicinal Use: Internal—Leaves and stem bark used for stomach upset; bladder irritations; fevers; headaches. External—Poultice of wilted leaves used for breast pain.

Description: A deciduous, climbing, and woody vine with tendrils that may reach 35 feet in length and may sprawl over nearby vegetation. Trunk of mature vines may be 6 inches across, with reddish-brown bark that peels in strips. Lower leaves are white and hairy, with visible veins.

Habitat: Sandy soils along rivers and streams; dry, rocky, and upland woods.

Distribution: Top half of the state, patchy in other parishes.

Plant Status: Native.

Vitis riparia

Other Names: Riverbank grape, frost grape.

Medicinal Use: Internal—Some Indigenous peoples used the juice of *V. riparia* for coughs and colds. External—Leaves applied to sprains and bruises.

Description: The vine may grow up to 75 feet long, has reddish-brown bark that shreds into narrow strips, and heart-shaped, three-lobed leaves with toothed margins. Small clusters of fragrant, pale-green flowers appear in the spring, followed by clusters of bluish-black fruits in late summer and fall.

Habitat: Disturbed areas of lower and upper woodlands, dunes, thickets, riverbanks, abandoned fields, and along railroads.

Distribution: Spotty throughout the northern half of the state.

Plant Status: Native.

Vitis rotundifolia

Other Names: Muscadine, scuppernong, bullace-grape.

Medicinal Uses: Cardiovascular complaints, elevated blood cholesterol and triglycerides, hypertension; cancers (including lung, colon, breast, prostate, liver and others).

Description: The climbing vine is deciduous and has simple tendrils, and length depends on surrounding support. Bark is smooth, nonexfoliating, and is greenish to greenish-brown. Small, greenish-yellow to white flowers bloom in panicles from May to June. Leaves are large, green, shiny, and broad with blunt teeth and a heart-shaped base. Berries are large with thick skin, and are shiny purplish-black to bronze, ripening in fall. They appear singularly and not in clusters

Habitat: Dry upland forests with especially sandy or rocky soil, swamps, roadsides, and thickets.

Distribution: Much of the state, except for extreme southeast parishes.

Plant Status: Native.

Vitis vulpina

Other Names: Frost grape, fox grape, wild grape, winter grape, chicken grape.

Medicinal Uses: Internal—Fevers; diabetes; bladder irritations; headache; liver support. External—Poultice for breast tenderness.

Description: Lower leaf green. Teeth smaller, all same size. Hairs on and between veins, base of leaf with U-shaped sinus.

Habitat: Low woods, stream banks, riverbanks, and thickets.

Distribution: Spotty throughout the state, more concentrated in northern and eastern parishes.

Plant Status: Native.

For All Species, Parts Used: Whole fruit, skin, leaves, and seed.

Medicinal Properties: Plant parts of species listed above have been shown to have antioxidant, antiaging, cardioprotective, antihyperlipidemic, anticancer, chemopreventive, and antihypertensive properties.

Uses: Grape juice and wine can decrease blood-glucose levels, improve cholesterol status, lower triglycerides, and prevent blood clotting. Grape leaf has been used for attention deficit hyperactivity disorder (ADHD); chronic fatigue syndrome (CFS); diarrhea; heavy menstrual bleeding, uterine bleeding; canker sores. Grape seeds (and grape seed extract [GSE]) have been used to support healthy hearts, joints, blood sugar, brain function, cell function, immunity, and sexual function, and to alleviate a wide range of health concerns including headaches, conditions related to aging, fatigue, menopause, and more. Fruit enhances nonspecific immunity and helps to prevent several diseases. Also, fruits are nutrient packed and have all the properties listed for other plant parts.

Risks: Consuming large quantities of grapes might cause diarrhea. Some people have allergic reactions to grapes and grape products. These reactions might include cough, dry mouth, and headache.

Animal Use: Fruits of wild grapes are eaten by more than eighty species of birds and mammals, including bobwhites, cardinals, catbirds, crows, ducks, quails, ring-necked pheasants, ruffed grouse, wild turkeys, black bear, deer, coyote, red and gray foxes, opossums, rabbits, raccoons, and skunks. Deer will browse leaves, and some species of birds will use vines and foliage for nesting material.

Natural History: Grapes appear to have been part of the Indigenous North American diet for over ten thousand years. They have been found in sites of this age, including the Dust Cave site in northwestern Alabama, which dates to the Late Paleoindian period (8500–8000 BCE). Native grapes were found in North America by the first European settlers and are prized for their cold-hardiness and disease resistance.

Designation: Edible, herb of commerce, Cajun traiteur remedy, Native/Indigenous food and remedy, Ayurvedic herb, African American home remedy.

Cultivation: Many *Vitis* species prefer deep, fertile soils and can tolerate warmth and humidity. They do not like calcareous soils or soils with poor drainage.

Remedy Form: Edible, tincture, tea, wine, jams and jellies, extract, poultice.

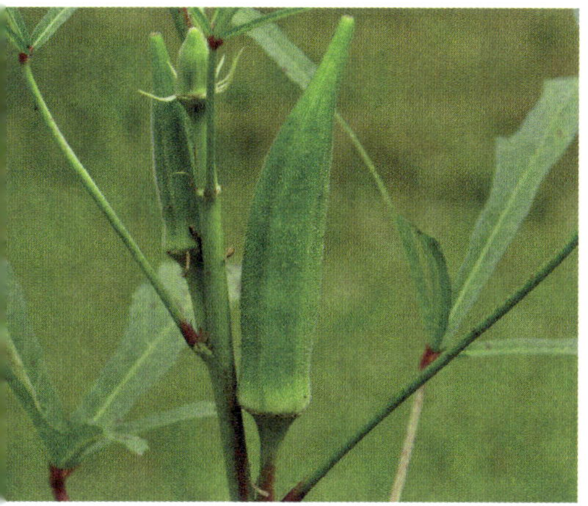

Photo by mumemories (1103651942) on Unsplash

OKRA & NANETTE'S GUMBO

SUMMER

Okra
(*Abelmoschus esculentes*)

I was never a big fan of okra. As a child, I didn't notice that it was in the rich and tasty dishes my mom cooked. In her gumbo, it was there—but after half a day of cooking down with other vegetables and the roux, all I could recognize were the small, pale, rounded seeds floating in the brothy part of the dish. And since there was crabmeat in the seafood gumbo, I vaguely registered them and thought maybe they were crabs' eyes. That was kind of a disgusting idea, but a child growing up in the Deep South learns early that you're going to eat just about everything that nature offers up, so it didn't bother me. But okra by itself was just a little too much like caterpillars—fuzzy on the outside, slimy on the inside. It wasn't until I was a much older adult that I finally began to appreciate the vegetable. Eating it fried, I could ignore the slimy bit—and having it mixed with something as yummy as maque choux, I could concentrate on the shrimp and corn. But once I heard about how many health benefits there are in consuming the plant, I was grudgingly interested. Then, as an herbalist, I learned about the numerous healing properties of a natural mucilage, and that tugged me over the line.

According to Dr. James Duke, an international authority on medicinal plant use, okra has been found to be useful for over five hundred health problems. The USDA-run online website Dr. Duke's Phytochemical and Ethnobotanical Database lists many of the plant's healing properties. It notes that the plant is antihypertensive, anti-inflammatory, anti-insomniac, antimigraine, antineurotic, anti-Raynaud's, antishingles, antiseptic, anti-asthma, cancer-preventive, hepatoprotective, and on and on and on. Along with other Mallow family members, okra has been found to reduce the risk of some serious health threats including heart disease, cancer, kidney disease, digestive tract disorders, and type 2 diabetes. It is also known to alleviate nervous system conditions such as anxiety, depression, Alzheimer's disease, and migraines.

Which leads me back to gumbo. It's been said that gumbo is the heart of Louisiana cuisine. Like any Louisiana child, I often had gumbo at family gatherings. Growing up, I learned that there were a few different kinds. Seafood gumbo was my favorite, but I also loved chicken and andouille gumbo. And on special occasions, one grandmother or the other would prepare "gumbo z'herbes." This was made with a blend of many kinds of greens and traditionally was eaten on Holy Thursday, supposedly to fortify the diners in preparation for fasting on Good Friday. And then, there was the issue of tomatoes! Our mom never used tomatoes, but I know that some folks insist that they're supposed to be part of the stew. A little research on that question turned up a suggestion that a Cajun cook would not include tomatoes, but a Creole cook would. I guess it depends upon your cooking teacher or your family origins as to "yay" or "nay" on the tomatoes issue.

But the one ingredient that never wavered, at least in our family, was okra! As it turns out, that is probably a very wise thing. With so many health benefits, okra should definitely be a permanent staple in a southern diet. I think it was my cousin Nanette who changed my stance on this vegetable. Not only is it a regular addition to her delicious gumbo but she served me a dish once of maque choux with okra in it, and I was sold.

Which leads me to the issue of gumbo recipes. Growing up, I just figured that my mom's gumbo was the (delicious) norm. But it turns out that cooks are very particular about their recipes, and each batch of gumbo, even made by the same cook, will have some variations. Nanette's gumbo has turned out to be one of my favorites, and several years ago she shared some of her secrets with me. But the main thing, she said, was the process of making the dish. You don't just throw the ingredients together—you have to pay attention, take your time. It's the layers and timing that matter—one stage done, then the next, with nothing ignored. Every step is all love and attention, details and patience, and savoring. In the end, the flavors seep into each other, settle into something nourishing and rich, each effort different from the last.

I like thinking about it that way. And even though I am still a little wary of okra, I love knowing some of its many healing properties and am always very glad to sit down to one of my favorite ways to enjoy the herb—in a big bowl of (healing) gumbo.

Other Names: *Abelmoschus esculentus,* lady's fingers, ochro.

Parts Used: Pod/fruit, leaves, seeds.

Medicinal Properties: Antibacterial, anti-inflammatory, antimicrobial, antiviral, antioxidant, promotes cellular regeneration, demulcent, detoxifying, laxative, reduces cholesterol, supports mucous membranes.

Uses: Alzheimer's disease; heart disease; cancer; high cholesterol; constipation and indigestion; kidney disease; anxiety, depression, migraines, nervous irritability; coughs, colds, flu, respiratory disorders, sore throat; skin repair; blood sugar imbalances.

Risks: Should be avoided if taking Metformin; avoid in presence of gastrointestinal diseases or kidney stones. Okra's high vitamin K content may interact with blood-thinning medications such as Coumadin (warfarin). Excess consumption may have a laxative effect.

Description: The species is a perennial, often cultivated as an annual in temperate climates, often growing to around 6 feet tall. Leaves are 3–8 inches long and broad, palmately lobed with five to seven lobes. The flowers are 1.6–3 inches in diameter, with five white to yellow petals, often with a red or purple spot at the base of each petal. Fruit is a capsule up to 7 inches long with pentagonal cross-section, containing numerous seeds.

Habitat: Okra likes warm to hot temperatures, grows well in a variety of soil types, and prefers full sun. It is sometimes found near old garden sites.

Distribution: Commonly cultivated, occasionally escaping into surrounding areas, especially in northern parishes.

Plant Status: Introduced.

Animal Use: Rabbits, voles, deer, woodchucks, and squirrels consume leaves and fruits. Aphids, stinkbugs, corn earworms, snails, and slugs use various parts of the plant.

Natural History: The genus name *Abelmoschus* is derived from Arabic and means "father of musk." The species name *esculentus* is Latin and means being fit for human consumption. The first use of the word "okra" appeared in 1679 in the Colony of Virginia, deriving from the Igbo word *ókùrù.* The word "gumbo" was first recorded in the American language around 1805, deriving from Louisiana Creole, but supposedly originates from either the Umbundu word *ochinggômbo* or the Kimbundu word *ki-ngombo.* Despite the fact that in most of the United States the word "gumbo" often refers to the dish, many places in the Deep South still use it to refer to the okra pods and plant as well.

Designation: Edible, African American remedy.

Cultivation: Start okra in mid-spring when soils have warmed. Soak seeds overnight in warm tap water to soften the hard seed coats. Plant the seed about 0.25–0.5 inch deep, and space plants 15–18 inches apart in well-developed rows with only moderate soil fertility. Soil pH should be 5.9–7.2. Start with a fertilizer of lower nitrogen and higher phosphorous and potassium, and side-dress this long-term crop every month, but avoid overfertilizing. Keep plants well picked to extend pod-setting growth. Harvest pods every other day and pick when small. In midsummer, plants may be cut back to 18 inches to regrow to a workable height.

Remedy Form: Edible; also used as an "okra water." After soaking fresh pods in water overnight or up to twenty-four hours, squeeze any leftover sap from the pods and combine it with the infused water. The okra water reportedly should be drunk first thing in the morning on an empty stomach.

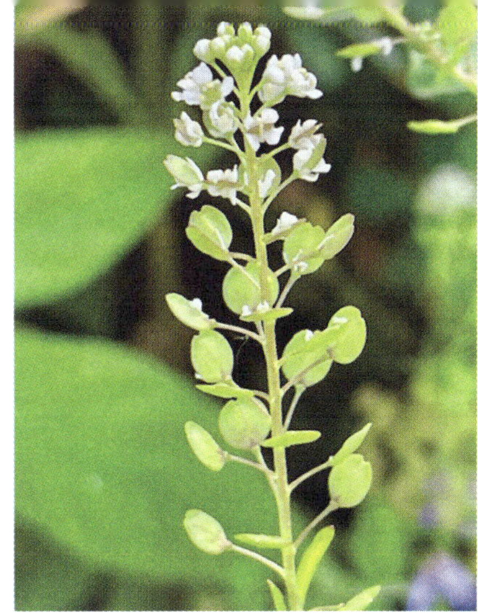

PEPPERGRASS & THE RESILIENT WRENS

SPRING

Peppergrass
(*Lepidium virginicum*)

Today the Carolina wrens are back, and I'm out early to see them and to catch the sunrise. It's a two-orb morning—the fat, full, translucent moon is sliding down the western sky just as the sun slips up beyond the marsh. And then the birds begin to sing.

I've noticed in the past year or two that just about the time the wrens start their nesting chores, the peppergrass is blooming in the fields and thriving in the newly warm sun. I'm so happy to see them both—the wrens, because they have returned to their carport roof-beam home after two years of halting hurricane repair, and the peppergrass, because it's a familiar herb ally. And it turns out that I can use it both as a nutritious edible and also as an herbal remedy.

I got to know the wrens before the latest big hurricane. They had worked for days at nest building—flitting in and out of one end of a metal pipe, depositing dried grasses and leaves and bits of fluff, then heading back out for more material. I loved having them as wild neighbors—they'd sit at one of the open ends of the pipes and chat, then sing and sing as one or the other sailed away for food. They were pretty resilient and had gotten used to the mower guy who went in and out of the shed whenever he mowed the yard. They didn't seem to mind me sitting out on the patio under their nest, either. And even after the hurricane, the wrens stuck around when the repair crew started tearing things apart. I think they really wanted to stay. Pretty soon, though, they abandoned the nesting work, and even the newly laid eggs, as the roof was torn off to make way for a new one. But suddenly they're back, just as the peppergrass is returning, too.

My first introduction to peppergrass was in herb school. On one of our walks around the school, I spotted what I thought was shepherd's purse (*Capsella bursa-pastoris*), a well-known herb for various issues, especially for heavy bleeding after birth or during menstrual cycles. But on closer examination, it turned out that what I had thought were the heart-shaped seed pods of *Capsella* were actually round instead. And though the flowers of both herbs were small and white, our teacher noted that there were definite differences in the herbs, and we should learn to recognize which was which.

I was intrigued to find that peppergrass had its own medicinal properties, and I did some exploration. It turned out that *Lepidium virginicum* has a history of use not only by U.S. Indigenous tribes but also as an Ayurvedic remedy, a Chinese medicine herb, and a helpful plant in the folk medicine of Mexico. The leaves contain generous amounts of vitamin C, and the unripe seed pods have a spicy flavor that can add zest to salads or cooked dishes. Medicinally, the plant is known to be useful for asthma and cough and has proven to be a gentle cardiac tonic and a mild anti-inflammatory for rheumatic pain. It has also been used supportively to help balance blood sugar in diabetes. Externally, the crushed leaves can be used on poison ivy rashes. They can also be applied to the chest as a remedy for a deep cough, wheezing, and the hoarseness of croup. In addition, it is used to treat impetigo, a highly contagious skin infection that causes red sores.

I've also heard that in Ayurvedic medicine, one of the herb's uses is to fight off fatigue or weakness. Since my last year with Bodi was pretty rough, ending in his passing away recently, I've felt pretty weak as I try to reorient my life without him. Maybe that's one reason I'm suddenly fascinated by peppergrass.

It also turns out that peppergrass is closely related to a recently popular herb called maca (*Lepidium meyenii*). As an herbal medicine, maca has been used to improve sexual function and overall energy and health. According to the Phytochemical and Ethnobotanical Databases of Dr. James Duke, a well-respected ethnobotanist who worked with the USDA before his death, maca has 367 reported uses for healing. That cousin of peppergrass also has a number of other medicinal properties, but its reputation for boosting libido and increasing fertility have markedly increased its sales in the herbal marketplace. I don't think that peppergrass shares those same properties, but I'll have to do a little more research to find out.

I stop to watch the moon disappear into the horizon over the fields, and as the sun gets higher, I take a couple of peppergrass photos and begin to make a harvest of the plants. A few mosquitoes dive-bomb me, and I wish I could rally the wrens to take care of the skeeters. I pick for a while, swatting at the bugs for as long as I can stand it, and then head on back at a speedy pace.

At home with my little bundle of peppergrass, I pour boiling water over the herb, then wait for it to steep. I nibble a few sprigs of the stems and seed pods and taste the sharp, peppery flavor that gives the plant its name. It's a pretty impressive taste, but not unpleasant, and I can imagine tossing a few sprigs into a salad for an added zest. Siting on the sunporch, I watch the wrens finish up their nest building for the day and begin their mating ritual. I guess they're eager to get on with their spring work of ushering in new life, just as those of us who are struggling after the latest big storm are hoping to heal and rebuild and move on.

All in all, I'm happy to have the wrens back, I'm eager to try my cup of peppergrass tea, and I'm grateful for resilience and whatever the future brings.

Other Names: *Lepidium virginicum,* Virginia pepperweed, poor man's pepperweed, poor man's pepperwort, Virginian peppercress.

Parts Used: Whole plant.

Medicinal Properties: Anthelmintic, antiasthmatic, antiscorbutic, antitussive, cardiotonic, detoxifying, diuretic, nutritional edible (contains vitamin C).

Uses: Internal—Acute bronchitis, asthma, colds, coughs, chronic respiratory conditions, croup; cardiovascular support; diabetes; fatigue/weakness; intestinal parasites; rheumatism. External—Impetigo, poison ivy rash.

Risks: May cause digestive irritation if eaten in large amounts. Peppergrass is a hyperaccumulator of minerals. If the soil is contaminated with toxic metals, peppergrass will absorb them, so be careful where you harvest the plants.

Description: Grows 6–20 inches tall. Stems branch from the base and are short-haired. Plant has a peppery smell and taste. Flowers are very small, white, and have four petals. The outer parts of the flowers are narrow, commonly slightly reddish, and not very obvious. Leaves are alternate, with the ones lowest on the plant soon falling, making the plants appear wiry at the base. Central and upper leaves are stalkless, lance-shaped or toothed. Seed pods are round to oval, with small notches at the end. Plant is said to resemble a little bottle brush.

Habitat: Fields and other disturbed habitats, sandy soils, dry or moist soils, gardens, roadsides, and waste places.

Distribution: Most of the state.

Plant Status: Native.

Animal Use: Eaten by Canada geese, quail, and other grain-eating birds; white-tail deer eat the foliage. Goats, sheep, and cattle will graze on new growth. The plant is pollinated by a variety of insects and bees.

Natural History: The Acadian French name for peppergrass is *cresson,* which is standard French for watercress. It is found in disturbed soils in Louisiana and southern and central Texas.

Designation: Native American remedy, Ayurvedic herb, traditional Mexican medicine, Chinese medicine.

Cultivation: Not often cultivated due to its weedy distribution. If you choose to cultivate to use as an edible herb, plant seeds thickly in spring and reseed biweekly for fresh greens.

Remedy Form: Edible, tea, tincture, poultice, wash.

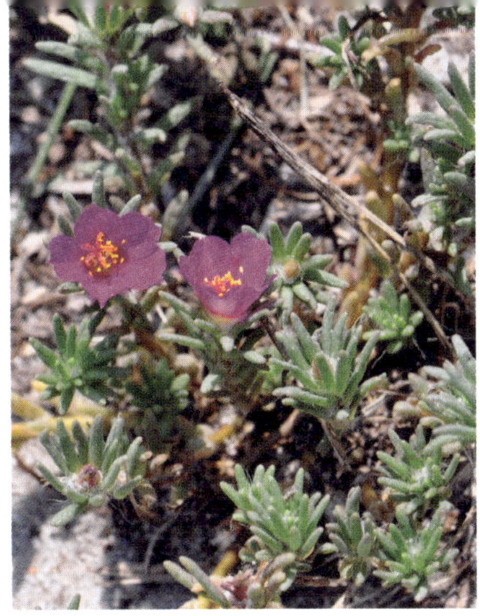

PURSLANE & THE DROUGHT

SUMMER

Purslane
(*Portulaca* sp.)

It's been a hard year for the garden, a hard year for the land and for the wild creatures who depend upon puddles for their daily drink. Everyone I know is complaining. Shocked, worried, not sure what to do. This place that is known for being saturated with water—in fact, in danger of drowning—is parched. Dry as a bone. Brutal heat and relentless humidity have broken many a garden this summer, and many a gardener's heart. Northern wildfires in the state are unstoppable, it seems. And fields that we are used to seeing green and lush are parched, brown, turning to dust. It's hard to know what to do.

Sometimes, when things are hard, when everything seems out of control, I like to turn simple—get back to basics. I need food. I need water. And even if the benefits are immeasurable, I need small beauties to remind me that life is still good, there is still hope, and I can find my way despite the heart-wrenching state of the planet and of our home ground.

When things seem too painful and impossibly complex, simple just seems like a good idea. Which brings me to purslane. What could be simpler? It's always underfoot. It doesn't require much of me. In fact, it just gets on with its daily task of surviving and finding a place to live. And it's easy to use.

I've known purslane forever, it seems. As a child, my sister and I puttered around in my mom's flower garden, supposedly helping out. Mostly we made mud pies when she watered the lawn, or chopped up bits of fallen flower petals to make our "gumbo." But we learned to identify some of what our mom considered weeds—those things she hadn't planned on growing, but that volunteered and often seemed hardier than the pretty flowers she was intending to grow. Purslane was one of the most consistent weedy visitors. The *Portulaca* cousins popped up everywhere. I kind of liked them because (a) they had pretty flowers and (b) it was fun to squish the leaves and rub the slime that oozed out of them all over my skin. But never would I have imagined then that I'd learn to love purslane later in life because of its healing properties.

When attending herb school, I was enthralled to learn that the *Portulaca* were prized plants. For one thing, they are packed with nutrients. Apparently, both species of the plant that grow in Louisiana contain more nutrition than many of the greens and veggies we include in our daily diets. High amounts of calcium, iron, beta-carotene, vitamin E, and omega-3 fatty acids are stored within this common plant. And as all Louisiana gardeners know, this is no shy or wimpy weed. The seeds are viable for up to twenty-five years. The plants also have numerous medicinal properties. Useful for a variety of health issues, the plant parts have been employed for immune system support, heart health, weight loss, cancer prevention, gastrointestinal health, good vision, strong bones, healthy circulation, and for reducing cholesterol, triglycerides, and LDL. And at that time, as the mother of a child with asthma, I was so grateful to find that it was also anti-inflammatory to respiratory membranes and could be useful for various lung conditions. According to the World Health Organization, purslane has been used in folk medicine since ancient times and is one of most widely used medicinal plants in the world.

With all of that in mind, instead of weeding out the feisty herb from my garden beds, lately, I'm giving it some space. And instead of buying six-packs of the ornamental *Portulaca* from the big-box stores' garden sections, I'll be encouraging the two Louisiana species of purslane that grow in the wild to think of my garden as home. In these dry and brutally hot times, that will decrease my need to water the flower beds, and I'll have fewer weeding chores—since I'll be nurturing the weeds!

Since I haven't used purslane yet for healing, I think I'll start by adding it to my diet first. On hot days, I like to make salads with a variety of textures and colors and tastes. I think the fleshy, slightly salty young *Portulaca* leaves might be interesting to toss in with some frilly lettuces and freshly snapped green beans and a few nuts and dried fruits. With a little olive oil (heart healthy), a splash of aged balsamic vinegar (also packed with antioxidants and other healthy compounds), and a few crumbles of goat cheese, I'll be well on my way to my own personal purslane healing. And I'll be helping to heal my garden space by encouraging native plants where I used to grow fancy cultivated things that took a lot more work.

Which takes me back to simplicity. Maybe if more of us take a simpler approach to noticing and appreciating the natural lands around us, and to managing our gardens by letting some of the wily plants that volunteer stay right where they are, we'll be doing our teensy part toward helping to create a less troubled world—one tiny, dirty step at a time.

Species: Two species of *Portulaca* that grow wild in Louisiana and have been shown to have medicinal properties include:

Portulaca oleracea

Other Names: Little hogweed, purslane, common purslane, akulikuli-kula, duckweed, pursley, wild portulaca, garden purslane, pigweed, verdolaga.

Parts Used: Whole plant.

Medicinal Properties: Analgesic, antiasthmatic, antibacterial, anxiolytic, anti-inflammatory, antifungal, antioxidant, antiscorbutic, antiseptic, antitussive, cardiovascular tonic, depurative, diuretic, febrifuge, immunomodulatory, muscle relaxant, neuroregenerative, neuroprotective, and lowers blood lipids.

Uses: Asthma; high cholesterol and high triglycerides; bone fractures, bone strength, osteoporosis, pain relief; type 2 diabetes; insomnia, nervous system disorders. Helpful as a gargle for oral lichen planus symptoms and for inflamed gums and sore throat.

Risks: Purslane contains oxalic acid and should not be consumed by those with kidney disease or high uric acid. The plant may be laxative if eaten in large quantities.

Description: An annual succulent that has smooth, reddish, mostly prostrate stems and alternate fleshy oval leaves. Leaves tend to be clustered at joints and stem ends. Flowers are small (0.25 inch), yellow, and have five heart-shaped petals that can appear any time of year.

Habitat: Grassy slopes, dunes, salt marshes, gardens, and other disturbed sites throughout Louisiana and most of Texas. Often found growing through cracks in the sidewalk.

Distribution: Found in much of the state.

Plant Status: Introduced, native.

Animal Use: Numerous species of flies, bees, and beetles visit flowers. At least two species of sawflies eat the leaves. Sparrows, other songbirds, and mice eat the seeds.

Natural History: Native to Central Asia, the Near East, Europe. Reportedly, purslane has been eaten for at least two thousand years. Cultivated in ancient Egypt and eaten by ancient Romans and Greeks. Can be found throughout the temperate and tropical regions of the world. The young leaves are edible raw or cooked. When eaten raw the leaves have a mucilage quality, much like okra. Seeds can be used as flour. Acadians sometimes pickle the stems.

Designation: Indigenous remedy, folkloric herbal treatment, Native American remedy.

Cultivation: Grow from seed sown directly in the ground or started indoors 4–8 weeks before last chance of frost for earlier bloom. Barely cover the tiny seeds whether sown indoors or out, and plant in full sun. Light is believed to benefit germination.

Remedy Form: Edible, tea, tincture, powder.

Portulaca pilosa

Other Names: Kiss me quick, chisme, hairy pigweed.

Parts Used: Whole plant.

Medicinal Properties: Analgesic, antibacterial, antidiabetic, anti-inflammatory, anticancer, antioxidant, antiulcer, diuretic, hepato-protective, neuroprotective, antibacterial, and wound healing.

Uses: A flower extract of the plant has been used medicinally as a salve to treat wounds for hundreds of years. It has also been used for its anti-inflammatory properties. Traditional Chinese medicine uses the extract as an antidote to bee stings, snakebites, and sores.

Risks: Contains oxalates and should be avoided by those with kidney stones. May also have laxative effects if used in large quantities.

Description: A prostrate, fleshy, branching plant with small, pink or purplish flowers at the end of branches with tufts of whitish hairs in the leaf axils.

Habitat: Dry, sandy soil, disturbed areas.

Distribution: Spotty throughout the state.

Plant Status: Native.

Animal Use: Squirrels, other rodents, and deer will eat the leaves.

Natural History: Existence of this plant is reported around four thousand years ago. The succulent stems and fleshy leaves indicate that it may have originated and adapted to desert climates of the Middle East and India. It is reported to have been Mahatma Gandhi's favorite food. It can be found in Europe, Africa, North America, Australia, and Asia.

Designation: Indigenous medicinal practice, Chinese medicine, Native American remedy, folkloric herbal treatment.

Cultivation: The species is very adaptable and can be propagated by seed, root division, and from bits of stem. The prostrate plant spreads quickly, creating a dense mat covering the ground. Purslane's abundant seeds sprout readily in summer when soil is warm and moist or when disturbed soil exposes buried dormant seeds to light.

Remedy Form: Edible, compress/poultice, tea, tincture, wash.

PURSLANE AND FETA CHEESE SALAD

- 2 cups purslane sprigs, rinsed and patted dry
- 2 diced tomatoes
- 3–4 cipollini onions, sautéed
- 1 cup coarsely chopped flat leaf parsley
- 1 tablespoon dried oregano
- 1 tablespoon fresh lemon juice
- 1/4 to 1/3 cup extra-virgin olive oil, to taste
- Cracked black pepper to taste
- Kalamata olives
- 1 cup crumbled feta cheese

1. Combine purslane, tomatoes, cipollini onions, parsley, and oregano in a serving bowl.

2. Whisk lemon juice and olive oil together. Pour over the salad and sprinkle with the pepper and olives.

3. Lightly toss everything together; sprinkle with feta cheese. Serve with pita bread.

(http:cms.herbalgram.org-herbclip.news.122)

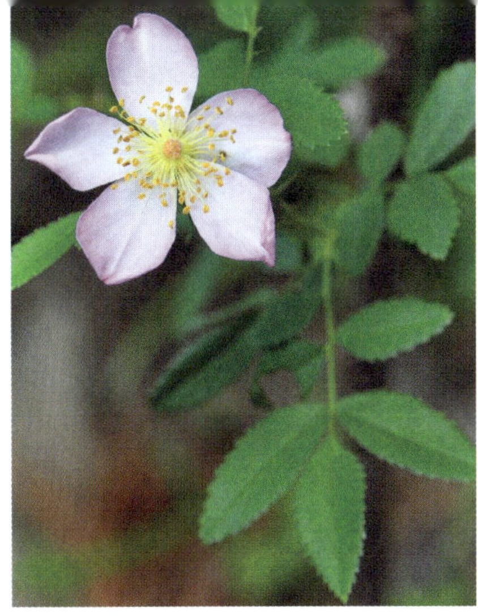

ROSES & UNCLE JIMMY'S YARD

SPRING

Rose
(*Rosa* sp.)

At 5:45 a.m., the early sky blushes rose and lavender, then settles into blue. The air is cold, with a feisty wind, and the outside thermometer registers only 40 degrees. Bodi is still snoring when I get up, but once I'm dressed and ready to go, he's eager to be out. Lately, with his increasing age, any walk with him is slow. But he is still curious, sniffing every scent trail, and happy for an adventure. I wonder, again, about the end—his end, and how I will know when it's time. For today, though, he is still here, still curious, and happy to be prowling new ground.

On the levee, the crows are back again after the latest storm. Hundreds of them gather on the power lines and then take off, squawking, dozens at a time. They fly over the batture and settle into the recently wounded woods. Bodi and I pass so many broken trees. They are shoved back against a ditch—piles and piles of them. Recently, the town crews have come by to start cleaning up. The trees that are left standing look lonely. Old oaks are missing limbs, sycamores are splintered, and what's left of a few ragged pines trembles in the wind.

Walking away from the sad mess, we take a new trail and end up exploring land that one cousin has said belonged to Uncle Jimmy. He kept horses in the nearby field and lived here for decades.

While Bodi sniffs, I check to see what's growing underfoot. I spot the usual clovers, plantain, and yellow dock. Then I see something interesting and make my way to what turns out to be a tall, rangy, old rose bush. It has climbed up into one of the broken sycamores and, oddly enough, is blowsy with blooms. White, fragrant flowers are bright against the backdrop of messy trees. I lean close to sniff up their perfume. I wonder if these were planted here by Uncle Jimmy and his wife, or if they arrived here decades ago in some flood and then took up residence, hoping to thrive in a new place. And if they've been here for generations, did Uncle Jimmy and his wife welcome the roses right into their garden? Their old house is gone now, and plans are in development for a new library here. I think Uncle Jimmy would like that idea—his land, cared for again, and housing a place for learning and exploring. Maybe, once the library is built, I can offer to make a little healing herb trail around the place, with signs listing the traditional use of each plant. That could be a sweet way to share knowledge and give back to the community. For now, I fill a pocket with petals to take with me for tea, then nudge Bodi across the ditch and head on home.

One of my very favorite herbal memories is driving to the coast every summer, to where the seaside roses bloom wild, and harvesting petals. I'd try not to disturb the plant, would just wrap fingers gently around the flower and pull. When my baskets were filled with the petals, I'd drive home with the windows up so the flowers wouldn't blow away, and the whole car would fill with that amazing scent. Once home, I'd spread the petals out so they could dry. Old window screens propped up on tables or between chairs acted as drying racks in the dining room of the old farmhouse, and every day I'd walk past that beauty, that fragrance.

At home now, I make a rose petal tea as Bodi settles back into sleep, and I think again about roses and family and the feral land. I grab a few herb guides to refresh my memory of the many healing uses of today's find. Louisiana apparently has four species of *Rosa*—two of which are native, and the others introduced and described as invasive. I decide that the species I found climbing into the tree was *Rosa bracteata,* known commonly as prairie rose. It is often found in old pastures, so I guess its occupancy of Uncle Jimmy's abandoned field shouldn't be a surprise.

Roses have a respected position in the international herbal trade. One of the most well-known and researched members of the species is the dog rose, or *Rosa canina.* Ethnobotanist and author James Duke documented 564 medicinal uses for the plant worldwide. And many other rose species have been researched and utilized for healing. Roses have nutritional value as well. The rose "hip," or fruit of the plant, contains vitamins A, C, and E, along with many minerals. Various parts of the plant, especially the fruit, can be used for making jam or rose hip "leather," and can help to support the immune system and soothe digestion. And rose is one of the herbs that is just as useful externally as it is when consumed. Internally, the plant has been found to have antidepressant, antispasmodic, astringent, antibacterial, antiviral, antiseptic, and anti-inflammatory activities. And even smelling the rose flower can have healing effects. A recent report by the National Institutes of Health documented numerous healing properties of rose petal extract scent. Apparently, our olfactory receptors (those tiny, scent-perceiving organs that line the membranes of our noses and other tissues) detect the rose odors and relay the scent to the brain, beginning a chain of healing responses that can offer much benefit.

Rose is one of the oldest recognized medicinal plants in the world. Some fossils of the species have been determined to be over thirty million years old. Many species are celebrated for healing and beauty, and much research has been done to document their chemical properties and healing potential. Physical, emotional, and even spiritual maladies have been positively altered with the use of rose products. In traditional Chinese medicine, *Rosa chinensis* is used to cleanse the blood, increase bile production, regulate menses, stimulate digestion, and help alleviate the effects of stress. In Ayurvedic medicine, different rose species were commonly used to relieve spiritual ailments and clear the chakras. And all parts of the plants have been found to be useful. The first distillation of roses for their oil occurred in the late seventh century in Iran, and even in modern times, research continues to reveal important healing effects of the herb. Recent investigation of the external effects of rose hip oil application confirmed dramatic skin anti-inflammatory activity when applied to ultraviolet damage from the sun.

One of my favorite ways to use the roses, though, is as a simple tea—of either the rose hips, or petals, or both. It's a comforting feeling, because I know I'm getting not only the delicate, slightly tangy flavor but I'm also soaking up the nutrients and breathing up the scents that will calm my mind and spirit and relax my body.

Reviewing all the benefits of the *Rosa* family makes me more excited about using some of Uncle Jimmy's roses for healing. I've recently found a recipe for making rosewater spray for the skin, and I'm eager to try that. In fact, I'll bet I can talk a couple of cousins into experimenting with me.

Then we'd have a lovely homegrown product to use and a reminder of Uncle Jimmy and the lush land he once called home.

Species: Several species of *Rosa* grow in the wild in Louisiana and have been shown to have medicinal properties. These include:

Rosa bracteata

Other Names: Cherokee rose, McCartney rose, prairie rose, evergreen rose, wild rose, *Rosa blanda*.

Medicinal Uses: Fevers, colds; acid reflux.

Description: Evergreen, thorny, climbing, or trailing shrub that grows up to 10 feet in height. Plants often grow in clumps. Stems are arching canes with recurved thorns. Leaves are alternate, pinnately compound with serrated margins. Leaflets are 1–3 inches long. Flowers are white with five petals and occur in small clusters. Fruits are small green to red rose hips, growing 0.25–0.4 inch in diameter.

Habitat: Waste places, ditches, and pastures.

Distribution: Much of the state.

Plant Status: Introduced.

Rosa carolina

Other Names: Carolina rose, pasture rose.

Medicinal Uses: Edible—provides rich source of vitamins, minerals, essential fatty acids. Helps relieve digestive complaints; fruit may reverse the growth of some cancers.

Description: Low-growing shrub that is generally upright but may sprawl if plants grow taller than 3–4 feet. In early summer it bears an abundance of 2–3-inch-wide, bright-pink flowers with yellow centers. Leaves are strongly serrate and dark green, and stems are prickly with straight, needlelike thorns. A deep taproot makes this rose very drought-tolerant. It also produces shallow rhizomes and can spread vegetatively to form small colonies.

Habitat: Dry prairies, disturbed areas, sandy open woods, thickets, roadsides, and pastures.

Distribution: Northern, central, and eastern parts of the state.

Plant Status: Native.

Rosa laevigata

Other Names: Cherokee rose.

Medicinal Uses: Internal—Diarrhea, digestive upsets; elevated cholesterol; infertility, menstrual irregularities, urinary tract disorders, uterine prolapse. External—Skin irritations, sun damage.

Description: A climbing evergreen rose that may grow to 6–20 feet long on arching stems armed with hooked thorns. May also occur as a sprawling, freestanding shrub. Stems have trifoliate dark-green leaves with coarsely toothed leaflets. Single, fragrant, white flowers are up to 4 inches in diameter with scalloped petals and yellow stamens. Flowers are followed by large, bristly, orange-red hips that are up to 2 inches long.

Habitat: Roadsides and low woods.

Distribution: Spotty throughout the state, approximately two dozen parishes.

Plant Status: Introduced, naturalized.

Rosa multiflora

Other Names: Multiflora rose, Japanese rose, many-flowered rose, seven-sisters rose, Eujitsu rose, rambler rose.

Medicinal Uses: Internal—Inflammation, pain. External—Abrasions, insect bites, minor burns, rashes.

Description: A multistemmed, bushy shrub with long, arching, thorny canes that form dense thickets and reach heights of 10–15 feet. The branches are covered in sturdy, curved prickles. Leaves are alternate, pinnately compound and divided into five to eleven leaflets. Stiff, backward-curved thorns with wide bases and sharp, narrow points extend along the length of the stems.

Habitat: Fencerows, pastures, thin woodlands. Rarely found in dry pastures, prairies, margins of woodlands, roadsides, rocky, open wooded hillsides, and stream valleys.

Distribution: Primarily in northern half of the state, a couple of southern and central parishes.
Plant Status: Introduced.

For All Species: Parts Used: Flowers/petals, fruit, leaves, bark, essential oil.
Medicinal Properties: Antidepressant, antifungal, anti-HIV, anti-inflammatory, antioxidant, antiseptic, antiviral, antitumor, bacteriostatic, cardioprotective, digestive stimulant, immune system support, lipid-lowering, menstrual regulator, renal protective, cardiovascular protective. Also provides nutrients including vitamins A, B1, B2, B3, niacin, K, and E, potassium, and iron.
Uses: Internal—Blood sugar irregularities, diabetes; colds, fevers, flu; inflammation; dysmenorrhea; depression, fatigue, insomnia, irritability, mood swings, stress, seizures; indigestion, acid reflux, stomach acid deficiency, gallbladder ailments, gallstones; menstrual irregularity, cramps, menopausal symptoms; renal support, kidney disease; diseases associated with aging; skin repair. External—Abrasions, minor burns, cuts, heat rashes, minor wounds, sunburn. Also used cosmetically to rejuvenate skin. Essential oil used in aromatherapy.
Risks: Side effects of overuse include digestive upset, nausea, or diarrhea. Avoid if sensitive to oxalates and prone to kidney stones or use with a health practitioner's guidance. Avoid if allergic to roses. Should be avoided by those with sickle cell disease, hemochromatosis, thalassemia, sideroblastic anemia. Drug interactions may occur if taking the following medications: Demeclocycline, doxycycline, eltrombopag, fleroxacin, gemifloxacin, levofloxacin, lymecycline, minocycline. Dosage should be limited to two to three cups of tea daily.
Animal Use: Attracts birds and is valuable to native bees and bumblebees. Also provides nesting materials/structure for native bees.
Natural History: Rose species have been documented to have evolved between thirty-five and seventy million years ago, with some fossils proven to be around thirty-five million years old. Garden cultivation of roses began approximately five thousand years ago in China, where various parts of the plant were utilized for food and to treat various

health conditions and to increase qi, or life energy. Roses were widely cultivated during the Han Dynasty (141–187 BC). In Iran, the damask rose has been consumed and utilized for healing since the seventh century, and the first documented production of rose oil began there. In the Middle East, China, and India, flowers are routinely added to jams and pastries. Approximately 150 species of *Rosa* grow throughout the Northern Hemisphere. Roses from different regions of the world hybridize readily, giving rise to types of the plant that overlap the parental forms and making it difficult to determine basic species.

Designation: Herb of commerce, folkloric herbalism remedy, African American herb, Indigenous/Native healing plant, Chinese medicinal herb, Ayurvedic healing remedy, flower essence remedy.

Cultivation: Seeds of roses are generally dormant when fresh. Often, this can be overcome by scarification followed by cold/moist stratification for 60–120 days at 41 degrees Fahrenheit. Seeds germinate while being stratified. Plant the seeds 0.5 inch deep at temperatures between 68–86 degrees Fahrenheit. If growing rose for its medicinal and/or nutritional value, it is best to plant species that are determined to be native in the state, or in North America. This is because the effects of hybridization on the medicinal compounds in a cultivated rose are difficult to ascertain. Also, many cultivated roses are heavily treated with hazardous chemicals to protect their beauty from insect or animal damage.

Remedy Form: Edible, tea, tincture, syrup, essential oil, salve, liniment, rose water, compress, poultice, flower essence.

ROSEWATER

2–3 cups of fresh rose petals, rinsed and cleaned
Wide pot or saucepan
Strainer
Glass spray bottle or jar
1/2 gallon distilled water

1. Add clean rose petals to pot or saucepan.
2. Add enough distilled water to just cover the petals. (If you add too

much water, it will dilute the end product.)

3. Place the pot on the stove, on low heat.

4. Cover the pot with a lid and let it simmer for 30–45 minutes, and until petals lose their color.

5. Leave rose water in pot until cooled completely.

6. Strain water into a spray bottle or jar.

7. Refrigerate and use for up to a month.

8. For external use, spray on minor wounds such as minor burns and cuts, and can also be used to reduce the appearance of scars when used in high concentrations.

(https://www.healthline.com/health/beauty-skin-care/how-to-make-rose-water)

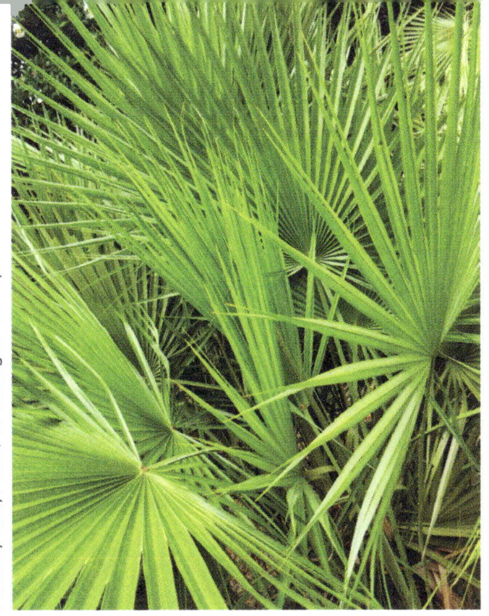

Photo by Larry Allain, US Geological Survey

SAW PALMETTO & THE HERBS OF COMMERCE

WINTER

Saw palmetto
[*Serenoa repens*]

Driving up beyond New Orleans in early winter to talk with a local herb group, I'm happy to get away from home for a while and to see a different landscape. I get out of the car at a little rest stop to explore and walk along the banks of what turns out to be the Pearl River. The ground under my feet is sandy, and out on the water a fishing boat putters by. In early winter, the surrounding trees are tawny with late-autumn colors. I walk over fallen leaves and fading vegetation and spot a small dust-colored snake who is so well camouflaged I almost step on her. I only see her as she suddenly coils up and slides down a dusty hole near my feet. It is kind of a thrill to see her, to be so close—I only wish I had noticed her features so I could try to identify her later. If Bodi had been here with me, he would have been curious for sure—which might not have been such a good thing.

At the edge of the beach is a plant that is quite familiar, though rare in this area. A couple of clumps of saw palmetto edge the thin woods that lead up to the beach and remind me of my early days in herb school when I was first introduced to this herb. It has an interesting history. Modern-day herbalists have high praise for the usefulness of this plant. It is one of the major herbs of commerce acknowledged by herbal researchers and practitioners and is often recommended for reducing the symptoms of benign prostatic hyperplasia (BPH)—a noncancerous enlargement of the prostate gland. Such symptoms as frequent urination and nighttime trips to pee are often alleviated with the use of this plant. It is also known to be helpful for chronic pelvic pain, hair loss, migraines, and to relieve symptoms of polycystic ovary syndrome (PCOS) in women. In the Ayurvedic medicine of India, the herb is recommended for male and female pattern baldness, underactive bladder, chronic pelvic pain, prostate cancer, asthma and chronic bronchitis, cold, cough, and migraines.

And it turns out that interest in *Serenoa repens* is not new. Between 1870 and 1950, the herb was a regular treatment for prostate and urinary tract problems. The first pharmaceutical-grade saw palmetto remedies appeared in Savannah, Georgia, in 1879. By the mid-1890s, saw palmetto products were offered by pharmaceutical companies including Parke Davis, Eli Lily, Merck, Sharp & Dohme, Squibb, and other turn-of-the-twentieth-century drug firms. But even before that, saw palmetto and some of its cousins were used by Native American tribes in the Deep South. The Houma, Chitimacha, and Choctaw people used fruits of both saw palmetto and dwarf palmetto for healing and for food.

I like knowing the history of herbal use. The transition of medicinal plants from Native and folkloric usage to modern-day practice has been an interesting road—one paved with oral history, experimentation, and increasing scientific investigation. When I was teaching about medicinal plants in a university nursing school, I'd often hear folks say that there was no research, or proof, of an herb's effectiveness. Nothing could be further from the truth. Between 1960 and 2019, over 110,000 studies of medicinal plant use were completed and published. In more recent times, over 5,000 research publications are released every year. And while herbs in the U.S. are now relegated to the "complementary medicine" category of remedies, medicinal plants have continued to be investigated and commonly used in European and Asian countries right alongside pharmaceutical drugs.

In 1992, the American Herbal Products Association endeavored to create a list of all common and scientific plant names used for products containing herbs. The "Herbs of Commerce" project was initiated to reduce confusion about labeling botanical ingredients and to establish a single standardized common name for each listed herb. The document was incorporated by reference in 1997 as the FDA initiated rulemaking to implement the Dietary Supplement Health and Education Act of 1994. Since the first edition, two more have been produced with the aim of expanding and updating each subsequent edition to reflect herbs presently on the market and in contemporary botanical nomenclature. The newly published third edition contains entries for over 2,800 separate plant species, over 1,000 botanical synonyms, over 300 Ayurvedic remedies, and over 700 pinyin (Chinese) names.

Around the same time, renewed interest in herbal healing in the U.S. was stimulated by the publication of *The Complete German Commission E Monographs* in English in 1998. The Commission E in Germany was a scientific advisory board of the Federal Institute for Drugs and Medical Devices and was composed of two dozen scientific experts who evaluated the safety and efficacy of herbal medicines. The work also included scientific research related to the approval of substances and products previously used in traditional, folk, and herbal medicine. Following the release of the *Monographs* in Europe, the American Botanical Council translated and edited the volume.

Since then, those monographs are being replaced in the European Union by EMA Community Monographs that are produced by experts from all over the European Union. But the original monographs are still regarded as accurate and relevant, and the ongoing efforts of many researchers, scientists, and practitioners continue to reveal more information about medicinal herbs. With approximately half a million vascular plants on the planet, and about 10 percent of them already reported to have medicinal properties and uses, I imagine it will continue to be an exciting, curious, and sometimes confusing journey. And I'm happy to be a tiny part of it.

I take a few photos of the saw palmetto clumps in front of me and examine the weathered fruits. The herb has been so overharvested that commercial harvesting licenses are required in some states. Because the plant is now considered rare in Louisiana, I'm thinking that it might be best to try growing my own crop on a bit of land closer to my home. According to the LSU AgCenter website, cultivating the herb isn't too difficult, and growing my own supply will reduce any increased harvesting pressures on the plant in Louisiana.

I head back to my car, keeping an eye on the ground underfoot, just in case the little snake has ventured out again. I'm glad to have spotted her, and glad to have seen the saw palmetto. And I'm grateful for the many curious and dedicated scientists and herbalists and healers who have devoted their lives to exploring the role of medicinal plants in health care and to helping us to see the world around us for the amazing healing gift it really is.

Other Names: *Serenoa repens.*

Parts Used: Fruit/berries.

Medicinal Properties: Adaptogen, antiseptic, anaphrodisiac/aphrodisiac, diuretic, expectorant, sedative, tonic, urinary tract support, uterine tonic.

Uses: Prostatitis, benign prostatic hyperplasia (BPH), urinary tract problems, irritable bladder impotence, debility in elderly men, and bronchial complaints associated with coldness. Used in Ayurvedic medicine for BPH, male and female pattern baldness, underactive bladder, chronic pelvic pain, prostate cancer, asthma, chronic bronchitis, cold, cough, and migraines.

Risks: Very rare side effects include headache, nausea, diarrhea, and dizziness. If taking for prostate issues, consult with a licensed health care provider to screen for prostate cancer prior to using the herb. Should not be used by pregnant or nursing women, or women who have had, or are at risk for, hormone-related cancers. Saw palmetto may interfere with the absorption of iron. Do not use this herb in combination with finasteride, or other medications used to treat BPH, or with antiplatelet and anticoagulant drugs (blood thinners). It may make oral contraceptives for women less effective.

Description: The herb is a fan palm that grows as a tree or shrub. It can reach heights of 10 feet. Leaf clusters grow up to 2 feet or more, and the plant has a creeping, horizontal growth pattern. Lush, green, saw-toothed leaves fan out from thorny stems. White flowers produce yellow berries that turn brownish-black when ripe. The plants emerge from subterranean or low-growing stems, and each plant is capable of producing thickets up to 18 feet in diameter.

Habitat: Mesic flatwoods, wet flatwoods, dry flatwoods, scrubby flatwoods, scrub, hardwood hammock.

Distribution: Orleans and St. Tammany Parishes, though can be cultivated throughout the state.

Plant Status: Native.

Animal Use: Larval host for the palmetto skipper. A variety of mammals, reptiles, and insects consume the fruit and use the thickets to hide from predators. Blooms are a good source of nectar and pollen and are attractive to European honeybees and many native pollinators.

Natural History: The species Latin name was given in honor of Sereno Watson, an important nineteenth-century American botanist who worked mostly in the Western Hemisphere tropics before becoming a curator of the botanical collection at Harvard University. The common name, saw palmetto, is based on the leaf stalks, which are armed with saw-like teeth. In recent years medical science has been able to verify some claims about the herb's benefits, and organized harvesting is now common in areas where the plant is native. Saw palmetto plants live for a long time, with some estimated to be five hundred to seven hundred years old.

Designation: Herb of commerce, African American herb, Native American remedy, Chinese medicine, Ayurvedic healing herb.

Cultivation: Saw palmetto may be propagated by seed or can be transplanted. The best time to transplant or plant a palm is from late April through August, when the soil is warm and encourages the roots to grow vigorously, though many palms are not very tolerant of transplanting when they are young. Container-grown palms are generally smaller and will have their entire root system intact. Although smaller, they grow faster initially than palms that are field-grown and dug.

Remedy Form: Tincture. Tea can be used, but some of the most important anti-inflammatory compounds in the fruit are not readily extracted in water.

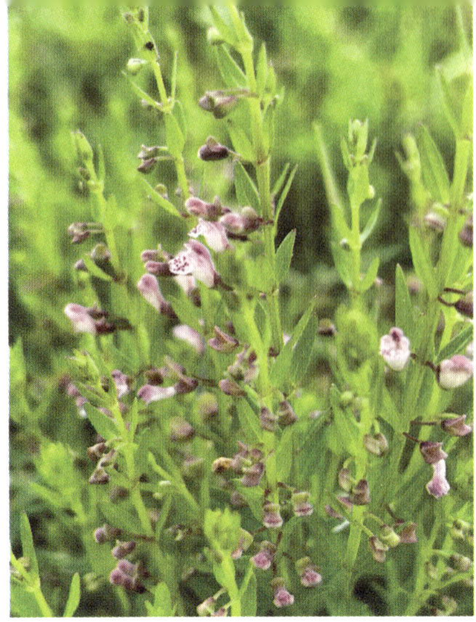

SKULLCAP & THE BROKEN MOWER

SPRING

Skullcap
(*Scutellaria racemose*)

On a cold and gusty March morning, I have two walks, the first one solo. My little labradoodle, Bodi, at almost sixteen years old, prefers to sleep in lately, so I tuck his blanket around him and head on out. Under the still-dark sky at 6:30 a.m., I'm grateful for my warm jacket and hat and gloves. We are having a sudden cold snap after a nice period of spring warmth, so the songbirds are busy keeping nests comfortable and eggs warm, and the hawks haven't started their morning hunt over the batture woods yet. The leftover moon, a thin but huge crescent, hangs in the sky above the river, and a few filmy clouds turn rose and then orange. I take some photos and then walk through the long back field in the pale first light.

And I'm thrilled again, with so much lush and surprising growth. The lawn mower—well and often used—has been in the repair shop for several weeks now, and in just that little time the grass has grown longer and thick, and so many plants I don't normally see have shown up in the lawn. The violets are stupendous this season, and every walk is a tasty treat. The usual cast of earthy characters is here, too—chickweed and cleavers, mock strawberry and henbit and lyreleaf sage. The spiderwort that I normally only see at the edges of the road are flowering right in the middle of the yard and have grown tall and thick. And the wild *Geranium* is blooming, so I've already made several harvests of them.

But there are a few new things I've discovered in the longer grass. The delicate corn salad, or *Valerianella,* is near flowering now, and I nibble a few tender leaves as I pass by. And a plant I've identified as wild chervil has sprung up just about everywhere. Seeing so much of it, I've researched the plant to see if it has any medicinal properties, but so far I've only found that it can be used as a wild edible. I pick a crinkly leaf and pop it into my mouth. It tastes like very mild parsley, and I can see why it would be used for seasoning.

My favorite discovery, though, is a plant that I've used for healing for many years—skullcap. The species I've used before in the Northeast is *Scutellaria laterifolia,* which is fairly tall. But this skullcap is tiny, and pinker than the herb I'm used to seeing. And it's so low-growing that I have probably walked over it many times lately before I stopped to peer more closely. My guidebook notes that this is *Scutellaria racemosa*—or South American skullcap. Now that I've finally seen and identified it, I'm finding many sizable colonies of it all across the lawn. Apparently, this species is typically six to twelve inches tall, but in my patchwork yard, it is about four inches in height.

In herb school, we learned about *Scutellaria*'s usefulness for supporting and toning the nervous system and for helping the body adapt to stress. I've used it for anxiety, tension, insomnia, and along with other herbs for women going through menopause, and also for reducing pain. A nervous system tonic, the herb can be taken for longer periods of time without having to worry about a negative reaction. In the last decade or so, much research on the skullcaps have targeted *Scutellaria baicalensis,* often used in Chinese medicine, as the most effective species. But I've also found that modern research reveals *S. racemosa* has much to offer in terms of nervous system support, and that over 360 species contribute bioactive compounds that show promise for supporting various biological activities. And across the world, the *Scutellaria* are widely used in local communities as a natural remedy. With my tiny skullcap colonies so newly thriving in the yard, I'm eager to transplant some into a spot in my garden where they can make themselves at home before the mower returns.

I reach home after my first and very gusty walk and then make tea and snuggle with Bodi as he finally wakes from his long sleep. On our way back out, I plan to visit the little skullcap colonies again. Bodi will be happy to sniff scent trails in the field, and I'll be grateful for the luxury of wild gifts and abundant spring growth on a cold spring day, and for the broken mower that introduced me to so many "volunteer" healing plants I wouldn't have seen otherwise.

Then, just as I step out the door, I get a phone call from the repair shop. The mower is fixed. So there will go the newly found yard herbs—*Valerianella* and skullcap, lyreleaf sage and betony, bacopa and wild onions. I guess this is progress. But it does make me wonder about things—about how much our idea of progress depends on mowing over, tilling under, "managing," and even sometimes destroying our wild plants and surroundings.

I guess I will always want a simpler life, even as I try to keep up with all the complexity of living in this ultramodern world. I'm not sure if we will ever know how much we lose, every day, of the thriving, throbbing, resilient, and vulnerable web of life and liveliness all around us. But it helps me to know that all these little wonders are in the soil, even if the mower whacks away at them on a regular basis. They're still out there, just waiting for another chance to bloom.

Species: There are several *Scutellaria* species in the state. Some have medicinal properties and a history of use for healing. These include:

Scutellaria elliptica

Other Names: Hairy skullcap.

Medicinal Uses: Nervous system conditions, insomnia; menstrual irregularity, recovery from childbirth; chills, diarrhea, fevers, sore throat.

Description: Skullcap is a mint-family member, with square stems and opposing leaves. Flowers are snapdragon-like, tubular and hooded, two-lipped, and blue-purple. Plant will grow 12–18 inches tall. Leaves, stem, and flowers all have hair. Fruit is a two-parted capsule containing four nutlets.

Habitat: Dry upland woods and thickets; mixed deciduous woodlands and road banks.

Distribution: Concentrated in west-central part of the state, some clustered populations in other areas.

Cultivation: Plant prefers partial shade in rocky to average to sandy soils with some organic material in a woodland-type setting. It needs well-drained soils, can tolerate drought, and doesn't do well in standing water.

Plant Status: Native.

Scutellaria ovata

Other Names: Heartleaf skullcap, eggleaf skullcap, forest skullcap.

Medicinal Uses: Used in some healing traditions for anxiety, and may help with food allergies, Alzheimer's disease, and Parkinson's disease.

Description: *S. ovata* is a mint-family plant with square stems and opposing leaves. Flowers are snapdragon-like, tubular, two-lipped, blue-purple (with whitish lower lips), and bloom May to September in branched terminal racemes up to 6 inches long atop square pubescent stems clad with ovate, crenate-serrate, rugose, heart-shaped green leaves (up to 4 inches long). Plants typically grow 16–24 inches tall.

Habitat: Open woodlands, along roads, and on brushy slopes. Grows in moist sand, loam, clay, or limestone.

Distribution: Patchy throughout the state (about two dozen parishes).

Cultivation: Grow in dry to medium, well-drained soil in full sun (though plant can tolerate some shade). Drought-tolerant. Plants may go dormant after bloom in hot, dry summer weather.

Plant Status: Native.

Scutellaria parvula

Other Names: Small skullcap.

Medicinal Use: Used in traditional folk medicine for anxiety, inflammatory conditions, and bacterial infections. Also known for its antispasmodic and tonic properties. The dried roots have been used in China to treat diarrhea, insomnia, dysentery, respiratory infections, and inflammation. Native Americans used a leaf tea to transition young girls to womanhood. Infusions of the roots were used to treat diarrhea, kidney problems, and breast pains.

Description: The plant has opposite, sessile leaves and bluish, two-lipped flowers borne in the axils of the leaves. The stem and leaves are glandular-pubescent. The rhizome produces tubers. The plant does not have a fragrance. Plant grows 3–9 inches tall. Sometimes it branches from the base; otherwise, the stems are unbranched. The stems are light green, four-sided, and slightly to moderately hairy, especially along the angles of the sides. Pairs of opposite leaves occur along the stems. The leaf blades are 0.5–.075 inch long and about one half that size across; they are lanceolate, ovate, or oval, while their revolute margins are smooth to crenate with a few blunt teeth. Generally, the upper leaves are more slender and less likely than the lower leaves to have teeth. The upper leaves are sessile; the lower leaves have short petioles. The upper-leaf surface is medium green and hairless to sparsely pubescent; the lower surface is pale green and sparsely to densely pubescent.

Habitat: Low woods, fields, upland prairies, woodlands, limestone ledges, rocky sandy soils.

Distribution: Primarily western half of the state, scattered in other areas.

Cultivation: Spreads by short rhizomes. Tolerates sun or shade.

Plant Status: Native.

Scutellaria racemosa

Other Names: South American skullcap.

Medicinal Use: Melatonin and serotonin have been scientifically detected in *Scutellaria racemosa* and may contribute to its neuroprotective activity. Also has significant antioxidant activity that was statistically consistent with the commercially utilized *Scutellaria* species (that is, *S. baicalensis* and *S. lateriflora*).

Description: The herb is a perennial and forms large colonies from slender rhizomes. The stems are erect to ascending, 6–12 inches in height, square in cross-section, frequently branched, glabrous, and green or purplish in color. Leaves are opposite, short-petioled, triangular to ovate or lanceolate in outline, entire except for one lobe on one or both sides at the base, glabrous or minutely pubescent along the veins and the margin. Flower produced singly in the axils of the upper bract-like leaves. The flowers are pubescent exteriorly, two-lipped, and pinkish-lavender in color with spots of purple on the lower lip. The fruit is a nutlet.

Habitat: The plant grows in moist areas in forest and woodland and as a garden weed, occurring in flower beds and lawns, along lake and stream margins, on golf courses, in roadside ditches, and along railroads.

Distribution: Found in a few scattered parishes in the state. (Allen, East Baton Rouge, Lincoln, Livingston, Ouachita, St. Tammany, Tangipahoa).

Cultivation: Prefers well-draining soil and medium to wet conditions. Can tolerate full sun to partial shade.

Plant Status: Introduced.

For All Species, Parts Used: Aerial parts.

Medicinal Properties: In general, *Scutellaria* species offer antibacterial, anti-inflammatory, anxiolytic, anticonvulsant, antioxidant, and antiviral activities, and have beneficial effects on cardiovascular and cerebrovascular diseases as well as providing hepatoprotective and neuroprotective effects. Various research studies have proven the plants to have antitumor properties and have shown strong anticancer activity against certain cancer cells including human malignant glioma, malignant breast cancer, and human prostate cancer.

Uses: Anxiety, insomnia, neurological problems, pain; cancer; cirrhosis, hepatitis, jaundice.

Risks: Some species of skullcap can increase the effect of drugs that have a sedating effect, including anticonvulsants, such as phenytoin (Dilantin) and valproic acid (Depakote), and barbiturates and benzodiazepines, such as alprazolam (Xanax) and diazepam (Valium).

Animal Use: Most skullcaps are visited by bees, butterflies, and hummingbirds. However, the plant seems to be unpalatable to deer, rabbits, and geese.

Natural History: Various species have been used for centuries by Native Americans to treat menstrual disorders, nervousness, and digestive and kidney problems. The name "skullcap" refers to the flower's resemblance to helmets worn by European soldiers.

Designation: Herb of commerce, Native/Indigenous healing traditions, African American remedy, traditional Chinese medicine remedy.

Cultivation (For All Species): Most species prefer some moisture but can tolerate occasional drought conditions. Rich, acid soils with good drainage are best, though some species can tolerate more moisture. *Scutellaria* can tolerate varying degrees of sun and shade. Propagation can be done by seed, cuttings, or division. Maintenance requirements are minimal.

Remedy Form: Internal—Tea, tincture, powder, capsules. External—poultice, compress, wash.

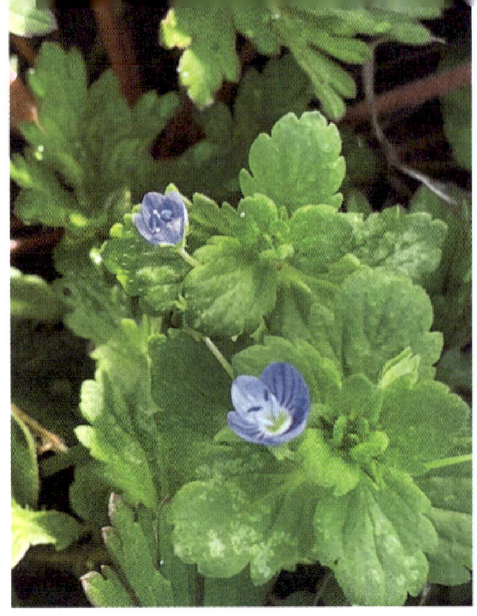

SPEEDWELL & THE HAWKS

SPRING

Speedwell
(*Veronica* sp.)

I'm out for an early walk this morning, before the sun rises up over the river. The air is warm, and the yard is damp already with dew. So many small herbs are popping up where the mower can't reach. The yellow flowers of snake berry are opening lately, the violets are purple and tasty, the cranesbill leaves are spread out in dark-green rosettes and getting ready to bloom, and the first of blackberry flowers are unfurling at the edge of the woods. On the levee, all the growth is lush, and even though I've taken loads of photos already, I can't help but stop and say hello to all the plants, tasting a leaf here and there.

As I walk, I keep an eye on the red-shouldered hawks overhead. Lately, they're busy with mating and nesting, screeching raucously to each other across the fields. Even when they're out of sight, their piercing calls ring over the woods. I try to follow their flight path to see where they're headed. Spotting what seems like a nest in one tall tree, I move closer to figure out if this is a real nest or just another squirrel "patio." But the birds are not happy with my presence, so I move away. This nest at the edge of the woods seems like a fairly vulnerable spot—high in the crotch of an old oak, exposed to wind and rain. But the hawks are nothing if not resilient, and I'm pretty sure they know what they're doing.

Red-shouldered hawks are a vital part of Louisiana's diverse ecosystem. The male and female apparently mate for life and work together at nest building and feeding chicks. And they help to keep other species from overtaking a place—feeding on a variety of small mammals, songbirds, amphibians, and reptiles. But they are facing challenges as the state loses land due to development, so I'm happy to see them thriving here.

In addition to the hawks, one of my favorite things to see this time of year are the pretty, delicate blossoms of tiny speedwell—a beautiful species of *Veronica.* Three species grow in Louisiana, and they often grow together. I'm partial to one of the introduced species because of its cerulean-blue blossoms, but all species have similar healing properties and uses. These days, thick clutches of the speedwells line the levee trail, poke up in the yard, and edge neighborhood sidewalks. Though not an official herb of commerce, the plant has much history of use. I thought that its name might indicate healing possibilities, but apparently the "speedwell" refers to the fact that if picked, its flower petals will drop off very quickly. And its genus name, *Veronica,* is linked to the belief that a young girl whose name was Veronica approached Jesus during his crucifixion and wiped his bloody face with healing speedwell and her veil. A lovely story, and while it's impossible to verify, it's certainly an indication of the ages-old healing potential of the plant.

Though the various species have pretty flowers, they're mostly tiny plants, and not very flashy. And even though they have numerous healing properties and uses, they're not really thought of as important herbal remedies. But that doesn't mean they're insignificant. According to the U.S. National Institutes of Health, the *Veronicas* have antibacterial, antimicrobial, antifungal, anti-inflammatory, antiviral, antiparasitic, antioxidant, anticancer, and neuroprotective activities. And various cultures have used different species for such problems as respiratory tract conditions, gastrointestinal inflammations, arthritis, and urinary tract issues. It has also been proven to help calm anxiety and to aid in restful sleep when taken internally and has been used externally to soothe small wounds and irritated eyes.

I pick a few flowery stems to taste, careful that the blossoms don't fall off immediately, and manage to get them into my mouth. Probably if I tried to carry a bundle of them home, the petals would start to let go, so when I decide it's time for a *Veronica* harvest, I'll bring a basket with me to ensure that I capture all the parts. For now, one more tasty flower tip is enough, and I head on home.

On the way, I pass by the little post office where three of the hawks continue to screech and dive and carry on overhead. Several customers pause, and we all marvel at the hawks. We stand for minutes, watching their antics and smiling. After a while, the birds head toward the woods and quiet down. But we are all still curious and thrilled long after they leave.

I think about these species that surround us—like the *Veronica* and the hawks—that help to make up the matrix of life in which we humans knit our own place. They are often so familiar we stop noticing them until something calls them to our attention. But they are always there, helping to keep the balance of this remarkable and threatened state. From now on, I'll know that each spring, when I start to notice the nesting hawks, I'll be likely to find *Veronica* nearby, and can start my speedwell harvest for the season.

Species: Three species of *Veronica* grow in Louisiana and share similar healing properties. These include:

Veronica arvensis

Other Names: Corn speedwell, rock speedwell, wall speedwell, common speedwell, corn sperry.

Description: Plant is hairy, erect to almost recumbent, 3.5–15.5 inches tall. Leaves are opposite and arranged in pairs around the stem and are 0.5–1 inch in length. Flowers are pale blue to blue-violet, less than 0.25 inch in diameter, and four-lobed with a narrow lowest lobe. Fruit capsules are heart-shaped.

Habitat: Moist open-wooded slopes, fields, sandy flatwoods, roadsides, moist meadows.

Distribution: Most parishes in the state.

Plant Status: Introduced.

Veronica peregrina

Other Names: Neckweed, purslane speedwell.

Description: Plant has erect, hairless stems that are up to about 11 inches tall. Leaves vary in shape from linear to lance-shaped to spoon-shaped with smooth or serrated edges. Blossom is a loose raceme of flowers and lance-shaped bracts. Flowers are generally white and less than 0.25 inch wide.

Habitat: Moderately moist meadows, stream banks, shores of lakes and ponds.

Distribution: Most parishes in the state.

Plant Status: Native.

Veronica persica

Other Names: Persian speedwell, winter speedwell, birds-eye speedwell.

Description: Plant has short-stalked leaves that are broadly ovate and have coarsely serrated margins. Leaves are 0.5–0.75 inch long, are paired on lower stems, and are alternate on the upper parts. Weak stems form a dense, prostrate groundcover, and tips of stems often grow upright. Flowers are 0.4 inch wide and are sky-blue with dark stripes and white centers. They are solitary on long, slender, hairy stalks in the leaf axils. Fruit is heart-shaped with two widely separated lobes.

Habitat: Waste ground, lawns, fields, and roadsides.

Distribution: Southern half of the state, and spotty in other areas.

Plant Status: Introduced.

For All Species, Parts Used: Whole plant.

Medicinal Properties: Antibacterial, antimicrobial, antifungal, anti-inflammatory, antiviral, antiparasitic, antioxidant, anticancer, and neuroprotective activities.

Uses: Internal—Anxiety, insomnia; arthritis; coughs; urinary tract inflammations. External—Irritated eyes, small wounds.

Risks: None known when used in moderate dosages. Heavy use may cause nausea.

Natural History: Most species worldwide are noted to be edible and nutritious and are reported to have a flavor similar to watercress. In 1769, Joseph Banks and Daniel Solander collected plants in the Southern Hemisphere that were later published in the genus *Veronica,* such as *Veronica pubescens* and *Veronica stricta.* Although another genus, *Hebe,* was established in 1789, few botanists initially accepted it, continuing to use *Veronica.* Native Americans used *Veronica* species as an expectorant tea for bronchial congestion, asthma, and allergies. *Veronica* species have been used in traditional Australian and New Zealand medicine for supporting the nervous system, respiratory tract, cardiovascular system, and overall metabolism. Various species of the herb have been used in Chinese medicine for mild respiratory and arthritis conditions, sore throat, and skin problems. In Ireland and other countries, it was considered to be a good luck charm and was sewn into clothes before a journey to protect against accidents.

Designation: Native American remedy, European traditional healing herb, Korean medicinal plant, Afghani healing plant.

Cultivation: *Veronica* plants prefer well-drained, loamy soil with plenty of organic matter. They grow in slightly acidic, neutral, and slightly alkaline soil (pH 6.0–8.0). Once established, the plants tolerate drought and need little supplemental watering. Freshly harvested seeds germinate well.

Remedy Form: Edible, tea, tincture.

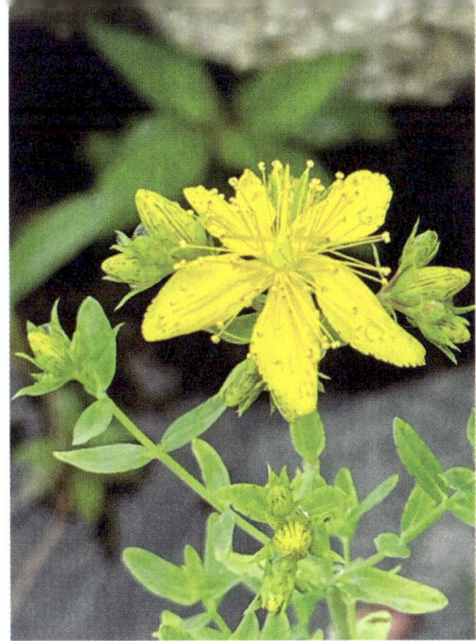

St. Johnswort
(*Hypericum perforatum*)

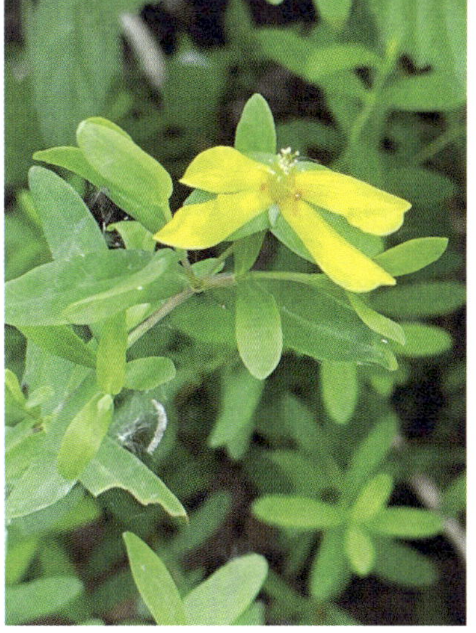

St. Andrew's cross
(*Hypericum hypericoides*)

ST. JOHNSWORT & THE GRAND DÉCOURAGEMENT

SUMMER

It's damned hot. It's another damned hot day. Lately, we all stay inside most of the time, then sneak out after the latest rainstorm to check the struggling gardens, fill the birdbaths again, let our dogs out with booties on so the scorching road tar won't burn their feet. And we all pray that the power doesn't go off with the heavy electricity demand in these midsummer days. And it's getting even hotter. New Orleans had its hottest summer on record last year, and its hottest recorded day ever. The state had more than six hundred wildfires in addition to extreme drought conditions.

We live in complicated times. We live with confusion and concern, trying to figure out how to take in what's important about the changes, and how to make whatever adjustments we can without just giving up and walking away. Because how could we do that?

Louisiana folks are no strangers to challenges, of course. In fact, you could say that struggles and adaptability are baked right into our souls. It's kind of hereditary. In the mid-1700s, in what is known as the "grand dérangement," thousands of French Catholics were expelled from Nova Scotia because they would not swear allegiance to Great Britain and the king. Whole families, having already survived the transition from France, where farmland was hard to find, to Canada's Maritime Provinces, where they could establish a new home, were then expelled to various areas of the U.S. East Coast. Several thousand settled in Louisiana, becoming the first Cajuns (aka Acadians) in the U.S. Many folks whose families have lived in southern Louisiana for generations have roots that go back to that "grand dérangement." One branch of my own family tree has been here now for seven generations.

And once again, here we are, faced with the prospect of another great upheaval—this time, not caused by governmental injunction but by the wrenching changes of fierce weather and rising waters. A recent report, *Louisiana 2050,* has proposed that within the next two dozen years, 30 percent of the state—especially the coastal areas—will be underwater. Already, we are facing the new version of that relocation event in what I've begun to call the "grand découragement"—a great discouragement—as we come to the reluctant, sad acceptance that soon, home ground may become untenable.

One of my ninety-year-old cousins has noted that he won't go down to Cocodrie anymore because it is just too sad. Some of the offshore islands where he used to go fishing with family are now gone. Underwater. And small towns down the bayous are emptying out—schools, businesses, homes—just abandoned, with the rise of water and the increasing severity of storms.

I have no doubt that if or when people go, they will take that sense of family and community with them. That, at least, is too strong to be washed away. In a recent history I read about that first eviction from their home ground, one proposed reason why the Acadians were so successful at settling into their new Louisiana home centuries ago was that "their sense of themselves as a people was undiminished. As far as it lay in their power, they attempted to re-create the same self-contained and independent life they had had before 1755. . . . A place called Acadia no longer existed, but it was still possible to be an Acadian in North America."

I believe that will continue to be true, no matter what choice people make now, or what direction they take.

And, after all, the worst hasn't happened yet, and some things here are still good. Despite the fiery heat, my garden is raggedy but okay. The cukes are bursting out of their skins, and the onions were good this year, so I'll settle in later to make salad and to start a batch of pickles. And the

St. Johnswort has taken over its patch in the flower bed and is leaning into the yard, begging to be picked.

St. Johnswort has been one of the most sought-after and important plants in modern herbalism, both in this country and in others. Known for its potential for relieving anxiety, depression, mood fluctuations, and also acting as a strong antiviral, the plant has been recognized for its healing properties since the first century AD. It has been popular in Europe for several centuries and rose to "celebrity status" in the U.S. in 1997 after an article on the herb's usefulness for depression was published in a popular magazine. Much research continues on the healing compounds of the herb and on its usefulness for various conditions. I'm always happy to see it, and today I'll be making my first harvest for the season.

Recently, in the garden, I noticed that the flowers were bright, deep yellow. Today they have started to seed, and some of the lower, smaller leaves are turning red—a sure sign that the important healing compounds are growing stronger in the plant.

I walk out to the garden, cut some of the lush *Hypericum* flowers and leaves and seeds, and bundle them up to take inside. Some of these will get hung up on the sunporch to dry and will later be used either for tea or to make the infused oil that the old-timers called "red oil" when they used it on bruises or aches and pains. And I'll make another batch of fresh plant tincture, too, to use for low mood or anxiety—something we might all be experiencing.

Inside the air-conditioned house, I settle in for a little herb work—turn the radio on to Mavis Staples and sing along with her. I strip the leaves and flowers from the stems and pack them into a large glass jar. A few tiny insects take off across the countertop, and I brush them into my hand and drop them outside the back door.

By the time I've chopped up today's haul and packed the flowers and seeds into a jar, my fingertips are dark purply-red and the pale countertop is smudged. I pour just enough grain alcohol over the plant parts to cover them, press them down with a wooden spoon, and close the jar. Within a half hour or so, the mixture will turn a dark, deep-red color as healing compounds are leached out into the liquid.

The most commonly used species of St. Johnswort, *Hypericum perforatum,* doesn't grow naturally in Louisiana. But some other species have proven to contain varying degrees of the same compounds found in that herb. Some research has suggested that several primary chemicals found in the plants could have antidepressant, anxiolytic, and antiviral effects. But it's complicated to figure out which species to use, and how much of any particular compound you're ingesting with the native versions of the herb. That's why I'm growing the "official" St. Johnswort in my home garden, right alongside some of the native species. This will give me a chance to experiment a bit, and also to make tincture and oil from the species that is traditionally used.

According to horticulture instructor Jennifer Blanchard at LSU in Baton Rouge, *Hypericum perforatum* is not too challenging to grow. She reports that the seeds can be stratified in the refrigerator for three to four weeks, then planted and lightly covered with soil. The seeds should germinate in one to two weeks, she says. This species likes full sun and well-drained or sandy soils.

In any case, I'll soon have tincture to keep on hand, and that'll be a good thing. In times like these, we could all use a little support—to lighten the anxiety, stave off gloomy thoughts, and gain a little clarity and courage for the times ahead. Luckily, we have many of nature's healers to help us get through hard times, especially the many species of St. Johnswort that make their home in Louisiana.

Obviously, it will take a lot more than a few doses of *Hypericum* to help us manage the challenges. But a little lift, a little lightening up, doesn't hurt. And maybe, as we sip our St. Johnswort tea, or rub the deep-red oil into our tense and aching muscles, we'll remember to thank nature, once again.

It's a good thing, this herb work.

It's a beautiful place we've inherited.

Now we just have to figure out how to take care of it.

Species: Twelve species of *Hypericum* grow in Louisiana. Some have been documented to have medicinal uses, while others have yet to be researched but may share similar healing properties. These include:

Hypericum cistifolium

Other Names: Round-pod St. Johnswort.

Description: Typically 2–4 feet tall, but may grow much taller in certain conditions. Many main stems are woody, with peeling bark. Leaves are opposite, grow in alternate directions, are often needlelike, and are 0.5–1 inch long. Leaves have a papery texture with a clasping base and a keeled mid-nerve, and edges are often rolled down. Flowers are bright yellow and have five petals that are 1 inch wide, with many pollen-tipped stamens. Seed pods are rounded, and dark rusty-red in color as they mature.

Habitat: Savannas, ditches, low pinelands, sandy soils.

Distribution: In only nine parishes, scattered around state, mostly in central and very northern areas.

Plant Status: Native.

Hypericum crux-andreae

Other Names: St. Peterswort, Atlantic St. Peterswort.

Medicinal Uses: Choctaw people used the root as an analgesic for colic and the leaves as a wash for sore eyes.

Description: A small, upright shrub that grows 1–3 feet tall. Brilliant lemon-yellow flowers with four petals occur at its branch tips. Sepals are of unequal size. Leaves are oblong-elliptic; the upper leaves are clasping, opposite, pale green, oval-to-oblong leaves about 0.75 inch wide. Older wood has shedding bark. Seed capsules are small, brown, and clam-shaped.

Habitat: Prefers partial sun and is adaptable to various soils, though often found in sandy areas.

Distribution: Western half of the state, a few central and eastern parishes as well.

Plant Status: Native.

Hypericum densiflorum

Other Names: Bushy St. Johnswort.

Description: Shrub may grow up to 6 feet tall with a spread of 3–6 feet.

Shrub is densely branched and has coppery bark. Numerous slender branches are slightly angled and branchlets are two-edged. Leaves are 1–2 inches long and 0.15–0.3 inch wide. Yellow flowers have five petals that are 0.4–0.6 inches wide. Seed capsules are 0.14–0.25-inch-long, cone-shaped pods that split in the fall and persist all winter.

Habitat: Low boggy places, seepage slopes, pond and lake borders, wet meadows, stream banks, roadside ditches, moist pinelands, moist bottomlands, edge of swamps and marshes. Tolerates a variety of soil types and moisture levels.

Distribution: Scattered throughout western half of the state, also some eastern and central parishes.

Plant Status: Native.

Hypericum drummondii

Other Names: Nits and lice, Drummond's St. Johnswort.

Description: Approximately 1–1.5 feet tall, with several branching stems in the upper part of the plant. Leaves are opposite, very narrow, and entire. They are abundant and erect and are about 0.5 inch long. Flowers have five yellow petals that are borne in the leaf axils and rotate (generally to the right) like airplane propellers; the flowers terminate each branch.

Habitat: Dry woods, fields, and roadsides, in sandy or gravelly soils in fallow fields, open scrub oak and cedar-oak flatwoods, forest edges, prairies, and weedy pastures.

Distribution: Most of the state, excluding lower southeastern tip.

Plant Status: Native.

Hypericum fasciculatum

Other Names: Peelbark St. Johnswort, sandweed.

Medicinal Uses: Menopause; moderate depression. Seminole used roots as a cathartic for blocked bowels and urination.

Description: Plants may be up to 10 feet tall, though are often much shorter. Leaves are simple, opposing, needlelike, with entire or revolute margins. Stems are multibranched with reddish bark that flakes off in papery sheets. Flowers are bright yellow, five-petaled, with conspicuous yellow-orange stamens. Fruit is an inconspicuous capsule that is oval in shape.

Habitat: Wet places about ponds and lakes, in low pinelands and along forested streams and cypress pools.

Distribution: Found in about a dozen parishes, mostly central-west and east of the state.

Plant Status: Native

Hypericum galioides

Other Names: Bedstraw St. Johnswort.

Description: Plant height is up to 5 feet and is slender and branching. Leaves are linear, roughly 6–14.5 inches long, and very narrow. Flowers are small and bright yellow with five petals. Leaves are up to 6 inches long.

Habitat: Low wet pinelands, prairies, swamps, depressions around ponds and lakes, and along ditches.

Distribution: Central, eastern, and western parishes.

Plant Status: Native.

Hypericum gentianoides

Other Names: Orangegrass, pineweed, pineweed St. Johnswort.

Medicinal Uses: The Cherokee used the plant to promote menstruation, to help relieve diarrhea, and to reduce fevers. Used externally as a poultice.

Description: Plant has scaly leaves on erect, wiry branches, and grows up to 20 inches in height, appears leafless, and has wiry ascending opposite branches. Leaves have a citrus scent when crushed. Tiny yellow flowers only open in sun, and seed capsules are red.

Habitat: Fields, roadsides, rock outcrops, and dry or gravelly or sunbaked sandy soil.

Distribution: Found in about two dozen parishes in top two-thirds of the state.

Plant Status: Native.

Hypericum gymnanthum

Other Names: Clasping leaf St. Johnswort.

Description: Plant is woody, grows up to 2 feet tall, and is unbranched except toward the apex, where the flowers occur. Pairs of opposite leaves occur at intervals along the stem. Leaves are up to 1 inch long and 0.7 inch across. Each leaf clasps the stem at the base and tapers gradually to a blunt tip. Flowers are yellow, small, with four petals.

Habitat: Bogs, savannas, in sandy soils in barrens or low ground.

Distribution: Western half of the state, also a few eastern-central parishes.

Plant Status: Native.

Hypericum hypericoides

Other Names: St. Andrew's cross.

Medicinal Uses: Used by several Native American tribes for such disorders as pain, colic, diarrhea, and as a pain relief in childbirth. Also used for kidney and bladder support, and externally for skin irritations.

Description: May be confused with *Hypericum crux-andreae*, which is the only other prairie species with four petals. Plant may grow 2–4 feet tall and 3 feet wide. Leaves are oblong-elliptic. Small yellow flowers have four narrow petals and four unequal sepals that form an X. Bark is exfoliating and reddish. Flowers are borne in axils and have four unequal sepals. Leaves may be linear, elliptic or ovate, and are opposing. Stems are branched and reddish-brown. Fruits are ovoid capsules.

Habitat: Pinelands, dry or moist rocky soil.

Distribution: Most of the state, except for extreme southeastern tip.

Plant Status: Native.

Hypericum nudiflorum

Other Names: Pretty St. Johnswort, early St. Johnswort, naked St. Johnswort.

Description: Deciduous shrub grows to about 2–3 feet tall and has a moderately branched look with a rounded overall shape. Leaves are broadly elliptic to ovate and are about 1.5–2 inches long. Flowers are small, slightly rounded, and occur in clusters at the tips of branches. Flowers are bright yellow and about 0.5 inch wide.

Habitat: Moist sandy or low woods, thickets, swamps, or stream banks.

Distribution: Top half of the state.

Plant Status: Native.

Hypericum perforatum

Other Names: St. Johnswort, Klamath weed, goat weed.

Medicinal Uses: Anxiety, mild to moderate depression, pain relief, nervous system support; inflammation; menopause symptoms; neuropathy; viral infections. There are over six hundred documented activities for this species, including but not limited to antidepressant, anxiolytic, analgesic, antiretroviral, antiseptic, antispasmodic, aromatic, cholagogue, diuretic, digestive stimulant, nervine, sedative, stimulant, vermifuge, vulnerary. The National Institutes of Health have documented the following activities for preparations of the herb: antibacterial, antiviral, anticancer, antioxidant, neuroprotective, anti-inflammatory, wound healing, and reducing opium dependence.

Description: Erect, multistemmed plant grows 1–3 feet tall and has slender stems that are often reddish and woody at base. Leaves are 1–2 inches long and 0.25 inch wide, are stalkless, and oblong or linear with round tips. Leaves have scattered translucent dots that make the leaf look perforated when held up to the light. Numerous flowers are symmetrical around a central point and occur in flat-topped clusters. The short-stalked flowers are yellow and are about 1 inch wide. Petals are peppered with black dots around the edges. Seed pod is a three-sectioned capsule that is dark reddish-brown when mature.

Habitat: Prefers full sun or partial shade. Grows well in moist, well-drained soils.

Distribution: Does not occur in the wild in Louisiana.

Plant Status: Can be cultivated.

Cultivation: Can be propagated by seed, division, or softwood cuttings. Requires well-drained or sandy soil and prefers full sun. Seeds can be stratified in refrigerator for 3–4 weeks before spring and then planted on top layer of soil and lightly covered. Keep moist. Should germinate in 1–2 weeks.

Hypericum prolificum

Other Names: Shrubby St. Johnswort.

Description: A small, mound-shaped, deciduous shrub growing 2–4 feet tall, with dense, upright branches. Lower stems are woody with shredded gray-brown bark; the upper stems are green. Dark-green, lance-shaped leaves are 2–3 inches long and turn yellow-green in fall. Bright-yellow, five-petaled flowers are up to 1 inch and have numerous yellow stamens. Stamens are bushy to the point of partially obscuring the petals. Each flower is replaced by a cone-shaped seed capsule about 0.3–0.5 inch in length, which splits in autumn to release black seeds.

Habitat: Rocky or sandy open woods, meadows, seepage slopes, swamp margins, dry or damp sandy or rocky thickets.

Distribution: Sparsely scattered throughout upper half of the state.

Plant Status: Native.

Hypericum punctatum

Other Names: Spotted St. Johnswort.

Description: Plant grows 1–3 inch tall. Leaves are simple, opposite, and stalkless to somewhat clasping, oblong to oval elliptic, 0.75–2.25 inches long, 0.3–0.5 inch wide. Flowers are deep yellow, 0.3–0.5 inch wide, with five oval to oblong petals that have blunt tips and conspicuous lines of black dots. Flowers occur in dense clusters at the tips of stems and branches. Fruit is an upright, oval to ellipsoid capsule 0.175–0.25 inch long, and reddish to deep purple in color.

Habitat: Moist or dry soil, fields, open woods, ditches, roadsides, thickets, edge of woods and fields.

Distribution: Top third of the state, scattered in other areas.

Plant Status: Native.

For All Species, Parts Used: Aerial parts.

Medicinal Properties: See above for individual species.

Uses: Many species have been used internally for nervous system support, and for treating afflictions such as anxiety, mild to moderate depression, menstrual pain and mood changes associated with menopause. (See above for specific uses.) Also used for inflammation, coughs, fevers, pain, viral infections, and support in HIV. Externally, the herb has a historic use for minor wounds and insect stings.

Risks: Minor side effects of some Hypericum species include digestive upset, diarrhea, dizziness, and restlessness. These usually resolve quickly once herb use is halted. Large doses of the herb may cause severe skin reactions with exposure to sunlight. Some medications may interact with Hypericum, including birth control pills (use additional protection if taking St. Johnswort), Xanax, Cyclosporin, or Digoxin. Consult with health care practitioner if pregnant, nursing, or taking prescription medications.

Animal Use: *Hypericum* species in the state provide nectar and pollen for bees and many other types of pollinating insects and are well-suited for use in pollinator restoration habitats. The plants are toxic for dogs, sheep, and cattle, and result in photosensitization. Most herbivores (including deer) avoid consuming the plant.

Natural History: The genus name *Hypericum* is possibly derived from the Greek words *hyper,* meaning "above," and *eikon,* meaning "picture," in reference to the tradition of hanging the plant over religious icons in the home. The common name St. Johnswort comes from the fact that its flowers and buds were commonly harvested at the time of the Midsummer Festival, which was later renamed St. John's Feast Day, on June 24. It was believed that harvesting the flower at this time made its healing and magical powers more potent. The herb would be hung on house and stall doors on St. John's Feast Day to ward off evil spirits and to safeguard against harm and sickness to people and livestock.

Designation: Important herb of commerce, edible, Indigenous remedy, traditional Chinese medicine plant, Greek and Islamic traditional medicinal herb, European phytotherapy medicinal plant.

Cultivation: General recommendations, for most species—Plant seeds indoors 6–8 weeks before the last frost, or outside after the danger of frost has passed. Press seeds into the soil, but do not cover them; the seeds will germinate better with light. Transplant seedlings when they are 2–3 inches tall. Plants will tolerate almost any soil conditions but prefer moist and light soils. Water only in prolonged drought. Prefers full sun or partial shade, and moist, well-drained soil. Space plants 2–3 feet apart and water regularly so that the soil is constantly moist but not sodden.

Remedy Form: Internal—Tea, tincture. External—Compress, oil, poultice, wash.

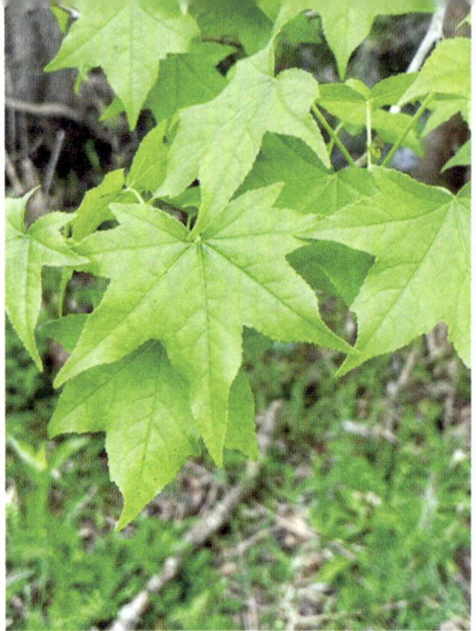

Sweet gum

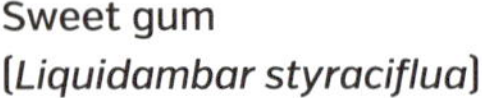

(*Liquidambar styraciflua*)

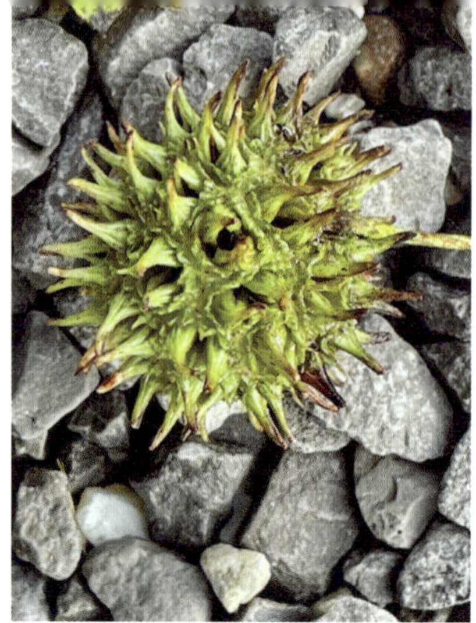

Sweet gum seed pod

SWEET GUM & THE BATTURE WOODS

SPRING

I'm out this morning a little late—after 7:00 a.m. It's a gray day, with no big sunrise event, no clouds, just a pale-gray sky. The usual yard birds are chatty, maybe because I'm so late putting out their seed. A small breeze sighs through the jasmine near the doorway, and a second bloom of blossoms is starting up, much to the joy of the neighborhood bees. The workers on the new house going up next door haven't arrived yet, so it's kind of quiet—until I get to the levee. There, for a third day in a row, the huge bulldozer–tree smasher machine is geared up and cutting into trees that line the woods. And not just the already-downed trees and shrubs but tall, healthy ones with new, green growth. The understory shrubs are all sheared right down to the muddy ground and shoved into a messy line. I thought at first that maybe the crew was clearing for a new road across the marsh and to the river, but now that I see how much, and how far, they've cut, that doesn't make sense.

But nothing about this makes sense—at least not to me. Aside from the fact that I love the woods, love the wild silence and hawks and eagles and egrets and herbs, there's the plain impracticality of it all. This area is prone to flooding. And if the batture is designed to help prevent flooding when the river is high or a huge storm rolls in, then why would you cut down the trees and vegetation that can soak up that water and help prevent floods? And in an area where summer heat is brutal, why would you cut down trees whose leaves provide "albedo"—reflecting heat from sunlight back into space, instead of absorbing it and raising air temperatures? And then there's how much we enjoy the beauty—no monetary or scientific value in that, I guess, but it's certainly what makes living here so lush and beautiful for us all.

I stand on the levee and watch, taking a few photos. I pray for the many trees that I've come to love—the tall sycamores, the big old oaks, the sweet gums that have just unfolded their bright-green, star-shaped leaves. Then the red-shouldered hawks rise up, screeching and circling. And the eagles follow, whistling and diving, confused and shocked and scared, I imagine. At this important nesting time, they probably have babies to protect. But what chance do they have against the machines?

I'm upset for the animals who are helpless against this onslaught—and I'm upset for myself. Just yesterday I discovered a huge, healthy sweet gum tree putting out its first spring leaves. I was hoping to use some of its resin to make an herbal salve, and to gather some of its leaves for tea.

I haven't used the tree for its healing properties yet, but I've heard much about its historic use. And it was not just important in the past. The trees produce much storax, a sweet-scented resin that continues to be useful for common ailments such as skin problems, coughs, and ulcers. In recent years, it's also proven to be a strong antimicrobial compound against multi-drug-resistant bacteria such as methicillin-resistant Staphylococcus aureus (MRSA). The leaves, bark, and seeds of sweet gum also possess helpful compounds such as shikimic acid, which is a precursor to the production of Tamiflu, an antiviral drug effective against several influenza viruses. Other extracts derived from sweet gum trees have shown potential as antioxidant, anti-inflammatory, and chemopreventive agents. And research has proven that both MRSA and E. coli were more sensitive to the extracts of one species of sweet gum than they were to traditional antibiotics such as penicillin. In addition, extracts from *Liqidambar styraciflua* show potential in the production of environmentally friendly pesticides and antifungal agents.

In a few days, maybe I can come back—once the machines have rumbled on down the road—and check out the wreckage, or as much as I can stand of it. I might be able to find a downed sweet gum tree that has already produced the resin it would have used to repair its wounds, if it had continued to live. And I can collect some to take home and turn into a healing salve, and maybe a tincture. At least then the tree can continue to offer something, even as it fades away.

Finally, I head home. I can still hear the hawks and eagles screaming, but soon the workers on the house next door arrive, and their construction noises drown out the tree-wrecking machines and the birds' distress calls. That's a tiny comfort, I guess. But in this case, ignorance is not bliss, just a small, momentary relief.

I'm sure there are good reasons for what's going on. But it just hurts my heart to see how easy it is for us humans to think of nature as a resource, a thing for us to use, instead of a collection of unique, throbbing, sensitive life forms that make up the matrix—the web of life—in which we all co-participate, and on which we all depend.

I recently heard a television program on the current state of the Earth during which the narrator remarked on how much nature has been negatively altered by our behavior. Humans, it turns out, just might bring about the next great devastation of the planet. I hope that doesn't prove to be true. I hope we can find ways to start limiting our negative impact and can contribute to the healing of the planet instead of its destruction. I imagine that it will be not one gigantic step we take but hundreds of thousands of tiny movements toward healing. As nature offers us so many ways to heal, maybe we can offer it something gentle in return. I am ever-hopeful.

Other Names: *Liquidambar styraciflua,* alligator tree, red gum, bilsted, star-leaved gum.

Parts Used: Bark, leaves, stems, resin.

Medicinal Properties: Antiseptic, anticonvulsant, antiviral, carminative, diuretic, expectorant, parasiticide, mild sedative, stimulant, vulnerary.

Uses: Internal—Asthma, coughs, sore throats; arthritis; colic, diarrhea. In traditional Chinese medicine, the seed balls are known as lu lu tong, and are used the treatment of nettle rash, rhinitis, rheumatic arthritis, bruises, missed menstrual periods, and low breast milk supply. External—Bruises, muscle aches, sores, skin and mucosal infections, wounds, hemorrhoids, ringworm, scabies.

Risks: Should not be applied to large open wounds. Avoid internal use if pregnant or breastfeeding.

Description: Sweet gum is a large tree with a long, cylindrical trunk and a pyramidal crown. Leaves are alternate, simple, star-shaped, with five (occasionally three or seven) lobes, 3–6 inches wide, and are deeply lobed. They are bright green and smooth, glossy above and pale underneath. Margins are toothed, and tips are long-pointed; leaves are slightly aromatic when bruised. Flowers appear in spring and persist into autumn or winter. Male blossoms have large numbers of tiny flowers gathered in clusters on a thick stalk and occur above the leaves. These produce large quantities of pollen. Female flowers are suspended as a single, spherical structure with masses of tiny flowers, and are found below the leaves. The curled, tubular structures covering the surface are the stigmas of the flower, and are sticky, which allows them to catch the pollen. In summer, the soft, delicate structure becomes a hard, prickly, complex fruit made up of seed capsules. Seeds are 1–1.5 inches large and occur in spiny balls that change from green to brown over late summer to fall.

Habitat: Low, rich woods, swampy woods.

Distribution: Most of the state.

Plant Status: Native.

Animal Use: Birds including goldfinches, purple finches, mallard ducks, wood ducks, bobwhite quails, Carolina chickadees, yellow-bellied sapsuckers, white-throated sparrows, towhees, Carolina wrens, mourning doves, quail, red-winged blackbirds, and others eat the seeds. Small mammals including chipmunks and squirrels will also eat the seeds. Beavers use wood for constructing dams. Sweet gum is a host plant for more than thirty species of butterflies and moths that feed on leaves, including luna and promethea moths.

Natural History: The first mention of any use of the resin or amber was described by Juan de Grijalva in Cuba in 1517. He told of gift exchanges with the Maya, "who presented them with hollow reeds . . . filled with dried herbs and sweet-smelling liquid amber which, when lighted . . . diffused an agreeable odour." In 1615, Spanish naturalist Francisco Hernandez described the species as a large tree producing a fragrant gum resembling liquid amber. The species was introduced in Europe in 1681 by John Banister, the missionary collector sent out by Bishop Compton, who planted it in the palace gardens at Fulham in London. In 1686 John Ray's *Historica Plantarum* referred to it as *Styrax liquida.* Acadians of south Louisiana called this tree copal, which was adapted from the Aztec term for resin. Native Americans and early settlers noted that injuries to the tree produced a sticky resin called copalm balsam, which they used as chewing gum and a medicinal. And Linnaeus gave the tree its genus name, *Liquidambar,* to reflect its viscous resin ("liquid amber"), and its species name, *styraciflua,* to refer to the property of "flowing with gum" (which was known as styrax or storax).

Designation: Herb of commerce, Chinese medicinal remedy, Indigenous healing herb, commercial source of styrax.

Cultivation: Harvest sweet gum balls and let them dry out on a sheet of paper. When seeds fall out, collect them and place inside a plastic bag filled with moist, sterile potting soil. Refrigerate for three months, then plant into a pot outside. (Also—to keep snails away from other garden plants, use discarded gum balls as a mulch.)

Remedy Form: Tea, tincture, salve, poultice.

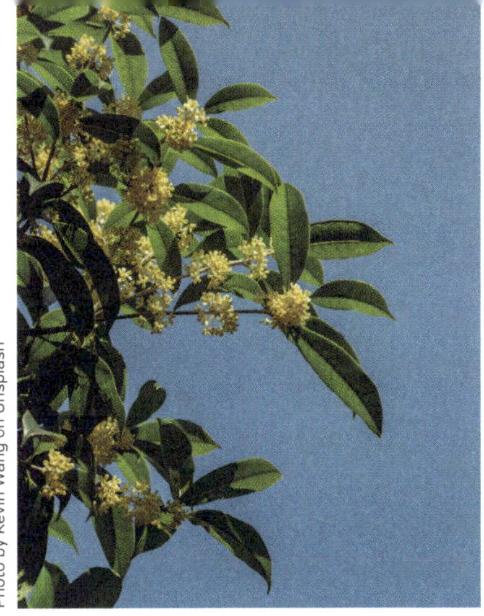

Photo by Kevin Wang on Unsplash

SWEET OLIVE & BELONGING TO A PLACE

SPRING

Sweet olive
(*Osmanthus* sp.)

It's a very damp morning, with a gray sky and puddles all over the soggy ground. But I'm grateful for the rain that started in the night after so many dry days. Along the levee path, I take photos of the slate-colored clouds. The usual egret hangs out at the shrinking batture pond, and all the weedy wildflowers are silvered with raindrops. Clovers and thistles and violets and wild *Geranium* are thick and healthy looking. I pass a slow-moving armadillo who skedaddles away from me, and I think about how much Bodi would have liked to see it. He loved being out walking and sniffing animal trails, and he loved the levee trail, especially when other folks were passing by. He was always hoping for a few head pats from fellow walkers. I'm missing him a lot lately, especially when walking around our favorite places or settling in for a rainy-day nap. But I feel that his little doggie self is still beside me, somehow.

Today, I'm not walking far. The light rain could turn heavy any moment now, so I check out what's growing, take a few photos, and head toward the town offices that are close to my home. Lately, I keep an eye on the little garden in front of the Planning and Zoning office. I recently discovered a few interesting plantings there and have thought about asking if they would like to grow some medicinal herbs for local folks to see. It turns out, though, that there are already some herbs in the landscape. A couple of small *Magnolia* trees and a native palmetto are thriving alongside a sweet-scented shrub that I didn't recognize at first glance. After a little investigation, though, I've discovered that it is the sweet olive that so many folks cultivate in their yards.

I've heard that there are two species of *Osmanthus* growing in Louisiana, and that they both have many medicinal properties. This particular shrub's Latin name, *Osmanthus fragrans,* testifies to one of its characteristics—the fragrance. We had one in our home yard when I was a child, and my mom and sister and I would make excuses to be out in the yard often so we could sniff up that scent. Little did I know then that it was a healing herb, especially beloved in Asian countries not only for its perfume but for its healing properties. Now I'm eager to get home and do a little more research on its uses. I pick a few sprigs from the flowery branches and head back to the house.

At home, while I wait for tea water to boil, I do a bit more reading on *Osmanthus.* I have a hard time finding much medicinal information on the native plant, *Osmanthus americanus,* but there are numerous documented uses for the species that people cultivate. Apparently, it is a highly prized herb in Asian countries that has been used for over 2,500 years. It is listed as one of the top ten flowers in China. Flowers, leaves, and fruit of the shrub are used in pastries, sweets, tea, and wine, and in tonics, condiments, and skin-care products. Also, research has proven that various parts of the shrub are anti-inflammatory and antioxidant, are helpful for balancing blood sugar, and are good for easing rheumatism, cough, and digestive disturbances. It's especially helpful for stress and anxiety when used as an inhalant, apparently. And it's an important healer in traditional Chinese medicine for boosting immunity and stopping the advance of some cancers. In fact, there are so many medicinal properties that I feel a little overwhelmed reading them all.

I decide that, for now, I'll start with a simple tea and see how it feels to me. And I'll try it in another way as well. Reports on the plant note that the flowery scent can bring relief from the effects of burnout, stress, and anxiety. I don't feel particularly anxious, but I recently bought myself a small vial of *Osmanthus fragrans* essential oil, thinking that it might help relieve a bit of the exhaustion that has settled into my body after such a hard time with Bodi's end of life. Now, I daub a little of the oil on my temples and behind my ears. And while I sip my newly brewed sweet olive tea, I sit on the front porch and gaze out at the road that winds through this small town where so many of my ancestors were born and raised.

I think back decades, to times when my grandmother and an aunt or uncle and I would sit on the front gallery and chat a bit before falling into a companionable silence. They'd know just about all the folks who were passing by—who was coming home from work, who was probably on their way to church, or who was likely to saunter by on a warm spring afternoon and sit down for a visit. They'd know, too, what plants would be starting their journey into flowering, or setting seed, or producing fruit, and what small animals would be wandering by in the night—because these are what made up their Home.

They had tended this place all their lives. They had paid attention, nudged it into a direction that they thought would be appealing or more productive, and made a sweet peace with it all. That's what it was like, then, to belong to a place—to be so familiar with your surroundings and neighbors that you could set your watch by them or know when it might be getting close to time to harvest something from the nearby field. It was a good way to live, I think. There was something about living close to a place, belonging to a place, that was comforting and humbling at the same time. We could remember that life, and our homeplace, wasn't just for us—it belonged to itself, really. We were just being gifted with its use. I still feel that way—I am just passing through, uplifted and supported and enlivened by this mesh of lands and waters and air, animals and plants and neighbors.

And while it's true that I have gone away, made another place, and then returned, this is still Home Ground—well known, and healing, and beloved. For that, I am ever glad.

Other Names: *Osmanthus fragrans*—Fragrant olive, tea olive, holly olive, false olive. *Osmanthus americanus*—*Cartrema americana,* devilwood, American olive, wild olive.

Parts Used: Flowers, leaves, stem bark, lateral roots.

Medicinal Properties: *O. fragrans* has been proven to have antibacterial, antioxidant, antitumor, anti-inflammatory, antihyperglycemic, antithrombotic, antimelanogenesis, antifatigue, antidrowsiness, neuroprotective, and hepatoprotective properties. In Chinese medicine, it is known to support the endocrine system, liver, and kidney. It is also an abundant source of nutrients such as minerals, proteins, vitamin E, fatty acids, polysaccharides, and sterols. *O. americanus* is assumed to have similar properties.

Uses: *O. fragrans*—Internal—Allergies, cough/whooping cough, respiratory infections, boosting immunity; cardiovascular support; dysmenorrhea/regulating menstrual cycles; cognitive enhancement; fatigue, drowsiness, insomnia, mood enhancement, stress reduction; hypertension, lowers blood lipid; rheumatism; stomachache, weight loss. External—Antiaging, boils, bruises, carbuncles, insect repellant, retinitis. Flowers are highly valued for their scent and are used in some of the world's most expensive perfumes. *O. americanus* has not been extensively researched, but many *Osmanthus* species have been proven to have similar medicinal uses. Indigenous healers in the southern states utilized parts of the plant for fevers and respiratory complaints.

Risks: Considered nontoxic, often used for food or as a food additive.

Description: *O. americanus*—An irregularly rounded and open shrub or small tree growing 15–40 feet with an equal spread. Long, evergreen leaves are olive green and leathery and are present throughout the year. Small, creamy-white flowers are extremely fragrant, and are followed by dark-blue fruit. Tree grows slowly. *O. fragrans*—A small, upright, evergreen tree or large shrub that will typically grow 10–15 feet tall in cultivation but may reach 20–30 feet tall in its native habitat in Asia (Himalayas, China, and Japan). Leaves are oval, leathery, glossy green, up to 4 inches long. Leaf margins smooth or finely toothed.

Habitat: *O. americanus*—Rich woods, swamps, maritime forests, and dry woods. *O. fragrans*—Forests, hillsides, along riverbanks. Also easily cultivated in ornamental gardens, parks, residential landscapes, containers, streets, patios, balconies, and large containers.

Distribution: *O. americanus*—East Baton Rouge, Sabine, St. Helena, St. Tammany, Tangipahoa, Washington Parishes. *O. fragrans*—Widely cultivated.

Plant Status: *O. americanus*—Native. *O fragrans*—Introduced and widely cultivated.

Animal Use: *O. americanus*—Bees, pollinators, songbirds. *O. fragrans*—Bees and butterflies. Plant is deer resistant.

Natural History: The genus name, *Osmanthus,* from the Greek words for "odor" and "flower," refers to the fragrant blossoms. *O. americanus* is often called devilwood because the fine-textured wood is difficult to split and work.

Designation: Traditional Chinese medicinal herb, folk medicine remedy, Native American use.

Cultivation: *O. americanus*—Prefers partial shade and rich, moist, well-drained soil, and can be pruned to maintain shape. *O. fragrans*—Plant in full sun to partial shade and in moist soils with good drainage. Afternoon shade is essential. Heavy clay soils are tolerated. Drought-tolerant once established, but needs supplemental watering in hot, dry months.

Remedy Form: Tea, tincture, compress, poultice, edible.

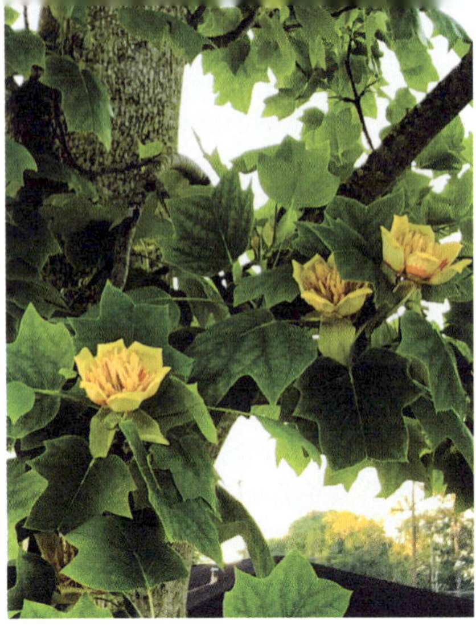

TULIP TREE & THE EOC

SPRING

Tulip tree
(*Liriodendron tulipfera*)

I'm out early to feed the birds and take a walk. It's a quiet morning, and the leftover translucent moon hangs in the branches of the live oak tree. The coming sun lights up hazy clouds over the river, so everything turns pink and orange and then fades into a quieter glow. On the dewy lawn, two bunnies hop away into the underbrush and several cardinals drop down to the feeder a few seconds after I hang it up.

But other than that, there's not much activity. It's a good time for a walk, and for scouting the edges of the woods for the blackberries that are ripening up lately. In the last few days, I've joined up with cousins for a trek into the tangled brush. We brought bowls and bags and stood not too far from each other as we stretched carefully to pick whatever blackberries we could reach. This year, the berries were late but worth the wait—huge, juicy, and sweet. In just a few minutes, each of us had a couple of boxes filled with the fruit. The only sounds were a shared word or two, or an occasional yelp as a hand got hung up in the prickly canes. Soon our fingers were purple, and we were swatting our berry-stained hands at mosquitoes that nagged us as we picked. It was fun working together under the warm sun, doing what people here do—work the land, harvest its fruits, catch up on how families are doing. I imagine that our long line of people has done this same thing, together, over decades and even centuries.

But today I'm out alone—no cousins, and no Bodi. Maybe that's a good thing, since he'd probably be chasing through the brambles after a possum or two. I take photos of the blooming wild onions, and of the newly seeding yellow dock, its tips ruddy red as the three-sided seeds color up. A yellow tree cricket hides under a hackberry leaf.

I tear myself away from the batture beauties and head for home with another plant visit in mind. Taking the shortcut across the parking lot at the town offices, I stop to check the tulip trees in front of the Emergency Operations Center (EOC) to see if the flowers have come yet. But though the trees are lush with new leaves, they aren't ready to bloom. I don't mind waiting, though, and am happy to keep an eye on the trees.

Apparently, *Liriodendron tulipfera* has a long history of medicinal use, and though I haven't tried it yet for any health problems, from what I've read, the tulip trees—along with their whole *Liriodendron* family—are strongly anti-inflammatory. They have proven to be useful for such conditions as arthritis and rheumatism, for autoimmune illnesses, for supporting the nervous system, and for stimulating circulation. And in an emergency, parts of the plant can be applied externally on wounds, burns, and achy joints. And all parts of the trees can be used.

I'd love to gather some of the flowers when they appear and try them as a tea. Obviously, I won't be taking bark from these town trees, and the bark is reported to be extremely bitter, so I probably wouldn't make a tea from that anyway. But the leaves are not too bad. I nibble at one now and am kind of surprised at how strong it tastes. First, there's a sharp astringent taste, and then the bitterness, and then something I hadn't expected—a deep flavor that reminds me of Vicks VapoRub! And it takes a while for that flavor to disappear. Next, I'll try the flowers when they come. I figure that if the bees love the scent and the nectar from the flowers, maybe they would taste a little more pleasant.

In the meantime, I worry about these trees some. Though they are native, they're normally found farther north in the state, in woodsy areas, growing in a clutch of their cousins. But these tulip trees are surrounded by the cement parking lot, and I wonder how deep their roots can go in this area. I'm happy that the town sometimes uses native plants in its landscaping, and I'm always glad to see the tulip tree flowers in late spring. I'm glad, too, to have learned some of the healing properties of tulip trees. I've read that it is a great "emergency medicine" healer, and that's kind of cool—because here they are, decorating the parking lot of the town Emergency Operations Center.

A few days ago, I was sitting on the sunporch when I suddenly heard the squeal of a car attempting to brake, followed by a loud crash. Peering out the window, I saw a large dump truck stopped in the road after having hit a car. The smaller vehicle was crunched into a utility pole and was lying on its side in the ditch. I immediately dialed 911 and reached an operator. She was very kind and straightforward and asked several questions about what I had seen of the event. Even before we finished talking, the first ambulance wheeled up to my house. I was pretty impressed at the speed and competency of the folks who responded to my call.

I pass by the Emergency Operations Center building several times a day but have never given it much thought. Mostly, I keep an eye on the tulip trees and other plantings nearby. And I guess I just kind of take it for granted that if something traumatic happens, the EOC will help us all get through it safely. But really, in a state so often threatened by potentially devastating storms, the sixty-four parish EOCs in the state are vital to our safety before, during, and after serious storms and other disasters.

Asking around, I find that the EOCs act as coordination centers for community responses to various types of emergencies including storms, security issues, and hazardous materials events. Specialists gather information and technology, head up communications, and facilitate cohesive parish responses to a crisis. In large-scale disasters, the EOC also acts as a liaison between local responders and the state.

I can't even begin to imagine what it must take for the EOCs to deal with all they do, but I've gained a great respect for their presence in our town. And I continue to be impressed by the tulip tree and its many offerings when it comes to healing. In fact, I'm thinking that if the tulip trees can grow in a concrete parking lot, I'm pretty sure that they'd feel right at home in my own yard. Apparently, it can be grown from seed, but it has a very low rate of germination. So I'll try a native plant nursery or a garden club sale. And when the flowers finally open up, I'll brew them into a tea and see how it tastes. And I'll dry some of the blossoms to have on hand for an emergency remedy.

In the meantime, I continue to be impressed by the tulip tree, and by its neighbor, the EOC. Nature offers so many remedies for some difficult health issues, just as the coordinated efforts of local folks at parish EOCs provide assistance and support during some of our most challenging times. We're so lucky to have all these amazing resources so close to home.

Other Names: *Liriodendron tulipfera,* tulip poplar, yellow poplar.

Parts Used: Bark, inner bark, buds, flowers, leaves, stems.

Medicinal Properties: Anthelmintic, anti-inflammatory, antimalarial, appetite stimulant, cardiac support, diaphoretic, diuretic, nervine, tonic, stimulant.

Uses: Internal—Autoimmune conditions, coughs, fevers, headache; gout, pain, rheumatism; indigestion, diarrhea, gastrointestinal distress, parasites; nervous system support. External—Boils, minor burns, small wounds, joint inflammation, and on fractures to help speed healing.

Risks: Generally safe for humans (though can be harmful for dogs).

Description: A very large tree with a long, clear trunk and a pyramidal crown. Tree may be up to 190 feet tall, though often slightly shorter. Leaves are alternate, simple, 4–6 inches long, and broad. Leaf tip is notched or V shaped at the center, with two lobes near the tip and two or four lobes on the lower sides. Margins are entire, and lobes are pointed. Leaves turn yellow in autumn. Flowers are pale green or yellow, with an orange band on the tepals or outer parts of flower. Blossoms produce large quantities of nectar and attract many species of bees.

Habitat: Low rich woods, stream banks, and waste places.

Distribution: Found in about thirty parishes in top two-thirds of the state.

Plant Status: Native.

Animal Use: A nesting site for many types of birds. Flowers attract hummingbirds and honeybees, and the tree is a larval host for eastern tiger swallowtail and tuliptree silkmoth. Deer browse on new sprouts, and squirrels eat seeds in early fall and midwinter.

Natural History: The genus name *Liriodendron* originated from the Greek words *leirion*, which means "lily," and *dendron*, meaning "a tree for the flowers." The species name *tulipifera* means "tulip," a description of its flowers that resemble tulips. The tree is sometimes called canoewood, referring to the fact that many Native American tribes used the huge tulip tree trunks for making large dugout canoes. Captain John Smith in 1612 described these canoes as being 40–50 feet in length and able to carry forty passengers. Members of many tribes used parts of the tree to treat parasitic worms, diarrhea, coughs, rheumatism, gastrointestinal upsets, fevers, and snakebites. Infusions made from bark were also used for poultices to treat fractured limbs, boils, and other skin problems.

Designation: Native American/Indigenous remedy, folkloric traditional herb, traditional Chinese medicine remedy, Ayurvedic medicine herb.

Cultivation: Prefers rich, moist soils. Seed is best sown in a shady place in a cold frame as soon as it is ripe. Stored seed requires 3 weeks warm followed by 12 weeks cold stratification, although only about 1 percent of the seed is viable. When seedlings are large enough to handle, set them out into individual pots and grow them in a greenhouse for at least their first winter. Plant them out into their permanent positions in late spring or early summer, after the last expected frosts.

Remedy Form: Internal—Tea, tincture, flower essence. External—Compress, poultice, salve, wash.

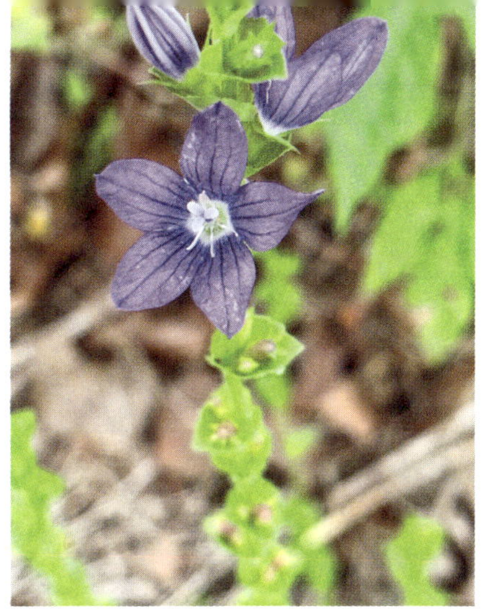

VENUS' LOOKING GLASS & THE EAGLES

SPRING

Venus' looking glass
(*Triodanis perfoliata*)

Spring! It's a time of welcoming the new, even as we release what's gone. This morning I'm thinking of little Bodi, who came to me in a dream just as I was waking up. He's been on my mind a lot lately, especially after so many noisy storms. Despite missing him, I was glad that when thunder rumbled and lightning flashed last night, he didn't have to tremble with fear. No midnight trip to the bathroom (his preferred safe spot), no piling of pillows and blankets that he could paw into a nest, no holding his quivering body until the noise was all over and he could fall into an exhausted sleep. I'm so glad he didn't have to suffer through one more storm.

And this morning, a gorgeous day begins. I'm out early enough to catch the colors before sunrise and to see layers of lit-up clouds. The early birds are excited, too—red-winged blackbirds, mockingbirds, red-shouldered hawks that are sparring as they enter into mating season. So much is unfurling and lush. All the clovers are thick and starting to flower, and the cleavers are prickly as they start to sprout up from the ground. Pecan trees are loaded with buds, and the sycamore leaves are just unfolding, knitted together this morning with spider silk that is beaded with leftover rain.

I head off down the levee, listening to the eagles whistle from the woods. I'd love to take a photo of them wheeling overhead, but so far they're staying hidden in their batture home.

After taking a few sky photos, I shift my gaze downward to the growth underfoot. Along the roadside, the fleabane is already tall, and its white and pinkish flowers are bright and open. Spiderwort is already on its second show of blue flowers and tender stems. The peppergrass is going crazy—

a foot tall, at least, and the hairy bittercress is delicate, lit up with first sun. And finally, the Venus' looking glass I've been keeping my eye on has stretched up over the clovers, and its first perfect purply-blue flowers are opening up. I love waiting for it to bloom. For a while, the stems get tall, and the little, rounded, cuplike leaves decorate the stems. But in late spring, their real show begins. It's a slow show, though, because the flowers seem a little shy. Only one or two blossoms will open at a time, even though the stem often has several buds. Still, it is kind of stupendous. And from what I've been reading lately, it's not only beautiful but full of healing potential as well.

According to the research, the plant has several medicinal properties and has been used by Indigenous cultures for various health problems. The chemical compounds in *Triodanis* are known to be anti-inflammatory, antimicrobial, antioxidant, decongestant, expectorant, and immune boosting, as well as calming for the nervous system. Lately, I've wanted to make a small harvest to try out the plant, and today, with no rain, I have a chance to do that. Breaking off a long flower-tipped stem, I nibble a leaf and find it to be tender and a bit sour, with a lingering taste. I've heard that it can be cooked up with veggie dishes, and I might decide to try that soon.

As I work at making a small harvest of the herb, I hear the eagles start their morning calls; suddenly, they're overhead! This morning, one adult and one juvenile sail by, but one day recently, I sat on the patio and watched as seven eagles soared over the levee in slow, loopy circles. Now, I'm so happy to be out in time to see them. Having them close to home is one of my favorite things about living near the river. I know that they were threatened not so many years ago, but Louisiana has done a good job of protecting them and their habitat, and their numbers are rising. That's a good thing for us all, I think.

By the time I've picked a small handful of the plant and turn to head home, my shoes are sopping wet from all the rain puddles, and the eagles have disappeared into the woods. But it's been a happy and productive morning, seeing two of my favorite bits of local wildness. I guess that, other than timing, the eagles and the Venus' looking glass don't have much in common. One is tiny, the other huge. One is abundant, and the other kind of rare. One could be ignored (at least until it blooms), and the other has a Big Place in the life of the batture woods. But they arrive at the same time, make their big push together, and give me yet another reason to love spring.

Other Names: *Triodanis perfoliata,* clasping leaf Venus' looking-glass, clasping bellwort, round-leaved *triodanis.*

Parts Used: Whole plant.

Medicinal Properties: Anti-inflammatory, antimicrobial, antioxidant, decongestant, expectorant, immune system support.

Uses: Internal—Bronchitis, colds, coughs, sore throat; bloating, digestive upsets; anxiety, stress; infections; inflammation. External—Minor skin irritations, wounds.

Risks: Generally safe, though should be used with a health care practitioner's guidance if taking antidepressants, or in the presence of liver disease.

Description: The herb may grow to a height of 4–18 inches. It has a central, unbranched, lightly hairy stem with alternate leaves that clasp the stem. Leaves are light green, rounded, up to 1 inch long. Leaf edges are scalloped and shell-shaped. Both the stem and the leaves contain a milky sap. On upper stem, one to three flowers emerge from leaf axils, although only one to two of flowers will be blooming at any one time. Flowers are wheel- or bell-shaped and have petals that are violet to blue in color, and approximately 0.5 inch wide. They have five-lobed corollas and are radially symmetrical. Plant produces a small, many-seeded capsule with two to three sections for fruit.

Habitat: Disturbed areas, sandy or gravelly soils, prairies, pastures. Fibrous roots have the capacity to stabilize disturbed soils.

Distribution: Most parishes, with exception of extreme southeast tip of the state.

Plant Status: Native.

Animal Use: Common visitors to the flowers include little carpenter bees, plasterer bees, green metallic bees, bumblebees, flies, small butterflies, and skippers. Small mammals may consume the seeds, but they are not an important food source.

Natural History: The common name supposedly originates from a tale about the goddess Venus, who misplaces her magic mirror, which ends up in the hands of a shepherd boy. He becomes so entranced with seeing his enchanted reflection that Venus has to wrest it back from him, and the mirror shatters, leaving shards everywhere, each one turning into a bellflower where it landed. Another tale is that the shepherd boy saw his reflection in one of the plant's tiny, shiny seeds.

Designation: Native American tribal remedy for Cherokee and Meskwaki. In plant symbolism, the herb is known for evoking beauty and love, inviting reflection and clarity, and protection against the evil eye.

Cultivation: Prefers well-draining, loamy soil, but can tolerate a range of soil types and thrives best in moderately nutrient-rich soil. Watering should be done sparingly. Does not like to be waterlogged and can tolerate dry conditions. Prefers full sun and moderate temperatures. To propagate, sow seeds by pressing directly onto the soil in early spring. The seeds require light to germinate, so do not cover them with soil.

Remedy Form: Tea, tincture, compress, poultice, salve, wash.

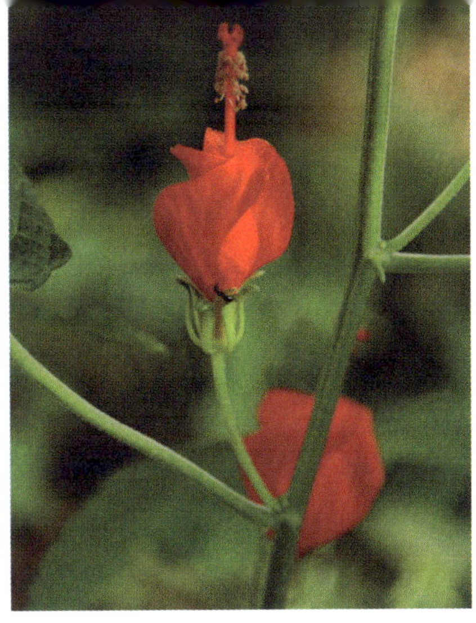

WAX MALLOW & THE PASSALONG PLANTS

SPRING

Wax mallow
(*Malvaviscus arboreus*)

I first heard about the "passalong plants" from my cousin Jara. I wasn't sure what she meant by the phrase, but then she pointed out some of the things in her garden that had come from someone else's yard as an example. I thought back to times when, as a child, I'd help my mom to garden, and how many of her flowers and shrubs had started out somewhere else. Grandma's rain lilies, Miss T's agapanthus, Dr. Allen's baby pines were right at home in our garden, where my mom helped them to take root and thrive in their new surroundings.

I liked the idea. I figured that most plants had originally started out in the wild, and so they should be good at reorienting and making a new home. They could draw on their ancient species memory and settle right in. And if I think about it, I've been doing that all my adult life as well. I envy the gorgeous color of an iris growing in a friend's yard and beg a few rhizomes for my own garden. One morning when I was out weeding in the hibiscus bed, a man driving by stopped to chat about his own hibiscus and then reached into his truck and pulled out a few babies he'd just dug up. He'd originally gotten the plant from Ms. Betsy, he said, and they'd done well, so he wanted to share. Even though she'd passed away, he was happy to keep her flowers going.

Apparently, passing along plants is a practice that gained popularity in southern states during the Civil War, when a shipping embargo limited access to other sources. But I imagine that sharing garden plants has been going on as long as people have been growing them intentionally. It's a way to share what we love and to keep another gardener's cherished plant alive and thriving even after they're gone. For decades, a tiny, all-green sweetheart rose hybridized by my grandfather and his sister was kept going in the yards of various cousins. I'm pretty sure I have a slip of one continuing on the tradition in my flower bed right now. And today, I'm off to "borrow" a snippet of my sister's Turk's cap hibiscus so I can introduce it into my garden and use it for healing in the future.

Even though it is early March; the air is chilly and the sky is gray, and wind gusts have us all wearing jackets. But despite the cold, I'm excited to be helping my sister in her garden. I've kept an envious eye on her very tall wax mallow "tree" for a couple of years. Though the branches are thin, the shrub towers over us and leans down across her yard. My sister would like it trimmed up a bit, and I've just recently learned more about the many medicinal properties of this herb. I am hoping to gather leaves to try for tea. But when we get out to the spot where it grows, we run into trouble. Apparently, the recent unusual freeze has stunned the shrub, and all the leaves are gone. I have heard that most of the time the plant can recover from cold spells, so I'm not too worried about this one. But I'll have to come back another time for leaves and flowers. And later in the year, once it produces fruit, I'll be over to gather a few of the small berries as well. Apparently, all parts of this *Malvaviscus* are not only medicinal but are nontoxic edibles as well. And they're loved by hummingbirds and other pollinators who are attracted to the bright-red, dangling blossoms—yet another good reason to introduce the tree to my yard.

Instead of gathering leaves, we set to work at trimming back the rangy branches. And instead of composting the bits we've cut off, I grab a handful to take home. Late spring and early summer are the best times to start cuttings, so even though I won't be getting leaves to use for tea, I'll have another job instead—tucking these bits of twigs into small pots of new soil and then waiting over the next couple of weeks for them to sprout.

Like many of its *Hibiscus* family relatives, *Malvaviscus* has several important healing properties and can be used for a number of physical conditions. Its demulcent, antibacterial, and soothing compounds make it useful for gastritis and other digestive disturbances internally, and externally a compress or poultice of crushed leaves and flowers can be used on burns, sores, and wounds. It has been proven to help relieve flu symptoms including fevers, sore throat, cough, and cold. And the plant has been used for helping to regulate blood sugar in diabetes and to help alleviate menstrual cramps and benign prostatic hyperplasia as well.

With so many healing properties, and such attractive flowers, I imagine that this beautiful native shrub will continue to be a beloved garden addition. It's nice to keep a native plant going in yards. And maybe once folks learn more about its healing properties, it will move toward the top of the list of popular "passalongs" in the state. I'm pretty sure it will become one of my favorites. And once this shrubby herb here starts its spring growth, I'm looking forward to brewing a drink of the flowers and leaves to use as an iced tea as the weather warms. For now, I've had a fun and productive time with my sister and gained an armload of small, thin twigs to take home and sprout—a pretty good outcome, I'd say. So, even on a gray and chilly day, there's healing all around.

Other Names: *Malvaviscus arboreus* var. *drummondii,* Turk's cap hibiscus, Drummond's Turk's cap, wax mallow, red mallow, Texas mallow, Mexican apple, manzanilla, sleeping hibiscus, bleeding hearts, ladies' eardrops, Scotchman's purse, wild fuchsia, manzanita-de-pollo.

Parts Used: Leaves, flowers, fruits, stems, roots.

Medicinal Properties: Antibacterial, anticancer, anticonvulsant, antidiabetes/antihyperglycemic, anti-inflammatory, antimicrobial, antioxidant, antiseptic, demulcent, emmenagogue, emollient, hepatoprotective.

Uses: Internal—Bronchitis, cough, colds, fevers, flu, sore throat, tonsillitis; diarrhea, dysentery, gastritis, liver and gallbladder issues, gallstones, stomachaches; kidney diseases, cystitis; hypertension; benign prostatic hyperplasia (BPH), menstrual cramps. External—Burns, canker sores, wounds, nosebleeds.

Risks: All parts of the plant are considered to be edible.

Description: A spreading shrub that grows 2–10 feet in height and is often as broad as it is tall. Blossoms are 2–3 inches long, bright red, and occur as pendant or drooping hibiscus-like flowers that are never fully open. Petals overlap to form a loose tube with the staminal column protruding. It is said to resemble a Turkish turban, leading to one of its common names. Leaves are alternate, stalked, broadly cordate to ovate-cordate, and are 2.3–4.5 inches long and up to 4 inches wide. Flowers are borne singly at leaf axils. Red fruit is smaller than 1 inch wide, matures in fall, and looks like a tiny tomato.

Habitat: Sandy, low ground near streams, limestone slopes around wooded creeks, palm groves, but will adapt to and thrive in many different sites, including full sun and heavy soil. Unremitting sun will cause its leaves to become rougher, smaller, darker, and puckered.

Distribution: Scattered around the state (in approximately thirty parishes), except for extreme southern parishes.

Plant Status: Native.

Animal Use: Visited by hummingbirds and butterflies. Resistant to damage by deer.

Natural History: A gallery forest species found at prairie forest interface. Grows on prairie soils of the southwest and in the northern part of the state. It ranges across the Gulf Coast from Florida to Texas.

Designation: Folkloric herbal remedy, South and Central American remedy. Many *Hibiscus* species have been found to contain medicinal properties and have a history of uses in many healing traditions.

Cultivation: Widely cultivated as an ornamental plant. Softwood cuttings taken in late spring or summer root easily. Prefers partial sun to shade and well-drained soil. Cut stems down to 6 inches above ground in late winter before spring growth begins. Can be pruned during the growing season. Drought-tolerant once established, and moderately salt-tolerant. Can also be started from seeds or root division.

Remedy Form: Tea, tincture, compress, poultice, wash, edible.

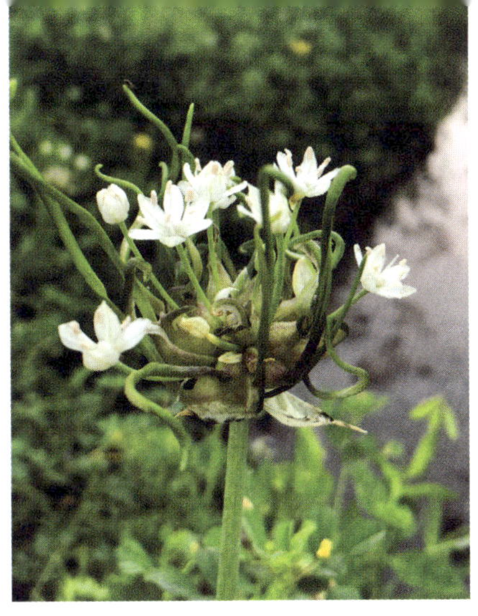

WILD ONION & THE NEIGHBOR'S KIDS

SPRING

Wild onion
[*Allium* sp.]

This morning, Bodi and I trek through the long, wet yard and up to the levee just as early light seeps into the sky. Pebbly clouds glow rose, then orange and fiery red. I stop to take photos while Bodi sniffs at nearby scent trails left by wild critters in the night. The air is cool, in the low fifties, and damp after spring rains. No walkers are out yet, so we have the place to ourselves. Red-shouldered hawks call to each other and then sail from nearby treetops toward the batture woods. The usual clovers are spongy underfoot and, lately, joined by wild *Geranium* and butterweed and the first wild onions. Soon the town mowing crews will start to pass by, and the air will smell like onions everywhere they cut.

Lately, the neighbor's two boys have been asking me if the wild onions are ready to pick. Their mother likes to use them for salads and soups, and there's a healthy crop of them lining my back field. The boys were hoping they could harvest bunches of them to give to their mom.

Knowing that there are some plants that look like wild onions but are actually somewhat toxic, I did a little research to make sure my onions were safe. According to field guides, there are several species of wild onions that grow in Louisiana, and they can look very much alike. One plant that is similar in appearance is known as crow poison, or *Nothoscordum bivalve.* But it has no garlic or onion smell when picked. And that is the biggest clue to that plant's potential toxicity.

This time of year, the wild onions look like tall, thin spikes of green. But later, the flowers and little bulbs will appear, making it a little easier to identify them.

Garden onions and garlic and their wild *Allium* cousins have numerous health benefits and have been used in many cultures and areas for their healing properties. I once had a woman from Panama in a class I taught, and she mentioned that her mother always had an "onion-honey syrup" going on the kitchen countertop. Instead of cooking the onions down in the honey, she just sliced the peeled vegetable into thin rounds, packed them down into a jar, and poured local honey over them. She put the lid on the jar, then set it aside, coming back every few days to stir the mixture. A week or two later, the juices from the onions had mixed with the honey, and if anyone in the family had a health issue—colds, the onset of flu, or coughs—they would be dosed by her mom with a teaspoon of the mix. It helped for many minor illnesses, the woman said, and the kids loved the taste. They often pretended to feel ill so they could have some.

And Panamanian culture isn't the only one to recognize the health benefits of the onion and garlic family. Traditional Chinese medicine and Ayurvedic healing both have much praise for and use of the *Allium.* And many Indigenous cultures included the plants in daily diets and in herbal remedies.

One of my favorite things about this plant family is how easy it is to use. Many times, when my children were sick with an earache, I'd just peel a small clove of homegrown garlic or a bulblet of the wild onion plant and insert it loosely in the afflicted ear. We'd let that stay in place for ten minutes or so and repeat this several times a day. The kids weren't that happy about having to lie in bed with a garlic clove in their ear and complained about smelling like spaghetti sauce, but the effects were pretty impressive.

In recent decades, medical science has proven that the *Allium* family of plants have many healing properties. Physicians and dietitians recommend that we consume onions and garlic and their relatives often in our daily meals and tout their many healing properties. Cardiovascular support, helping to lower cholesterol and other blood lipids, potential cancer prevention, antiasthmatic and decongestant properties, and antibacterial, antiviral actions are just a few of the proven healing effects of this family of plants. Really, thinking about all the health benefits the *Allium* offer makes me want to gather my own supply of the wild herbs in front of us and to add more onions and garlic to my daily meals.

As Bodi and I turn around to go home, the neighborhood boys race out to greet us. Bodi is ecstatic, and the boys are happy to see us and to romp with him for a while. I let them know that the wild onions will be ready soon. But they want to experiment right now! So I tell them how to make sure the plants are the right species (strong oniony smell and taste), then break off a few thin leaves. We stand around sampling the plants. We all decide that (a) it is definitely onion and (b) it's maybe a little too strong-flavored to consume raw and in large amounts. But they're eager to pick some for their mom, even before the little bulbs appear, and B and I leave them happily harvesting as we head into the house. Inside, I decide to start work on a big batch of onion soup for later today and to go back out again for another handful of these wild offerings to add to the pot. I can't wait to eat the "wild soup" once it's ready. I imagine it will be pretty tasty.

Species: Three species of *Allium—Allium canadense, Allium canadense* var. *canadense,* and *Allium canadense* var. *mobilensis*—grow wild in Louisiana and have been proven to have healing properties. All can be used interchangeably and are described together as follows.

Other Names: Meadow garlic, meadow onion, ail du Canada, wild onion, and Canada garlic have been used to describe all three species.

Parts Used: Whole plant.

Medicinal Properties: Antiasthmatic, antibiotic, antidiabetic, anti-inflammatory, antimicrobial (bacteria, fungi, viruses, and parasites), anti-obesity, cardioprotective, carminative, diuretic, expectorant, immune system support.

Uses: Internal—Cough, cold, croup, chest congestion or infection, headache; atherosclerosis; digestive disturbances; immune support. External—Ear infection, insect stings, coughs, colds.

Risks: Make sure that the plant is actually a wild *Allium*/wild onion or garlic. If your sense of smell isn't keen, have someone else check out the plant for you.

Description: All plants occur as sparse cluster of grasslike leaves that originate near the base. A flowering stalk of 8–12 inches rises from a bulb and is topped by a dome-like cluster of star-shaped, white or pinkish flowers. *A. canadense* has tight clumps of soft, linear, not hollow, keeled leaves with a distinctly onion-like smell. The bulbs are 0.3–1 inch long and have a fibrous outer coat with diamond-shaped spaces between the nerves. Flowers are white or pinkish and are often replaced by bulblets. *A. canadense* var. *canadense* has a round, smooth, flowering stem that grows up to 24 inches tall. Leaves are 6–15 inches long and curve upward and outward, supported by a keel on the blade. Leaves are flat except for the keel, solid and grasslike. Flowering stem is solitary, begins with a white, sack-like cover that splits open to expose rounded cluster of flowers and/or stalkless bulblets. *A. canadense* var. *mobilensis* has hollow stem 6–8 inches long and three or more basal leaves equally long and 0.125 inch wide. Flowers are pink, fading with age, and there are no bulblets. Each of the above should have a strong, onion-like odor.

Habitat: Open woods, prairies, meadows, thickets, fields, forests, and lawns.

Distribution: *A. canadense* and *A. canadense* var. *canadense,* most of the state; *A. canadense* var. *mobilensis,* concentrated in central, western, and northern parishes.

Plant Status: Native.

Animal Use: Bulbs and leaves are eaten by wild turkeys. Flowers produce nectar and pollen for many varieties of bees and flies. Cows may use the plants as forage, but this can affect the taste of milk or meat if used for food.

Natural History: *Allium* is an ancient name for garlic that is thought to be derived from the Celtic word *all,* which means "pungent."

Designation: Chinese medicine herb, African American remedy, Ayurvedic medicine remedy. In many healing traditions, the plant is felt to be edible and nutritious. Some Native American tribes used various species.

Cultivation: Start plants from bulblets, root division (in fall), and/or seeds. Larger bulblets germinate better than smaller ones.

Remedy Form: Internal—Edible, tea, syrup, tincture, capsules. External—Application of raw clove, oil, poultice, wash.

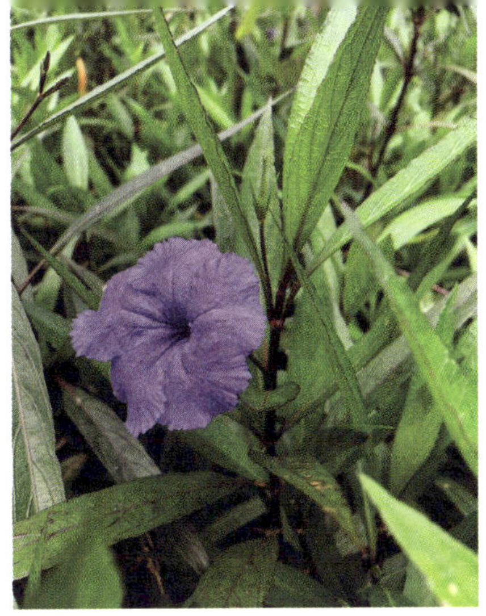

WILD PETUNIA & THE RAGGEDY GARDEN

EARLY FALL

Wild petunia
[*Ruellia* sp.]

There are some people who think a garden should be tidy. I agree, in theory. But it never happens at my house. No matter how hard I work at the beginning of the season, how much I plan and hoe and weed, my garden is always a tangle. By fall, it's hard to tell where any row once started and ended, or what exactly the primary crop was supposed to be, or what's worth saving and what isn't worth trying again. This summer's successes were dahlias and—chickweed! Neighbors came by often to pick the flowers, and some of the chickweed went into tinctures and teas; the rest of it was tumbled into the compost pile. It will certainly be back next year. The problem is, I can't bring myself to put poison on the plants I'm going to eat or use for healing, so I'm just stuck with messiness, I guess.

After decades of trying to get better at gardening, though, I've made some progress. I know how to prepare the soil. I know that if I do a better job of cleaning up the beds in autumn and layering in some compost to set through the cooler months, the spring garden will be healthier and new seedlings will get a good start. So I try. And I make some compromises. I told a neighbor recently that I've decided my garden is actually a lawn with some flowers and veggies thrown in, which is pretty much true. It turns out that my enthusiasm far outweighs my skill. And that might be okay.

This morning I trek out to see how things are going as we head into fall. The borage has given up trying to stand straight and is trailing over the side of its raised bed to tangle into the last of the green beans. The tired tomato vines are woven into the tall but fading dill, and what's left of the dahlias are shading the late basil that is getting ready to flower. The feral sunflowers are seeding into the squash bed. And the weeds—they're doing just fine.

And some other good things are happening. Despite my messiness, the bees are deliriously happy in the anise hyssop, the hummingbirds keep coming to feed on the fading *Lobelia* on their way down south, and the wild petunia is looking gorgeous.

I wrangled with what turned out to be *Ruellia* when I first returned to Louisiana. At that point, I was bent on having a tidy garden. I allowed a few "wildlings" to stay—the milkweeds could host monarch butterflies and the wild *Hibiscus* put on a colorful show, so they could stay put. But once I started weeding, I was intent. And that's when I discovered the nemesis of my garden plan. One weedy species kept coming back no matter how often I pulled it up. The leaves were kind of wrinkly, soft to the touch, but when I tried pulling the plant up by its roots, it wouldn't budge. Even when I yanked hard, the plant would just snap off at ground level and sprout back up again days later. Then, when I had been away from home for a short trip, I came back to find the plant sporting pretty lavender flowers. It turned out to be *Ruellia*—the wild petunia. Since the plant wouldn't go away, I did some research on it and was astounded by its numerous healing properties. And that's when I realized that the old adage about herbs appearing where and when you need them might indeed be true.

While not used in herbal commerce, *Ruellia* species have a long list of medicinal benefits. Research in various countries, over time, has proven the plant to have strong anti-inflammatory properties, and to be antioxidant, anodyne, antiseptic, diuretic, and diaphoretic. Its anti-inflammatory activity was noted to be similar to that of indomethacin, a well-known and commonly used drug for pain relief, and it has been shown to block the body's perception of pain. In various cultures, species of the plant have been used for bladder inflammation, bronchitis, constipation, fevers, and coughs. All of this is intriguing, especially as I struggle with arthritis in recent years. If this snarky and persistent "weed" just won't go away, I might try using it.

This experience made me decide to revisit my idea of what gardening is all about. Maybe a garden is not just something you create—it can also be something you discover. A garden has a life of its own, after all. It can't exclude nature but instead needs it, hosts it, includes it, in order to thrive. For who can imagine a garden without butterflies or bees, or all the surrounding vegetation and its host of soil?

I guess I have to get used to complexities. If science has only begun to examine and understand the many medicinal properties of some *Ruellia* species, and yet acknowledges that they offer much promise and healing, how can we imagine that we can totally understand and "manage" the lands that give space to our gardens?

Sometimes there are things we just don't know.

For now, I'm happy to host the pushy wild petunia—give it its own space and wait to see how this garden journey goes. Maybe instead of a tidy plot, I'll have a half-wild garden, where bees and butterflies and other tiny creatures can go about their own natural ways. Maybe I can learn how to cultivate a garden where every plant, and every critter, can feel at home. It sounds kind of complicated, and pretty messy, and probably not even very practical. But I'm willing to try.

Species: Several species of *Ruellia* occur in the state and will occasionally interbreed, making exact identification challenging. Those species with documented medicinal properties include the following:

Ruellia caroliniensis

Other Names: Carolina wild petunia.

Description: An unbranched, spreading perennial producing a profusion of trumpet-shaped, petunia-like, light-purple flowers borne in axillary clusters of two to four. Blossoms have a slender corolla tube and five petal-like lobes. Leaves are distinctly petioled and spreading.

Habitat: Dry woods, sandy fields, and rock crevasses.

Distribution: Top two-thirds of the state, scattered otherwise.

Plant Status: Native.

Cultivation: Prefers full to partial shade and grows best in well-drained soils. Very drought-tolerant. May be propagated by seed or cuttings and readily reseeds itself.

Ruellia humilis

Other Names: Prairie petunia, fringeleaf wild petunia, low ruellia, hairy ruellia, low wild petunia.

Description: Upright or slightly sprawling plants grow up to 1 foot tall, occasionally branching. Stems are light green and covered with white hairs. Opposing leaves are up to 2.5 inches long and 1 inch wide, and broadly lanceolate, deltoid, or ovate in form. They are light green to green, with smooth margins, and are covered with white hairs on both the upper and lower sides. The leaves also have hairy petioles. Flowers are light lavender or purple, funnel-shaped with five spreading lobes, and are 1.5–2 inches long. The short, tubular calyx has five long, linear teeth, and is green and hairy, like the leaves.

Habitat: Open forests, savannas, prairies, and old fields.

Distribution: Throughout Louisiana (except in the Mississippi River floodplain and the coastal parishes) and the eastern parts of Texas.

Plant Status: Native

Cultivation: Plants grow best in dry, sandy soils with a pH of 6–7.5. Seeds germinate easily in cold/moist or cold/dry stratification. Pods or stems can be collected in late summer and placed in paper bags. Plant seeds fresh in the fall or store dry seeds in a refrigerator and plant in early spring. Cuttings taken in late spring and summer should be dipped in rooting hormone and rooted under mist or in shade.

Ruellia noctiflora

Other Names: Nightflowering wild petunia.

Description: A perennial herb with slender, hairy, purplish stems 12–16 inches tall. Leaves are 1.5–2 inches long, opposite, oval with pointed tips, and with very short or no leaf stalks. Flowers are up to 4 inches across, glistening white, with five spreading petals; the tube and throat are more than 3 inches long; sepals are 0.5–1 inch long, very narrow, persisting around the base of the fruit as it develops. Flowers open at night, then fall off by midmorning. Fruit is an oval capsule, 0.8 inch long, with a long, persistent style. The plant is considered globally vulnerable and is listed as endangered in Florida. Its primary threats are fire suppression and habitat loss.

Habitat: Moist to wet flatwoods and savannas, low, wet hammocks.

Distribution: St. Tammany Parish.

Plant Status: Native. The plant is considered critically imperiled due to very low occurrence both in the state and in the U.S. It should not be harvested or removed from its site.

Cultivation: Prefers full sun to partial shade and moderate moisture. Can tolerate a variety of soil types, including clay, sand, or loam, and can be propagated by seeds, stem cuttings, or division.

Ruellia nudiflora

Other Names: Violet wild petunia.

Description: Plants are erect, 1–2 feet tall, with few branches. Leaves are opposing, 2–5 inches long, narrowed at the base, on short stems. Gray-green leaves have curly or wavy-toothed margins. Atop the plant are several trumpet-shaped, purplish blossoms that are nearly 2 inches across at the opening. Terminal panicle of flowers.

Habitat: Dry to moist soils, weedy roadsides.

Distribution: Concentrated in southeastern tip, and also in a few scattered parishes (Jefferson, Lafayette, Lafourche, Morehouse, Natchitoches, Orleans, Plaquemines, Pointe Coupee, St. Bernard, St. Charles, St. John the Baptist, Vermilion).

Plant Status: Native.

Cultivation: It will grow almost anywhere and has been used as a groundcover because of its hardiness and tolerance of a broad range of growing conditions. It is easily transplanted, requires no fertilization, and grows well in dry to moist soil and in shade, partial shade, or full sun. Spreads extensively by seed and can become quite aggressive and is often considered a weed.

Ruellia pedunculata

Other names: Stalked wild petunia.

Description: Leaves are dark green, opposite, lance-shaped, about 6–12 inches long, and approximately 0.5–1 inch wide, veins prominent below, margins smooth or wavy. Flowers are pedunculate, trumpet-shaped, 1.5–2 inches wide, and are solitary or borne in clusters at the tips of the stems, usually purple, but white and pink forms exist.

Habitat: Dry or rocky upland woods, open woods, and along streams.

Distribution: Top two-thirds of the state, also a few central and eastern parishes.

Plant Status: Native.

Cultivation: Plant seeds fresh in the fall or store dry seeds in refrigerator and plant in early spring. Cuttings taken in late spring and summer should be dipped in rooting hormone and rooted under mist or in shade.

Ruellia simplex

Other Names: Softseed wild petunia, Britton's wild petunia, Mexican petunia.

Description: The plant is an herbaceous perennial that is shrubby with a woody base and somewhat aggressive. Plant grows to 3–4 feet tall in the wild. It has linear, dark-green leaves that are not hairy and may be tinged with purple, and measure 6–12 inches long and 0.75 inch wide. Flowers are petunia-like, lavender to violet, and only last one day. It is evergreen in warm climates.

Habitat: Grows in a wide variety of habitats but produces more capsules in wet areas.

Distribution: The plant is widely cultivated and naturalized in the state.

Plant Status: Introduced.

Cultivation: Readily reseeds and spreads by rhizomes. Easily propagated but should not be included in restoration or native plantings. It is frost-intolerant, and temperature limits its range. It can become weedy and should be avoided even as a garden perennial.

For All Species, Other Names: Various species may be known as wild petunia.

Parts Used: Whole plant.

Medicinal Properties: Analgesic, antidiabetic, antihyperlipidemic, antihypertensive, anti-inflammatory, antinociceptive, antioxidant, gastroprotective, hepatoprotective.

Uses: Internal—Arthritis, pain; asthma, bronchitis, colds, coughs, fevers, respiratory infections; bladder inflammation, cystitis; blood sugar imbalances; cardiovascular support; antihyperlipidemic; constipation; eczema; fluid retention, influenza.

Risks: Should be avoided in pregnancy.

Animal Use: In general, *Ruellia* species are attractive to long-tongued bees, butterflies, and hummingbirds. Somewhat unpalatable to deer, rabbits, and cattle. Squirrels, tortoises, and chickens may feed on leaves and flower petals.

Natural History: Native to Central America and naturalized in numerous countries in tropical South Asia and Southeast Asia. The genus *Ruellia* was named for the French physician and botanist Jean Ruelle (1474–1537), herbalist and physician to Francis I of France and translator of several works of Dioscorides.

Designation: Folkloric herbalism, Ayurvedic medicine. Some species occur in Indonesia, Malaysia, Africa, Brazil, Central America, and Pakistan, and are used as medicinal plants.

Remedy Form: Internal—Tea, tincture. External—Compress, poultice, wash.

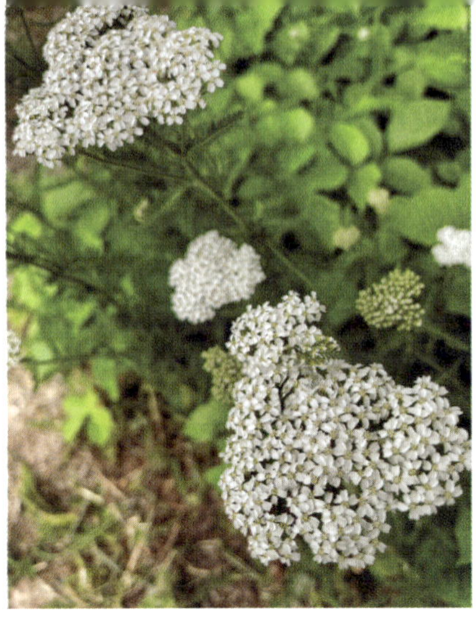

YARROW & THE PIG FARM

EARLY SUMMER

Yarrow
(*Achillea millefolium*)

It's a lovely early summer morning for a walk, with blue skies and the air not too hot yet, thanks to a slight breeze. Fog lies heavy over the fields but is rising with bright sun. A few cars pass by, and the air rings with birdsong—many newly hatched babies waiting to be fed. I'm off to explore a new side road I passed by recently but haven't had time to check out. Yesterday I spotted a small pig farm down the lane, and today I'm off to see if I can get closer for a visit.

The usual wildflowers and herbs are lush and blooming along the trail—horsetail is tall and thick, the ever-present cleavers tangle close to the road, much yellow flax is in flower, the vetch is deep purple with bloom. Many wild roses are open and fragrant, and in the midst of them, I spot one of the first plants I used as a student herbalist—yarrow, lush with flowers. I haven't seen this here often around my house, but my little trek to see the pigs has led me to it. I read somewhere that if you had to choose just one plant to use for healing, it should be yarrow.

My first experience of harvesting and using yarrow was for a moderately high fever. I had learned that yarrow was a diaphoretic and a febrifuge and would cause a mild sweat to help relieve that condition. Since the herb was also known as an anti-inflammatory, it seemed reasonable to me that it would work, so I tried it out as a tea. The brew was not terribly tasty—slightly bitter, but not too bad. And the results took only a few hours to occur.

Since then, I've learned about yarrow's other healing properties, and have used it both internally and externally for several health issues. As an antiseptic and wound healer, it's a great herb to use either as a compress or salve for cuts, wounds, minor burns, and insect bites. In fact, the plant's Latin name—*Achillea millefolium*—came from its reported history of use by the warrior Achilles, in Homer's *Iliad,* who applied the plant externally to wounds of soldiers and found it a good healing remedy. Internally, the plant has been used over centuries for helping with heavy menstrual cycles, gastrointestinal distress and ulcers, bladder infections, and muscle cramps and spasms. I pick a few flowering stems of the plant, hoping to bring them home to dry for tea.

In the cane field along the road, two men work side by side and stop to wave. As I get closer to the pig enclosure, I see that there are only about a dozen of them, probably one family's herd. One pig looks up as I get close—but none of them seem concerned about my presence. I guess if I had something interesting to eat, they might be more curious. Instead, they grunt and shove past each other in the squishy, dark mud, rooting around for whatever feed is left after the farmer's early visit. I feel a little bad for them—it seems that all their food is mud covered, and the low pond that is their only obvious water source looks scummy and foul. I wish I had something to give them to help out—I hate thinking that this might be the whole of their life.

I've always loved pigs, though I'm not sure why, since I've only actually met a few of them in person. But there's something about their kind of goofy "smile" that I like. I worked once with a woman who raised pigs for her family's food. She introduced me to a few—they were huge, pretty friendly, and very strong. I learned some surprising things about them from her. For instance, pigs have hair! Bristly hairs cover their rounded backs, supposedly to deflect the sun's intensity so they don't sunburn too badly. And pigs are very intelligent. The artist Jamie Wyeth, who had a pet pig, thought that he could teach them to type if he had a typewriter big enough. Also, pigs don't stop growing when they reach adulthood. If they're not slaughtered, they grow so huge that their legs can't support them and just give out. And pigs can be pretty friendly, if treated well—in fact, some species make great pets.

But pigs present me with a conundrum because I love bacon and ribs! I don't eat pork very often, but even in the years I was a vegetarian, I never stopped craving it. I guess this is what journalist Michael Pollan means by the "omnivore's dilemma." I'm hoping that the pigs I've discovered this morning don't know that about me; probably they're too busy trying to find their own food to care.

I wish I had bought something for them to snack on. Maybe I could offer them yarrow, but I'm not sure it is safe for them. I've read that it can be good forage for small rodent pets but can be toxic to horses. In any case, I wouldn't want to harm my newly discovered neighbors.

I bid the pigs goodbye and head up the road toward home. On the way, I will pick more yarrow to dry for tea and will see what I can find out about its possibility for pig forage. Maybe I could bring the pigs a small yarrow snack when I come next. For now, I am happy to have a little neighborly visit and grateful for the yarrow and all the healing that nature offers.

I think about how much I love these things, and why plants and animals and all of these natural gifts matter so much to us all. I guess there's something about nature's unconditional generosity, her unique beauties and workings, and her exquisite vulnerability that remind us constantly that we are all part of so many small miracles. I know I need them—the yarrow, the chatty birds trying to feed chicks, the waters and lands, and even the quirky pigs that make up this remarkable life on Earth. For all of these, I am forever grateful.

Other Names: *Achillea millefolium,* milenrama, milfoil, western yarrow, bloodwort, carpenter's weed, hierba de las cortaduras, plumajillo, milenrama, woundwort.

Parts Used: Aerial parts.

Medicinal Properties: Astringent, anti-inflammatory, antiseptic, antispasmodic, carminative, cholagogue, diaphoretic, digestive stimulant, emmenagogue, stimulant, tonic, vasodilator, vulnerary.

Uses: Internal—Loss of appetite, indigestion or heartburn; bladder infection or difficult urination; bleeding; fevers, inflammation; irregular menstrual cycle or cramps, muscle spasms; ulcers. External—Cuts, insect bites, minor burns, wounds.

Risks: Check with a health care provider if using with anticoagulant medications. Extended use of this plant can cause allergic skin rashes or lead to photosensitivity in some people. Yarrow may enhance the sedative effects of other herbs (such as valerian, kava, chamomile, hops) and sedative drugs. Possible sedative and diuretic effects from ingesting large amounts.

Description: The plant has a simple, upright, hairy stem, usually under 3 feet tall. Flowers are typically white but may be pinkish or pale purple. The petals are densely arranged in flattened clusters, and leaves are fernlike or feathery in appearance. Plants produce a distinctive rosette at the base of old stems during the fall.

Habitat: Disturbed soil.

Distribution: Spotty throughout the state, more common in northern parishes.

Plant Status: Introduced.

Animal Use: Visited by many pollinators including numerous species of bees, wasps, butterflies, moths, and beetles.

Natural History: The cultivated plant has escaped from gardens and now occurs in disturbed soil nearly everywhere in the lower forty-eight states. The genus name *Achillea* is thought to stem from the plant's mention as a medicine by the character Achilles in Homer's *Iliad.*

Designation: Herb of commerce, Cajun traiteur remedy, Indigenous/Native American remedy, folk medicine herb, edible.

Cultivation: Propagation by division is easy and best for small-scale production. For larger-scale plantings, seeds are a reliable method of establishment. Thrives in full sun and in average, dry, or medium moisture. Avoid rich, moist soils. Good drainage is necessary. Low-maintenance; drought-, heat-, humidity-tolerant; and deer- and rabbit-resistant.

Remedy Form: Tea, tincture, compress, poultice, wash.

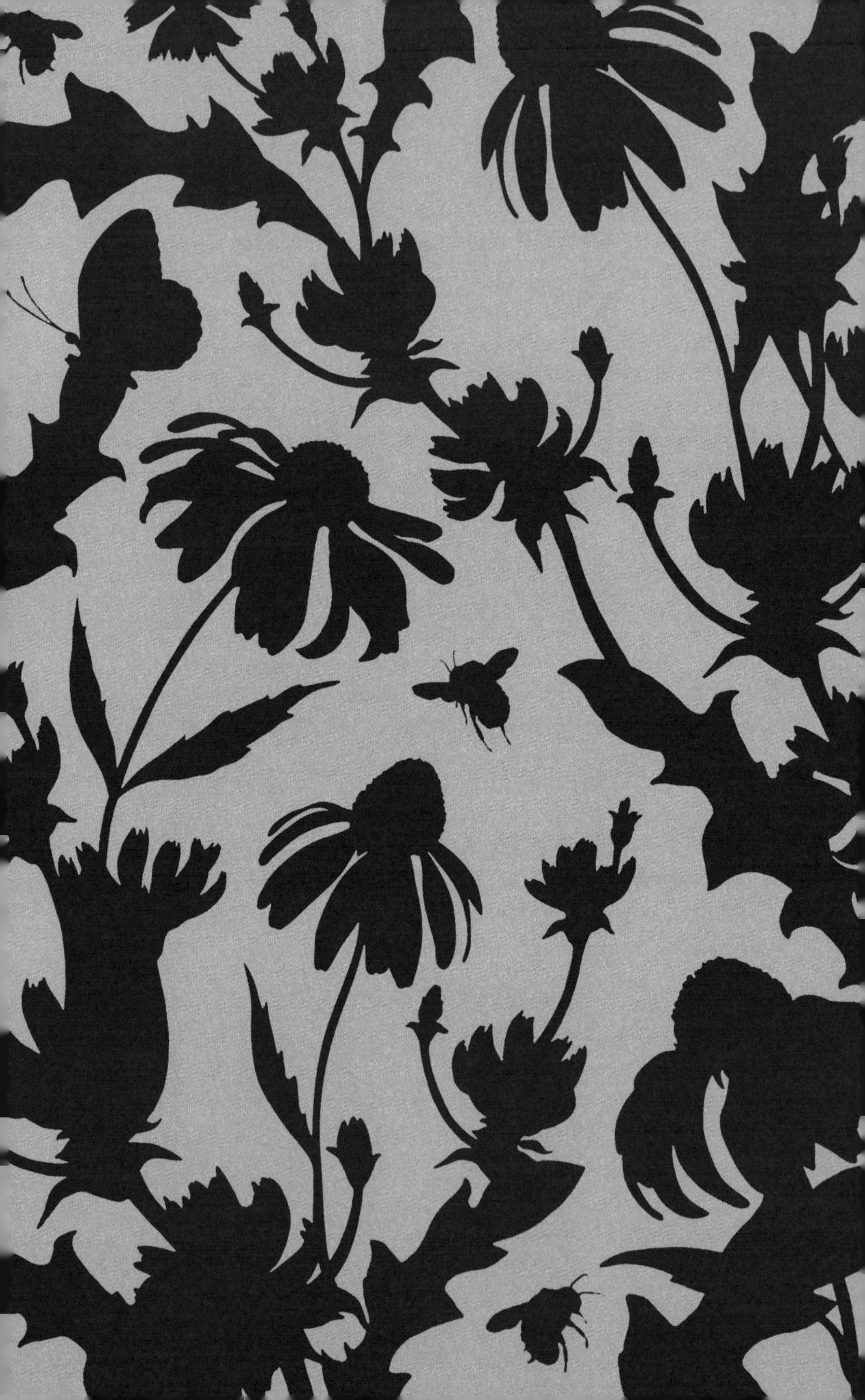

EPILOGUE

Jesuit's Bark and the Throwaway Coast

SPRING

At the end of the land in lower Montegut, I get out of the car and walk along the narrow road. Near a little bayou-side pond, dozens of shorebirds wade in shallow water, lift up in a cloud of feathers as I pass, then settle back down to feed. In the tattered rigging of an old shrimp boat, an osprey has built a nest that looks well-used and revisited. When I get close, the big bird shrieks at me, uncomfortable and edgy, so I move away.

A couple of fishermen stand in deep grass near the end of the land, tossing lines into the water. No luck so far, they say, but it's a good day to be out.

At the edge of the road, yellow sweet clover and giant ragweed and sow thistle are thick and lush, and orange lantana is blooming. Around my knees, Jesuit's bark is thick and tall. I'm happy to see it partly because it's a healing herb, but mostly because it helps to keep coastal soils in place.

I take a photo of the plants and soak up the wild silence, such a rare thing in these noisy, distracted times.

I stand on this narrow, sinking spit of land while the grasses shift in the breeze. I am happy, anxious, hopeful, sad. Before too long this place may crumble and wash away. But I will love it until its last salty breath, or until my own.

Amen.

GLOSSARY

Adaptogen—Moderates stress effects, increases resistance, and strengthens the immune system.
Alterative—Strengthens the body systems and restores health; assists in removing waste products.
Amphoteric—Helps to normalize functions of whole body or organ systems.
Analgesic—Relieves pain.
Anodyne—Mild pain reliever.
Antibacterial—Destroys bacteria.
Antibiotic—Kills or inhibits growth of bacteria or other organisms.
Anticoagulant—Inhibits the coagulation of blood.
Anticonvulsant—Reduces/relieves convulsions or spasms.
Antidepressant—Relieves or helps alleviate depression.
Antidiabetic—Helps to relieve diabetes.
Antidiarrheal—Helps to relieve diarrhea.
Antiemetic—Helps to stop vomiting.
Antifungal—Inhibits or kills fungi.
Antihistamine—Inhibits or neutralizes release of histamine.
Anti-inflammatory—Reduces inflammation of tissues.
Antilithic—Helps prevent and dissolve stones in the urinary tract.
Antimicrobial—Acts to kill or reduce microbes.
Antioxidant—Prevents cells from damage caused by free radicals, which may play a part in cancer, heart disease, stroke, and other diseases of aging.
Antipruritic—Prevents or relieves itching.
Antipyretic—Reduces fevers.
Antirheumatic—Reduces inflammation.
Antiseptic—Prevents sepsis or decay, usually by killing germs and microbes.

Antispasmodic—Reduces nervous or muscular spasms.
Antitumor—Reduces tumors.
Antitussive—Prevents or relieves cough.
Antiviral—Helps to reduce activity of a virus.
Anxiolytic—Reduces anxiety.
Aperient—Stimulates appetite.
Appetite suppressant—Reduces appetite.
Astringent—Constricts tissues, stops bleeding, draws wound edges together.
Ayurveda—India's traditional healing system, over three thousand years old. It is based on the understanding that health and wellness depend on an ever-shifting balance between the mind, body, and spirit.
Bach flower remedy—Solutions of brandy and water that contain extreme dilutions of flower material. System was developed by Edward Bach, an English homeopath, in the 1930s.
Bitter tonic—Stimulates appetite and digestive processes.
Blood purifier—Stimulates lymphatic system, prompting removal of waste products from bloodstream.
Calmative—Mild sedative.
Carminative—Relieves stomach or intestinal gas.
Cathartic—Promotes bowel movements.
Cholagogue—Stimulates gallbladder to release bile.
Counterirritant—Induces an inflammatory response in an area to promote healing.
Decongestant—Helps break up congestion.
Demulcent—Soothes irritated membranes (internal and external).
Depurative—Detoxifies body.
Diaphoretic—Increases sweating and may result in lowering fevers.
Digestive—Promotes the digestive process.
Diuretic—Stimulates urine flow.
Dysuria—Painful urination.
Eczema—Chronic skin disorder characterized by itching and redness.
Emetic—Induces vomiting.
Emmenagogue—Regulates menstruation.
Emollient—Soothes and protects skin.
Estrogenic—Promotes production of estrogen.

Expectorant—Helps to remove mucus from body.
Fatigue—Lingering tiredness that can be limiting and generalized.
Febrifuge—Reduces fevers.
Galactagogue—Increases production of breast milk.
Glycerite—Extract of an herb using glycerin as an extraction medium.
Hemostatic—Helps reduce flow of blood.
Hepatic—Affects liver function.
Herbs of commerce—Medicinal plants generally recognized as effective for various health issues and harvested or grown for sale in the herbal marketplace.
Homeopathy—Healing system based on the belief that the body can cure itself and that natural substances that would cause a symptom could actually heal it when used in tiny amounts.
Hyperglycemic—Raises blood sugar.
Hypertensive—Raises blood pressure.
Hypnotic—Nervous system relaxant that aids in restful sleep.
Hypoglycemic—Lowers blood sugar.
Hypotensive—Helps lower blood pressure.
Laxative—Loosens bowel contents, promoting evacuation.
Liniment—Topical preparation applied to skin for relief of pain and stiffness.
Lithotriptic—Helps break up urinary tract stones.
Lymphatic tonic—Aids in proper function of lymphatic tissues and system.
Mucilage—Naturally occurring substance in plants that soothes irritated and inflamed tissues.
Nervine—Supports nervous system.
Nutritive—Contains nutrients helpful for proper body system functions.
Oxytocic—Promotes production of oxytocin.
Purgative—Causes evacuation of intestinal contents.
Refrigerant—Cools body and thirst.
Relaxant—Relieves stress and muscle tension.
Resorbent—Promotes resorption of blood from bruising.
Rubefacient—Dilates local blood vessels and promotes blood supply in the area.
Sedative—Promotes soothing and relaxing effect.

Sialagogue—Induces saliva production.

Spasmolytic—Reduces spasms or cramps.

Stimulant—Increases organ or whole-body function over the short term.

Stomachic—Aids in stomach and digestive activity.

Styptic—Reduces bleeding when applied to a wound.

Sudorific—Induces perspiration.

Tonic—Supports proper function, strength, and tone of organ system or whole body.

Traditional Chinese medicine—Medical system from China that works to restore the body's balance and harmony through various methods, including the use of herbs and acupuncture.

Traiteur—Native Creole healer or a traditional healer of the French-speaking Houma Tribe, whose methods of treatment involve using prayer, laying on of hands, and medicinal plants.

Vasodilator—Dilates blood vessels.

Vermifuge—Expels intestinal worms.

Vulnerary—Acts to heal wounds.

REFERENCES

ASTER

Books

Moerman, Daniel E. *Native American Ethnobotany.* Portland, OR: Timber Press, 1998.

Shane, CoreyPine. *Southeast Medicinal Plants: Identify, Harvest, and Use 106 Wild Herbs for Health and Wellness.* Portland, OR: Timber Press, 2021.

Online

Orford, Emily-Jane Hills. "Homestead Stories: Beautiful Wild Asters Galore." *Insteading Blog,* September 6, 2023. https://insteading.com/blog/wild-asters/.

Rolnik, Agata, and Beata Olas. "The Plants of the *Asteraceae* Family as Agents in the Protection of Human Health." National Institutes of Health. March 16, 2021. https://pmc.ncbi.nlm.nih.gov/articles/PMC7999649/.

"*Symphotrichum dumosum*/Rice button aster." USGS.gov. https://warcapps.usgs.gov/PlantID/Species/Details/287.

"White Panicle Aster." Plants for a Future, Natural Medicinal Herbs. www.naturalmedicinalherbs.net/herbs/a/aster-lanceolatus=white-panicle-aster.php.

"Wild Asters Medicinal Uses." VI Farms. October 18, 2012. https://vifarms.wordpress.com/2012/10/18/wild-asters-medicinal-uses/.

BACOPA

Books

Bokelman, Jean M., M.D. *Medicinal Herbs in Primary Care: An Evidence-Guided Reference for Health Care Providers.* New York: Elsevier, 2022

Moerman, Daniel E. *Native American Ethnobotany.* Portland, OR: Timber Press, 1998.

Shane, CoreyPine. *Southeast Medicinal Plants: Identify, Harvest, and Use 106 Wild Herbs for Health and Wellness*. Portland, OR: Timber Press, 2021.

Online

Aguiar, Sebastian, and Thomas Borowski. "Neuropharmacological Review of the Nootropic Herb *Bacopa monnieri.*" NIH. August 2013. https://www.peirsoncenter

.com/uploads/6/0/5/5/6055321/rej.2013.1431.pdf#:~:text=This%20review%20synthesizes%20behavioral%20research%20with%20neuromolecular%20mechanisms,known%20as%20a%20neural%20tonic%20and%20memory%20enhancer.

"*Bacopa caroliniana.*" Florida Native Plant Society. www.floridaforaging.com/plant/bacopa-caroliniana.

Cheema, Amanpreet K., Laura E. Wiener, Rebecca B. McNeil, et al. "A Randomized Phase II Remote Study to Assess *Bacopa* for Gulf War Illness Associated Cognitive Dysfunction: Design and Methods of a National Study." National Institutes of Health. June 13, 2022. www.ncbi.nlm.niih.gov/pmc/articles/PMC9189930.

Martínez-García, Martha, et al. "Antioxidant, Anti-Inflammatory and Anti-Obesity Potential of Extracts Containing Phenols, Chlorophyll and Carotenoids from Mexican Wild Populations of *Bacopa monnieri.*" NIH. April 19, 2023. www.ncbi.nlm.nih.gov/pmc/articles/PMC10135869.

Shane-McWhorter, Laura. "*Bacopa.*" Merck Manuals Consumer Version. March 2024. www.merckmanuals.com/home/special-subjects/dietary-supplements-and-vitamins/bacopa.

BALD CYPRESS

Books

Moerman, Daniel E. *Native American Ethnobotany.* Portland, OR: Timber Press, 1998.

Online

Hsieh, Chung-Fan, Yu-Li Chen, Chwan-Fwu Lin, et al. "An Extract from *Taxodium distichum* Targets Hemagglutinin- and Neuraminidase-Related Activities of Influenza Virus *in vitro.*" *Scientific Reports,* October 31, 2016. www.nature.com/articles/srep36015.

Kolasa, Lindsay. "Late Fall Meanderings and Cypress Pine Pitch Salve." Lindsay Kolasa website. November 30, 2013. https://lindsaykolasa.com/2013/11/30/late-fall-meandereings-and-cypress-pine-pitch-salve/.

Singh, Ravikant, Jha Saket, Anand Pandey, et al. "Comparison of Antibacterial Activities of Essential Oils of *Juniperus communis* L., *Pinus roxburghii* Sarg. and *Taxodium distichum* L. Against *Klebsiella pneumoniea.*" *Journal of Emerging Technologies and Innovative Research* (JETIR), August 2018. www.jetir.org/papers/JETIR1808400.pdf.

BETONY

Books

Moerman, Daniel E. *Native American Ethnobotany.* Portland, OR: Timber Press, 1998.

Shane, CoreyPine. *Southeast Medicinal Plants: Identify, Harvest, and Use 106 Wild Herbs for Health and Wellness.* Portland, OR: Timber Press, 2021.

Online

Deane, Green. "Betony: Rich Root, Poor Root." Eat the Weeds. 2012. www.eattheweeds.com/florida-betony-150-a-pound/.

Tomou, Ekaterina-Michaela, Christina Barda, and Helen Skaltsa. "Genus *Stachys:* A Review of Traditional Uses, Phytochemistry, and Bioactivity." NIH. September 29, 2020. www.ncbi.nlm.nih.gov/pmc/articles/PMC7601302/.

Vickery, Natalie. "Florida Betony (*Stachys floridana*)." The Family Herbalist. December 2010. https://thefamilyherbalist.wordpress.com/2010/12/09/florida-betony-stachys-floridana/.

BLACK MEDIC

Books

Moerman, Daniel E. *Native American Ethnobotany.* Portland, OR: Timber Press, 1998.

Online

"Black Medic, an Underrated and Useful Wild Edible." The Planet. August 2022. https://eattheplanet.org/black-medic-an-underrated-and-useful-wild-edible/.

"Black Medic in Gardens: Tips for Growing Black Medic Herbs." Gardening Know How. 2022. www.gardeningknowhow.com/edible/herbs/black-medic/growing-black-medic-herbs.htm.

"Black Medick." Natural Medicinal Herbs. www.naturalmedicinalherbs.net/herbs/m/medicago-lupulina-black=medick.php.

"*Medicago lupulina.*" Plants for a Future. https://pfaf.org/user/Plant.aspx?LatinName=Medicago+lupulina.

Yadav, Girendra, Varsha Yadav, Ashwini Patel, et al. "Comprehensive Review on Traditional Uses, Phytochemistry, Pharmacological Properties and Metal Nanoparticles of a Leafy Vegetable, *Medicago polymorpha.*" *European Journal of Medicinal Chemistry Reports.* August 2024. www.sciencedirect.com/science/article/pii/S2772417424000360.

BLACK WALNUT

Books

Boyd, Eddie, and Leslie A. Shimp. *African American Home Remedies: A Practical Guide with Usage and Application Data.* Lafayette: University of Louisiana at Lafayette Press, 2014.

Moerman, Daniel E. *Native American Ethnobotany.* Portland, OR: Timber Press, 1998.

Shane, CoreyPine. *Southeast Medicinal Plants: Identify, Harvest, and Use 106 Wild Herbs for Health and Wellness.* Portland, OR: Timber Press, 2021.

Weed, Susun S. *Abundantly Well: The Complementary Integrated Medicine Revolution.* Woodstock, NY: Ash Tree, 2020.

Online

"Black Walnuts: A Nutritious Nut Reviewed." Healthline. March 29, 2019. www.healthline.com/nutrition/black-walnut#nutrition.

Ho, Khanh-Van, Kathy L. Schreiber, Danh C. Vu, et al. "Black Walnut (*Juglans nigra*) Extracts Inhibit Proinflammatory Cytokine Production from Lipopolysaccharide-Stimulated Human Promonocytic Cell Line U-937." NIH, Frontiers in Pharmacology. September 19, 1919. www.ncbi.nlm.nih.gov/pmc/articles/PMC6761373/.

"*Juglans nigra.*" Dr. Duke's Phytochemical and Ethnobotanical Database. USDA. https://phytochem.nal.usda.gov/ethnobotanical-plant-juglans-nigra.

Sharma, Munish, and Munit Sharma. "A Comprehensive Review on Ethnobotanical, Medicinal and Nutritional Potential of Walnut (*Juglans regia* L.)." NIH, Indian National Science Academy. September 22, 2022. www.ncbi.nlm.nih.gov/pmc/articles/PMC9510174/.

BLUE-EYED GRASS

Books

Armstrong, Johnny. *Rescuing Biodiversity: The Protection and Restoration of a North Louisiana Ecosystem.* Baton Rouge: LSU Press, 2023.

Moerman, Daniel E. *Native American Ethnobotany.* Portland, OR: Timber Press, 1998.

Online

"*Sisyrinchium angustifolium*—Mill." Plants for a Future. June 11, 2002. https://pfaf.org/User/Plant.aspx?LatinName=Sisyrinchium+angustifolium.

Washington, Betsy. "Blue-Eyed Grass Blooms for Bees and Butterflies." Virginia Native Plant Society. May 17, 2021. https://vnps.org/blue-eyed-grass-blooms-for-bees-and-butterflies/.

BLUE MIST FLOWER

Books

Bender, Steve, and Felder Rushing. *Passalong Plants.* Chapel Hill: University of North Carolina Press, 1993.

Online

Doucet, Patrice. "6 Medicinal Plants in Your Backyard." *Daily Iberian.* April 11, 2019. https://thedailyiberian.com/2019/04/11/6-medicinal-plants-in-your-backyard/.

"Mistflower." Gulf Specimen Marine Laboratories. https://gulfspecimen.org/mist-flower/.

BLUEBERRY

Books

Bokelman, Jean N., M.D. *Medicinal Herbs in Primary Care: An Evidence-Guided Reference for Health Care Providers.* New York: Elsevier, 2022.

Moerman, Daniel E. *Native American Ethnobotany.* Portland, OR: Timber Press, 1998.

Tyler, Varro E. *Herbs of Choice: The Therapeutic Use of Phytomedicinals.* Binghamton, NY: Haworth Press, 1994.

Online

Li, Hua, Hye-Mi Park, Hyeon-Seon Ji, et al. "Phenolic-Enriched Blueberry-Leaf Extract Attenuates Glucose Homeostasis, Pancreatic β-cell Function, and Insulin Sensitivity in High-Fat Diet-Induced Diabetic Mice." NIH PubMed. January 2020. https://pubmed.ncbi.nlm.nih.gov/31923607/.

"Metabolic Benefits of Drinking Blueberry Tea in Type 2 Diabetes." NIH ClinicalTrials.gov. April 2021. https://clinicaltrials.gov/study/NCT02629952.

Pimple, Bhushan P., and Sachin L. Badole. "*Vaccinium corymbosum:* Polyphenols in Chronic Diseases and the Mechanisms of Action." Science Direct. 2014. www.sciencedirect.com/topics/pharmacology-toxicology-and-pharmaceutical-science/vaccinium-corymbosum.

"*Vaccinium arboreum.*" Dr. Duke's Phytochemical and Ethnobotanical Database. USDA. https://phytochem.nal.usda.gov/phytochem/ethnoplants/show/16167.

"Vaccinium corymbosum." Plants for a Future. https://pfaf.org/user/Plant.aspx?LatinName=Vaccinium+cormbosum.

BOTTLEBRUSH

Books

Wrigley, John, and Murray Fagg. *Bottlebrushes, Paperbarks, and Tea Trees.* Sydney, Australia: Angus and Robertson, 1993.

Online

Arseniuk, Adam. "*Callistemon viminalis* and *Callistemon citrinus*—Weeping Bottlebrush and Lemon Scented Bottlebrush." Herbs from Distant Lands. June 24, 2020. http://herbsfromdistantlands.blogspot.com/2020/06/.

Laganà, Giuseppina, Davide Barreca, Antonella Smeriglio, et al. "Evaluation of Anthocyanin Profile, Antioxidant, Cytoprotective, and Anti-Angiogenic Properties of *Callistemon citrinus* Flowers." NIH PubMed. August 17, 2020. www.ncbi.nlm.nih.gov/pmc/artiles/PMC7465370/.

Rathore, Rinu, and Nitish Rai. "Pharmacological Action and Underlying Molecular Mechanism of *Callistemon:* A Genus of Promising Medicinal Herbs." NIH PubMed. March 2022. https://www.sciencedirect.com/science/article/abs/pii/S0944711322000915.

Salem, Mohamed Z. M., Mervat EL-Hefny, Ramadan A. Nasser, et al. "Medicinal and Biological Values of *Callistemon viminalis* Extracts: History, Current Situation and Prospects." *Asian Pacific Journal of Tropical Medicine.* March 2017. www.sciencedirect.com/science/article/pii/S1995764517303905.

BURDOCK

Books

Moerman, Daniel E. *Native American Ethnobotany.* Portland, OR: Timber Press, 1998.

Tyler, Varro E. *Herbs of Choice: The Therapeutic Use of Phytomedicinals.* Binghamton, NY: Haworth Press, 1994.

Weed, Susun S. *Abundantly Well: The Complementary Integrated Medicine Revolution.* Woodstock, NY: Ash Tree, 2020.

Online

İlgün, Selen, Gökçe Seker Karatoprak, Dery Çiçek Polat, et al. "Phytochemical Composition and Biological Activities of *Arctium minus* (Hill) Bernh: A Potential Candidate as Antioxidant, Enzyme Inhibitor, and Cytotoxic Agent." NIH PubMed. September 20, 2022. www.ncbi.nlm.nih.gov/pmc/articles/PMC9598467/.

Wang, Dongdong, Alexandru Sabin Badarau, Mallappa Kumar Swamy, et al. "*Arctium*

Species Secondary Metabolites Chemodiversity and Bioactivities." NIH PubMed. July 9, 2019. www.ncbi.nlm.nih.gov/pmc/articles/PMC6629911/.
"Why Burdock Root Is Better as a Food Than as a Supplement." Cleveland Clinic.com. August 11, 2023. https://health.clevelandclinic.org/burdock-root.
"Wresting Burdock Seed and Its Medicinal Uses." Northeast School of Botanical Medicine. November 2017. https://7song.com/wresting-burdock-seed-and-its-medicinal-uses/.

CARDINAL FLOWER

Books

Moerman, Daniel E. *Native American Ethnobotany.* Portland, OR: Timber Press, 1998.
Tyler, Varro E. *Herbs of Choice: The Therapeutic Use of Phytomedicinals.* Binghamton, NY: Haworth Press, 1994.

Online

Felpin, François, and Jacques Lebreton. "History, Chemistry and Biology of Alkaloids from *Lobelia inflata.*" Science Direct. July 2004. www.sciencedirect.com/science/article/abs/pii/S0040402004012943.
Folquitto, Daniela G., Juliane N. D. Swiech, Camila B. Pereira, et al. "Biological Activity, Phytochemistry and Traditional Uses of Genus *Lobelia* (*Campanulaceae*): A Systematic Review." NIH PubMed. April 2019. https://pubmed.ncbi.nlm.nih.gov/30664918/.
"*Lobelia cardinalis* (L)." Plants for a Future. https://pfaf.org/User/Plant.aspx?LatinName=Lobelia+cardinalis.
"What Is *Lobelia,* and How Is It Used?" Healthline. September 2024. www.healthline.com/nutrition/lobelia#what-it-is.

CHASTE TREE

Books

Bokelman, Jean M., M.D. *Medicinal Herbs in Primary Care: An Evidence-Guided Reference for Health Care Providers.* New York: Elsevier, 2022.
Perrin, Mary B., and Beverly Fusilier. *Healing Traditions of South Louisiana: Prayers, Plants and Poultices.* Opelousas LA, Andrepont, 2022.
Weed, Susun S. *Abundantly Well: The Complementary Integrated Medicine Revolution.* Woodstock, NY: Ash Tree, 2020.

Online

Rani, Anita, and Anupam Sharma. "The Genus *Vitex:* A Review." NIH. *Pharmacognosy Review,* July 2013. www.ncbi.nlm.nih.gov/pmc/articles/PMC3841997/.

"*Vitex agnus-castus,*" USGS Plants of Louisiana. https://warcapps.usgs.gov/PlantID/Species/Details/1446.

CHICORY

Books

Moerman, Daniel E. *Native American Ethnobotany.* Portland, OR: Timber Press, 1998.

Weed, Susun S. *Abundantly Well: The Complementary Integrated Medicine Revolution.* Woodstock, NY: Ash Tree, 2020.

Online

Pouille, Céline, Souad Ouaza, Elise Roels, et al. "Chicory: Understanding the Effects and Effectors of This Functional Food." NIH PubMed Central. February 22, 2023. https://pmc.ncbi.nlm.nih.gov/articles/PMC8912540/#:~:text=Industrial%20chicory%20%28Cichorium%20intybus%20var,antioxidant%2C%20anthelmintic%2C%20and%20prebiotic.

Street, Renée A., Jasmeen Sidana, and Gerhard Prinsloo. "*Cichorium intybus:* Traditional Uses, Phytochemistry, Pharmacology, and Toxicology." NIH PubMed Central. November 2013. www.ncbi.nlm.nih.gov/pmc/articles/PMC3860133/.

Thorat, B. S., and S. M. Raut. "Chicory, the Supplementary Medicinal Herb for Human Diet." *Journal of Medicinal Plants Studies.* 2018. www.plantsjournal.com/achives/2018/vol6issue2/PartA/6-2-4-808.pdf.

Weishaupt, Jeffrey. "Are There Health Benefits of Chicory?" WebMD. February 2024. www.webmd.com/diet/health-benefits-of-chicory.

CORN SALAD

Books

Moerman, Daniel E. *Native American Ethnobotany.* Portland, OR: Timber Press, 1998.

Online

"Common Cornsalad, *Valerianella locusta.*" Wild Flower Web, Aaron Kitching. 2025. www.wildflowerweb.co/uk/plant/2602/common-cornsalad.

"Valerian, the Sweet Salad That Is Good for You." Altamura. www.opaltamura.com/en/valerian-the-sweet-salad-that-is-good-for-you/.

"*Valerianella.*" Herbal and Natural Medicine. www.herbal-organic.com/en/herb/17507.

"*Valerianella locusta.*" Dr. Duke's Phytochemical and Ethnobotanical Databases. USDA. https://phytochem.nal.usda.gov/plant-valerianella-locusta.

"*Valerianella radiata* (Valerianaceae)." Dr. Duke's Phytochemical and Ethnobotanical Database. USDA. https://phytochem.nal.usda.gov/plant-valerianella-radiata.

CORYDALIS

Books

Armstrong, Johnny. *Rescuing Biodiversity: The Protection and Restoration of a North Louisiana Ecosystem.* Baton Rouge: LSU Press, 2023.

Moerman, Daniel E. *Native American Ethnobotany.* Portland, OR: Timber Press, 1998.

Online

Cooper, Dan. "Crazy for *Corydalis.*" The Frustrated Gardener. March 21, 2017. https://frustratedgardener.com/2017/03/21/crazy-for-corydalis/.

"*Corydalis.*" Science Direct, *Biomedicine & Pharmacotherapy.* 2021. www.sciencedirect.com/topics/medicine-and-dentistry/corydalis.

"*Corydalis micrantha.*" USGS Guide to Plants of Louisiana. https://warcapps.usgs.gov/PlantID/Species/Detals/919.

"Know Your Natives, Southern Corydalis." Arkansas Native Plant Society. April 25, 2019. https://anps.org/2019/04/25/know-your-natives-southern-corydalis/.

CRANESBILL

Books

Shane, CoreyPine. *Southeast Medicinal Plants: Identify, Harvest, and Use 106 Wild Herbs for Health and Wellness.* Portland, OR: Timber Press, 2021.

Weed, Susun S. *Abundantly Well: The Complementary Integrated Medicine Revolution.* Woodstock, NY: Ash Tree, 2020.

Online

Li, Jiyang, Hai Huang, Meiqing Feng, et al. "In Vitro and in Vivo Anti-Hepatitis B Virus Activities of a Plant Extract from *Geranium carolinianum* L." NIH PubMed Central. August 2008. https://pubmed.ncbi.nlm.nih.gov/18423640/.

CRAPE MYRTLE

Online

"Crepe Myrtle." Natural Medicinal Herbs, Plants for a Future. www.naturalmedicinal herbs.net/herbs/l/lagerstroemia-indica=crepe-myrtle.php.

"Health Benefits of Crepe Myrtle." Health Benefits Times.com. June 21, 2019. www.healthbenefitstimes.com/crepe-myrtle/

Judy, William V., Siva P. Hari, W. W. Stogskill, et al. "Antidiabetic Activity of a Standardized Extract (Glucosol™) from *Lagerstroemia speciosa* Leaves in Type 2 Diabetics: A Dose-Dependence Study." Science Direct, *Journal of Ethnopharmacology*. 2003. www.sciencedirect.com/science/article/abs/pii/S0378874103001223.

"*Lagerstroemia indica*." Dr. Duke's Phytochemical and Ethnobotanical Databases. USDA. https://phytochem.nal.usda.gov/?type=All&keyword=Lagerstroemia.

Yue, Ziwei, Yan Xu, Ming Cai, et al. "Floral Elegance Meets Medicinal Marvels: Traditional Uses, Phytochemistry, and Pharmacology of the Genus *Lagerstroemia* L." NIH PubMed Central. October 28, 2024. https://pmc.ncbi.nlm.nih.go/articles/PMC11548200/.

DAYFLOWER

Books

Armstrong, Johnny. *Rescuing Biodiversity: The Protection and Restoration of a North Louisiana Ecosystem.* Baton Rouge: LSU Press, 2023.

Online

"*Commelina erecta*." Dr. Duke's Phytochemical and Ethnobotanical Databases. USDA. https://phytochem.nal.usda.gov/phytohem/ethnoplants/show/16953.

"*Commelina erecta*." Useful Tropical Plants. October 13, 2024. https://tropical.theferns.info/viewtropical.php?id=Commelina+erecta.

"*Commelina erecta*." USGS Guide to Plants of Louisiana. https://warcapps.usgs.gov/PlantID/Species/Details/2333.

ECHINACEA

Books

Bokelman, Jean M., M.D. *Medicinal Herbs in Primary Care: An Evidence-Guided Reference for Health Care Providers.* New York: Elsevier, 2022.

Carpenter, Jeff, and Melanie Carpenter. *The Organic Medicinal Herb Farmer, Revised Edition.* White River Junction, VT: Chelsea Green, 2023.

Moerman, Daniel E. *Native American Ethnobotany.* Portland, OR: Timber Press, 1998.

Tyler, Varro E., ScD, and James E. Robbers. PhD. *Herbs of Choice: The Therapeutic Use of Phytomedicinals.* New York: Haworth Herbal Press, 1999.

Weed, Susun S. *Abundantly Well: The Complementary Integrated Medicine Revolution.* Woodstock, NY: Ash Tree, 2020.

Online

Aiello, Paolo, Maedeh Sharghi, Shabnam Malekpour Mansourkhani, et al. "Medicinal Plants in the Prevention and Treatment of Colon Cancer." *Oxidative Medicine and Cellular Longevity.* NIH PubMed. December 4, 2019. https://pubmed.ncbi.nlm.nih.gov/32377288/.

"Cone Flower—*Echinacea pallida.*" Natural Medicinal Herbs, Plants for a Future. www.naturalmedicinalherbs.nt/herbs/e/echinacea-pallida=cone-flower.php.

"Dosage Echinacea: Benefits, Uses, Side Effects, and Dosages." Health Line. March 9, 2023. www.healthline.com/nutrition/echinacea.

Miller, Sandra C. "*Echinacea:* A Miracle Herb Against Aging and Cancer? Evidence *In vivo* in Mice." NIH PubMed Central. September 2005. www.ncbi.nlm.nih,gov/pmc/articles/PMC1193558.

FUMITORY

Books

Moerman, Daniel E. *Native American Ethnobotany.* Portland, OR: Timber Press, 1998.

Online

"Fumitory—Uses, Side Effects, and More." WebMD. www.webmd.com/vitamins/ai/ingredientmono-451/fumitory.

Ward, Daniel B. "Contributions to the Flora of Florida: 5, *Corydalis,* Fumaria (Fumariaceae)." www.jstor.org/stable/4032650?seq=1.

Zhang, Ruifei, Qiang Guo, Edward Kennelly, et al. "Diverse Alkaloids and Biological Activities of *Fumaria* (Papaveraceae): An Ethnomedicinal Group." Science Direct. 2020. https://www.sciencedirect.com/science/article/abs/pii/S0367326X20302793.

GARDENIA

Online

Chen, Liping, Maoxing Li, Zhiqiang Yang, et al. "*Gardenia jasminoides* Ellis: Ethnopharmacology, Phytochemistry, and Pharmacological and Industrial Applications of an Important Traditional Chinese Medicine." NIH PubMed. April 28, 2020. https://pubmed.ncbi.nlm.nih.gov/3211486.

"Gardenia: Key Herb for Dispelling Dampness and Heat Via the Triple Burner." Institute for Traditional Medicine. September 2003. www.itmonline.org/arts/gardenia.htm.

"Gardenia—Uses, Side Effects, and More." WebMD. www.webmd.com/vitamins/ai/ingredientmono-1488/gardenia.

Zhang, Nan, Ying Bian, and Lei Yao. "Essential Oils of *Gardenia jasminoides* J. Ellis and *Gardenia jasminoides* f. *longicarpa* Z.W. Xie & M. Okada Flowers: Chemical Characterization and Assessment of Anti-Inflammatory Effects in Alveolar Macrophage." *Pharmaceutics.* NIH PubMed Central. April 29, 2022. https://pmc.ncbi.nlm.nih.gov/articles/PMC9145545/.

GERMANDER

Online

"*Teucrium canadense*—L." Plants for a Future. https://pfaf.org/User/Plant.aspx?LatinName=Teucrium+canadense.

"*Teucrium canadense.*" USGS Guide to Plants of Louisiana. https://warcapps.usgs.gov/PlantID/Species/Details/784/.

HACKBERRY

Books

Moerman, Daniel E. *Native American Ethnobotany.* Portland, OR: Timber Press, 1998.

Online

"*Celtis occidentalis.*" USGS Guide to Plants of Louisiana. https://warcapps.usgs.gov/PlantID/Species/Deetails/4004.

"*Celtis species.*" Dr. Duke's Phytochemical and Ethnobotanical Databases. USDA. https://phytochem.nal.usda.gov/ethnobotanical-plant-celtis-sp.

HAWTHORN

Books

Bokelman, Jean M., M.D. *Medicinal Herbs in Primary Care: An Evidence-Guided Reference for Health Care Providers.* New York: Elsevier, 2022.

Moerman, Daniel E. *Native American Ethnobotany.* Portland, OR: Timber Press, 1998.

Shane, CoreyPine. *Southeast Medicinal Plants: Identify, Harvest, and Use 106 Wild Herbs for Health and Wellness.* Portland, OR: Timber Press, 2021.

Tyler, Varro E., ScD, and James E. Robbers, PhD. *Herbs of Choice: The Therapeutic Use of Phytomedicinals.* New York: Haworth Herbal Press, 1999.

Weed, Susun S. *Abundantly Well: The Complementary Integrated Medicine Revolution.* Woodstock, NY: Ash Tree, 2020.

Online

Cloud, Alexa, Dwan Vilcins, and Bradley McEwen. "The Effect of Hawthorn (*Crataegus* spp.) on Blood Pressure: A Systematic Review." Science Direct, *Advances in Integrative Medicine.* 2019. www.sciencedirect.com/science/article/abs/pii/S2212958817301106.

"Hawthorn—Uses, Side Effects, and More." WebMD. www.webmed.com/vitamins/ai/ingredientmono-527/hawthorn.

"Herb of the Month: Shan Zha (Hawthorn Berry)." Stram Center for Integrative Medicine. September 2016. https://stramcenter.com/blog/blog-detail/herb-of-the-month-shan-zha-hawthorn-berry/.

Rababa'h, Abeer M., Omar N. Al Yacoub, Tamam El-Elimat, et al. "The Effect of Hawthorn Flower and Leaf Extract (*Crataegus* Spp.) on Cardiac Hemostasis and Oxidative Parameters in Sprague Dawley Rats." NIH Pub Med Central. August 22, 2020. www.ncbi.nlm.nih.gov/pmc/articles/PMC7452443/.

JOE PYE

Books

Armstrong, Johnny. *Rescuing Biodiversity: The Protection and Restoration of a North Louisiana Ecosystem.* Baton Rouge: LSU Press, 2023.

Moerman, Daniel E. *Native American Ethnobotany.* Portland, OR: Timber Press, 1998.

Shane, CoreyPine. *Southeast Medicinal Plants: Identify, Harvest, and Use 106 Wild Herbs for Health and Wellness.* Portland, OR: Timber Press, 2021.

Online

"*Eupatorium maculatum*—L." Plants for a Future. https://pfaf.org/User/Plant.aspx?LatinName=Eupatorium+maculatum.

"*Eupatorium purpureum.*" Dr. Duke's Phytochemical and Ethnobotanical Databases. USDA. https://phytochem.nal.usda.gov/ethnobotanical-plant-eupatorium-purpureum.

"*Eupatorium purpureum*—L." Plants for a Future. https://pfaf.org/user/Plant.aspx?LatinName=Eupatorium+purpureum

"Hummingbirds in Louisiana—Picture and ID Guide." Bird Advisors. www.birdadvisors.com/hummingbirds-louisiana/.

JUNIPER

Books

English, Camper. *Doctors and Distillers: The Remarkable Medicinal History of Beer, Wine, Spirits and Cocktails.* New York: Penguin, 2022.

Moerman, Daniel E. *Native American Ethnobotany.* Portland, OR: Timber Press, 1998.

Shane, CoreyPine. *Southeast Medicinal Plants: Identify, Harvest, and Use 106 Wild Herbs for Health and Wellness.* Portland, OR: Timber Press, 2021.

Online

Bolongaro, Kait. "An Uncanny Mixture: God, Alcohol and Even Cannabis." BBC News. October 27, 2016. www.bbc.com/news/business-37727458.

"*Juniperus virginiana* (Cupressaceae)." Dr. James Duke's Phytochemical and Ethnobotanical Databases. USDA. https://phytochem.nal.usda.gov/phytochem/plants/show/5909#act-label.

"*Juniperus virginiana*—L." Plants for a Future. https://pfaf.org/user/Plant.aspx?LatinName=Juniperus+virginiana.

"Pencil Cedar." Natural Medicinal Herbs, Plants for a Future. www.naturalmedicinalherbs.net/herbs/j/juniperus-virginiana=pencil-cedar.php.

LINDEN

Books

Moerman, Daniel E. *Native American Ethnobotany.* Portland, OR: Timber Press, 1998.

Shane, CoreyPine. *Southeast Medicinal Plants: Identify, Harvest, and Use 106 Wild Herbs for Health and Wellness.* Portland, OR: Timber Press, 2021.

Weed, Susun S. *Abundantly Well: The Complementary Integrated Medicine Revolution.* Woodstock, NY: Ash Tree, 2020.

Online

Begg, Graham S., Samantha M. Cook, Richard Dye, et al. "A Functional Overview of Conservation Biological Control." Science Direct. July 2017. www.sciencedirect.com/science/article/abs/pii/S0261219416303210.

Cárdenas-Rodríguez, María Eva González-Trujano, Eva Aguirre-Hernández, et al. "Anticonvulsant and Antioxidant Effects of *Tilia americana* var. *mexicana* and Flavonoids Constituents in the Pentylenetetrazole-Induced Seizures." NIH PubMed. August 13, 2014. https://pubmed.ncbi.nlm.nih.gov/25197430/.

"*Tilia Americana*—L., Plants for a Future." https://pfaf.org/user/Plant.aspx?LatinName=Tilia+Americana.

Zerdy, Joanne. "Six Herbs for Grieving and Healing." Heather Stang. May 9, 2019. https://mindfulnessandgrief.com/six-herbs-for-grieving-and-healing/.

MIMOSA

Books

Bender, Steve, and Felder Rushing. *Passalong Plants.* Chapel Hill: University of North Carolina Press, 1993.

Shane, CoreyPine. *Southeast Medicinal Plants: Identify, Harvest, and Use 106 Wild Herbs for Health and Wellness.* Portland, OR: Timber Press, 2021.

Online

"Albizia." Herb Reality: A Voice for Herbal Medicine, 2025. https://www.herbalreality.com/herb/persian-silk-tree/.

Sarris, Jerome, Erica McIntyre, and David A. Camfield. "Plant-Based Medicines for Anxiety Disorders, Part 1: A Review of Preclinical Studies." NIH PubMed. March 27, 2013. https://pubmed.ncbi.nlm.nih.gov/23436255/.

Turk, Max. "On Trauma, Grief, Finding Power and Being Joyful." Roots & Crowns. July 16, 2018. https://www.rootsandcrowns.com/blogs/recipes/on-trauma-grief-finding-power-being-joyful.

Zerdy, Joanne. "Six Herbs for Grieving and Healing." Heather Stang. May 9, 2019. https://mindfulnessandgrief.com/six-herbs-for-grieving-and-healing/.

MISTLETOE

Books

Moerman, Daniel E. *Native American Ethnobotany.* Portland, OR: Timber Press, 1998.

Tyler, Varro E., ScD, and James E Robbers, PhD. *Herbs of Choice: The Therapeutic Use of Phytomedicinals.* New York: Haworth Herbal Press, 1999.

Online

"American Mistletoe." RX List. www.rxlist.com/american_mistletoe/supplements.html.

"Mistletoe." Medicinal Herb Info. http://medicinalherbinfo.org/000Herbs2016/1herbs/mistletoe/.

"*Phoradendron serotinum.*" Dr. Duke's Phytochemical and Ethnobotanical Databases. USDA. https://phytochem.nal.usda.gov/ethnobotanical-plant-phoradendron-serotinum.

MOUNTAIN MINT

Books

Moerman, Daniel E. *Native American Ethnobotany.* Portland, OR: Timber Press, 1998.

Online

"*Phoradendron serotinum* ssp. *serotinum.*" USGS Guide to Plants of Louisiana. https://warcapps.usgs.gov/PlantID/Species/Details/4036.

"*Phoradendron serotinum* ssp. *tomentosum.*" USGS Guide to Plants of Louisiana. https://warcapps.usgs.gov/PlantID/Species/Details/4037.

"*Pycnanthemum virginianum.*" Dr. Duke's Phytochemical and Ethnobotanical Databases. USDA. https://phytochem.nal.usda.gov/ethnobotanical-plant-pycnanthemum-virginianum.

MUSCADINE GRAPE

Books

Boyd, Eddie, and Leslie A. Shimp. *African American Home Remedies, A Practical Guide with Usage and Application Data:* Lafayette: University of Louisiana at Lafayette Press, 2014.

Moerman, Daniel E. *Native American Ethnobotany.* Portland, OR: Timber Press, 1998.

Online

"Food as Medicine Update: Grape." Herbalgram.org. March 3, 2022. www.herbalgram.org/resources/herbalgram/volumes/volume-19/issue-3-march/news-and-features-1/food-as-medicine-update-grape/.

Greenspan, Phillip, John D. Bauer, Stanley H. Pollack, et al. "Antiinflammatory Properties of the Muscadine Grape (*Vitis rotundifolia*)." NIH PubMed Central. November 2005. https://pubmed.ncbi.nlm.nih.gov/16248541/.

Mellen, Philip B., Kurt R. Daniel, K. Bridget Brosnihan, et al. "Effect of Muscadine Grape Seed Supplementation on Vascular Function in Subjects with or at Risk for Cardiovascular Disease: A Randomized Crossover Trial." NIH PubMed Central. March 27, 2012. www.ncbi.nlm.nih.gov/pmc/articles/PMC3313487/.

Mendonca, Patricia, Ahmed G. Darwish, Violeta Tsolova, et al. "The Anticancer and Antioxidant Effects of Muscadine Grape Extracts on Racially Different Triple-

Negative Breast Cancer Cells." Anticancer Research. August 2019. https://ar.iiarjournals.org/content/39/8/4043.

Shi, Xiaonan. "Muscadine Health Benefits—An Interview with Dr. Patricia Gallagher, Wake Forest University School of Medicine." North Carolina State University. June 10, 2020. https://smallfruits.cals.ncsu.edu/2020/06/critical-article-muscadines-health-benefits/.

Singh, Jagdev. "5 Amazing Health Benefits of Muscadine Grapes (Vitis Rotundifolia)." *Ayur Times,* July 4, 2020. www.ayurtimes.com/muscadine-grapes/.

OKRA

Books

Van Wyck, Ben-Erik. *Food Plants of the World.* Portland, OR: Timber Press, 2006.

Online

Bauman, Hannah, and Allison Porter. "Food as Medicine, Okra (*Abelmoschus esculentus,* Malvaceae)." American Botanical Council. Herbalgram. 2014. www.herbalgram.org/resources/herbalgram/volumes/volume-12/number-8-august/food-as-medicine-okra-abelmoschus-esculentus-malvaceae/food-as-medicine/.

Chanchal, Dilip Kumar, S. Alok, M. Kumar, et al. "A Brief Review on *Abelmoschus esculentus* Linn. Okra." *International Journal of Pharmaceutical Sciences and Research.* November 22, 1917. https://ijpsr.com/bft/article/a-brief-review-on-abelmoschus-esculentus-linn-okra/.

Elkhalifa, A.E.O., Eyad Alshammari, Mohd Adnan, et al. "Okra (*Abelmoschus esculentus*) as a Potential Dietary Medicine with Nutraceutical Importance for Sustainable Health Applications." NIH PubMed. January 28, 2021. https://www.ncbi.nlm.nih/gov/pmc/articles/PMC7865958/.

Xia, Fango, Yu Zhong, Mengqiu Li, et al. "Antioxidant and Anti-Fatigue Constituents of Okra," NIH PubMed Central. October 28, 2015. https://pmc.ncbi.nlm.nih.gov/articles/PMC4632455/.

PEPPERGRASS

Books

Moerman, Daniel E. *Native American Ethnobotany.* Portland, OR: Timber Press, 1998.

Shane, CoreyPine. *Southeast Medicinal Plants: Identify, Harvest, and Use 106 Wild Herbs for Health and Wellness.* Portland, OR: Timber Press, 2021.

Online

"*Lepidium virginicum,*" Plants for a Future. https://pfaf.org/user/Plant.aspx?LatinName=Lepidium+virginicum.

"*Lepidium virginicum,* Wild Pepper Grass," Practical Plants. 2022. https://practicalplants.org/wiki/lepidium_virginicum/.

"Peppergrass, Abundant and with a Delicious Peppered Flavor." The Planet. March 2023. https://eattheplanet.org/peppergrass-abundant-and-with-a-delicious-peppered-flavor/.

PURSLANE

Books

Shane, CoreyPine. *Southeast Medicinal Plants: Identify, Harvest, and Use 106 Wild Herbs for Health and Wellness.* Portland, OR: Timber Press, 2021.

Weed, Susun S. *Abundantly Well: The Complementary Integrated Medicine Revolution.* Woodstock, NY: Ash Tree, 2020.

Online

Jalali, Jalileh, and Mahboobeh Ghasemzadeh Rahbardar. "Ameliorative Effects of *Portulaca oleracea* L. (purslane) and Its Active Constituents on Nervous System Disorders: A Review." NIH PubMed Central. www.ncbi.nlm.nih.gov/pmc/articles/PMC9790064.

"Portulaca oleracea," Plants for a Future. https://pfaf.org/user/plant/aspx?LatinName=Portulaca+oleracea.

"Purslane: Nutrition & Health Benefits." Organic Facts. July 23, 2021. www.organicfacts.net/health-benefits/vegetable/purslane.html.

Uddin, Kamal, M.D., Abdul Shukor Juraimi, Sabir Hossain, M.D., et al. "Purslane Weed (*Portulaca oleracea*): A Prospective Plant Source of Nutrition, Omega-3 Fatty Acid, and Antioxidant Attributes." *Scientific World Journal.* NIH PubMed Central. February 2014. www.ncbi.nlm.nih.gov/pmc/articles/PMC3934766/.

ROSE

Books

Bender, Steve, and Felder Rushing, *Passalong Plants.* Chapel Hill: University of North Carolina Press, 1993.

Carpenter, Jeff, and Melanie Carpenter. *The Organic Medicinal Herb Farmer, Revised Edition.* White River Junction, VT: Chelsea Green, 2023.

Online

"Benefits of Rose Water and How to Use It." Healthline. December 23, 2024. www.healthline.com/health/rose-water-benefits#soothes-digestionproblems.

Rivas-García, Lorenzo, José L. Quiles, Catarina Rama-Rodrigues, et al. "*Rosa* x *hybrida* Extracts with Dual Actions: Antiproliferative Effects Against Tumour Cells and Inhibitor of Alzheimer Disease." NIH PubMed Central. March 20, 2021. www.sciencedirect.com/science/article/abs/pii/S0278691521000521.

Yuan, G., and F. Du. "Studies on Chemical Constituents of the Fruits of *Rosa bracteata* var. *bracteate*." NIH PubMed. August 23, 2000. https://pubmed.ncbi.nlm.nih.gov/12575158/.

SAW PALMETTO

Books

Bokelman, Jean M., M.D. *Medicinal Herbs in Primary Care: An Evidence-Guided Reference for Health Care Providers.* New York: Elsevier, 2022.

Moerman, Daniel E. *Native American Ethnobotany.* Portland, OR: Timber Press, 1998.

Tyler, Varro E., ScD, and James E Robbers, PhD. *Herbs of Choice: The Therapeutic Use of Phytomedicinals.* New York: Haworth Herbal Press, 1999.

Weed, Susun S. *Abundantly Well: The Complementary Integrated Medicine Revolution.* Woodstock, NY: Ash Tree, 2020.

Online

"Saw Palmetto–*Serenoa repens*. Growables. www.growables.org/information/TropicalFruit/SawPalmetto.htm.

Thompson, Buster. "Saw Palmetto Berry Season in Full Swing." *Citrus County Chronicle.* September 18, 2022. www.chronicleonline.com/news/local/saw-palmetto-berry-season-in-full-swing/article_8f801bcb-4c91–5b49–9e8f-3dc366839027.html.

Ye, Zhangqun, Jian Huang, Liqun Zhour, et al. "Efficacy and Safety of *Serenoa repens* Extract Among Patients with Benign Prostatic Hyperplasia in China: A Multicenter, Randomized, Double-Blind, Placebo-Controlled Trial." PubMed. March 14, 2019. https://pubmed.ncbi.nlm.nih.gov/30880074/.

SKULLCAP

Books

Bokelman, Jean M., M.D. *Medicinal Herbs in Primary Care: An Evidence-Guided Reference for Health Care Providers.* New York: Elsevier, 2022.

Carpenter, Jeff, and Melanie Carpenter. *The Organic Medicinal Herb Farmer, Revised Edition.* White River Junction, VT: Chelsea Green, 2023.
Shane, CoreyPine. *Southeast Medicinal Plants: Identify, Harvest, and Use 106 Wild Herbs for Health and Wellness.* Portland, OR: Timber Press, 2021.
Weed, Susun S. *Abundantly Well: The Complementary Integrated Medicine Revolution.* Woodstock, NY: Ash Tree, 2020.

Online

Cole, Ian B., Jin Cao, Ali R. Alan, et al. "Comparisons of Scutellaria baicalensis, Scutellaria lateriflora and Scutellaria racemosa: Genome Size, Antioxidant Potential and Phytochemistry." ResearchGate. April 2008. https://pubmed.ncbi.nlm.nih.gov/18484546/.
Islam, M. Nurul, Frances Downey, and Carl K. Y. Ng. "Comparative Analysis of Bioactive Phytochemicals from *Scutellaria baicalensis, Scutellaria lateriflora, Scutellaria racemosa, Scutellaria tomentosa* and *Scutellaria wrightii* by LC-DAD-MS." Springer Nature. December 25, 2010. https://link.springer.com/article/10.1007/s11306-010-0269-9.
"*Scutllaria lateriflora.*" Dr. Duke's Phytochemical and Ethnobotanical Databases. USDA. https://phytochem.nal.usda.gov/ethnobotanical-plant-scutellaria-lateriflora.
"*Scutellaria lateriflora.*" Plants for a Future. https://pfaf.org/user/Plant.aspx?LatinName=Scutellaria+lateriflora.

SPEEDWELL

Books

Moerman, Daniel E. *Native American Ethnobotany.* Portland, OR: Timber Press, 1998.

Online

Fierascu, Radu Claudiu, Milen I. Georgiev, Irinia Fierascu, et al. "Mitorepressive, Antioxidant, Antifungal and Anti-inflammatory Effects of Wild-Growing Romanian Native *Arctium lappa* L. (*Asteraceae*) and *Veronica persica* Poiret (*Plantaginaceae*)." Science Direct, *Food and Chemical Toxicology.* January 2018. www.sciencedirect.com/science/article/abs/pii/S027869151730666X.
Salehi, Bahare, Mangalpady Shivaprasa Shetty, Nanjangud V. Anil Kumar, et al. "*Veronica* Plants—Drifting from Farm to Traditional Healing, Food Application, and Phytopharmacology." July 4, 2019. www.ncbi.nlm.nih.gov/pmc/articles/PMC6651156/
"Veronica." Rx List. www.rxlist.com/supplements/veronica.htm

ST. JOHNSWORT

Books

Armstrong, Johnny. *Rescuing Biodiversity: The Protection and Restoration of a North Louisiana Ecosystem.* Baton Rouge: LSU Press, 2023.

Bokelman, Jean M., M.D. *Medicinal Herbs in Primary Care: An Evidence-Guided Reference for Health Care Providers.* New York: Elsevier, 2022.

Shane, CoreyPine. *Southeast Medicinal Plants: Identify, Harvest, and Use 106 Wild Herbs for Health and Wellness.* Portland, OR: Timber Press, 2021.

Weed, Susun S. *Abundantly Well: The Complementary Integrated Medicine Revolution.* Woodstock, NY: Ash Tree, 2020.

Online

Freedman, Andrew, and Carlie Kollath Wells. "Louisiana Likely to Have Hotter-Than-Usual Summer." *Axios New Orleans.* April 26, 2024. www.axios.com/local/new-orleans/2024/04/26/louisiana-likely-hotter-than-usual-summer.

"*Hypericum perforatum*—L." Plants for a Future. https://pfaf.org/user/Plant.aspx?LatinName=Hypericum+perforatum.

Stojanovic, G., A. Dordevic, and A. Smelcerovic. "Do Other Hypericum Species Have Medical Potential as St. John's Wort (*Hypericum perforatum*)? NIH PubMed. 2013. https://pubmed.ncbi.nlm.nih.gov/23521674/.

SWEET GUM

Books

Shane, CoreyPine. *Southeast Medicinal Plants: Identify, Harvest, and Use 106 Wild Herbs for Health and Wellness.* Portland, OR: Timber Press, 2021.

Online

Foster, Steven. "Forest Gems: Exploring Medicinal Trees in American Forests." Herbalgram. Winter 2017. www.herbalgram.org/resources/herbalgram/issues/116/table-of-contents/hg116-feet-medtrees/.

Lingbeck, Jody M., Corliss A. O'Bryan, Elizabeth M. Martin, et al. "Sweetgum: An Ancient Source of Beneficial Compounds with Modern Benefits." NIH PubMed Central, *Pharmacognosy Review.* January 2015. https://pubmed.ncbi.nlm.nih.gov/26009686/

"*Liquidambar styraciflua.*" Dr. Duke's Phytochemical and Ethnobotanical Databases. USDA. https://phytochem.nal.usda.gov/phytochem/plants/show/5990#act-label.

Mancarz, Graziele Francine Franco, Carolina Laba Laressa, Elaine Cristina Pinto da Silva, et al. "*Liquidambar styraciflua* L.: A New Potential Source for Therapeutic Uses." NIH PubMed Central, *Journal of Pharmaceutical Analysis.* September 2019. https://www.sciencedirect.com/science/article/abs/pii/S073170851930158X.

SWEET OLIVE

Books

Moerman, Daniel E. *Native American Ethnobotany.* Portland, OR: Timber Press, 1998.

Online

"*Osmanthus fragrans.*" Dr. Duke's Phytochemical and Ethnobotanical Databases. USDA. https://phytochem.nal.usda.gov/ethnobotanical-plant-osmanthus-fragrans.

Wang, Baojun, Fei Luan, Yiwen Bao, et al. "Traditional Uses, Phytochemical Constituents and Pharmacological Properties of *Osmanthus fragrans:* A Review." Science Direct, *Journal of Ethnopharmacology.* July 15, 2022. www.sciencedirect.com/science/article/abs/pii/S0378874122003129.

Wang, Le, Nana Tan, Jiayao Hu, et al. "Analysis of the Main Active Ingredients and Bioactivities of Essential Oil from *Osmanthus Fragrans* Var. *thunbergii* Using a Complex Network Approach." www.ncbi.nlm.nih.gov/pmc/articles/PMC5745743/.

TULIP TREE

Books

Moerman, Daniel E. *Native American Ethnobotany.* Portland, OR: Timber Press, 1998.

Online

"*Liriodendron tulipifera.*" Plants for a Future. https://pfaf.org/uxer/Plant.as[x?lLatinName=Liriodendron+tulipfera.

O'Driscoll, Dana. "Sacred Trees in the Americas—The Magic, Medicine, and Uses of the Tulip Poplar (*Liriodendron tulipifera*)." The Druids Garden. April 2022. https://thedruidsgarden.com/2021/05/16/sacred-trees-in-the-americas-tulip-poplar-liriodendron-tulipifera/.

Quassinti, Luana, Filippo Maggi, Federica Ortolani, et al. "Exploring New Applications of Tulip Tree (*Liriodendron tulipifera* L.): Leaf Essential Oil as Apoptotic Agent for Human Glioblastoma." NIH PubMed. August 23, 2019. https://pubmed.ncbi.nlm.nih.gov/31444719/.

VENUS' LOOKING GLASS

Books

Moerman, Daniel E. *Native American Ethnobotany.* Portland, OR: Timber Press, 1998.

Online

Rose, Melody. "Identifying Wildflowers: *Triodanis perfoliata,* Venus' Looking Glass." Dave's Garden. July 22, 2017. https://davesgarden.com/guides/articles/identifying-wildflowers-triodanis-perfoliata-venus-looking-glass.

"7 Medicinal Health Benefits of *Triodanis perfoliata* (Clasping Venus)." Agric4Profits. October 29, 2023. https://agric4profits.com/7-medicinal-health-benefits-of-triodanis-perfoliata-clasping-venus/.

WAX MALLOW

Books

Bender, Steve, and Felder Rushing. *Passalong Plants.* Chapel Hill: University of North Carolina Press, 1993.

Online

Gazwi, Hanaa S. S., Nagwa A. Shoeib, Magda E. Mahmoud, et al. "Phytochemical Profile of the Ethanol Extract of *Malvaviscus arboreus* Red Flower and Investigation of the Antioxidant, Antimicrobial, and Cytotoxic Activities." NIH PubMed Central. November 18, 2022. www.ncbi.nlm.nih.gov/pmc/articles/PMC9686500/.

"*Malvaviscus arboreus.*" Dr. Duke's Phytochemical and Ethnobotanical Databases. USDA. https://phytochem.nal.usda.gov/phytochem/ethnoplants/show/11540.

"*Malvaviscus arboreus.*" Useful Tropical Plants. December 13, 2024. https://tropical.theferns.info/viewtropical.php?id=Malvaviscus+arboreus.

Vanta, Brindusa, M.D. "The Many Potential Benefits of Wax Mallow." Facty Health. March 14, 2023. https://facty.com/lifestyle/wellness/the-many-potential-benefits-of-wax-mallow/.

WILD ONION

Books

Moerman, Daniel E. *Native American Ethnobotany.* Portland, OR: Timber Press, 1998.

Shane, CoreyPine. *Southeast Medicinal Plants: Identify, Harvest, and Use 106 Wild Herbs for Health and Wellness.* Portland, OR: Timber Press, 2021.

Online

"*Allium canadense.*" Plants for a Future. https://pfaf.org/User/plant.aspx?Latin Name =Allium+canadense.

Keusgen, Michael, Reinhard M. Fritsch, Hikmat Hisoriev, et al. "Wild *Allium* Species (Alliaceae) Used in Folk Medicine of Tajikistan and Uzbekistan." *Journal of Ethnobiology and Ethnomedicine.* NIH PubMed Central. August 3, 2006. www.ncbi.nlm .nih.gov/pmc/articles/PMC1464120/.

Kothari, Damini, Woo-Do Lee, and Soo-Ki Kim. "*Allium* Flavonols: Health Benefits, Molecular Targets, and Bioavailability." NIH PubMed, *Antioxidants.* September 19, 2020. www.ncbi.nlm.nih.gov/pmc/articles/PMC7555649.

WILD PETUNIA

Books

Armstrong, Johnny. *Rescuing Biodiversity: The Protection and Restoration of a North Louisiana Ecosystem.* Baton Rouge: LSU Press, 2023.

Bender, Steve, and Felder Rushing. *Passalong Plants.* Chapel Hill: University of North Carolina Press, 1993.

Online

Afzal, Khurram, Muhammad Uzair, Bashir Ahmad Chaudhary, et al. "Genus *Ruellia:* Pharmacological and Phytochemical Importance in Ethnopharmacology." NIH PubMed. September 2015. https//pubmed.ncbi.nlm.nih.gov/26665388/.

Alam, M. Ashraful, Nusrat Subhan, M. Abdul Awal, et al. "Antinociceptive and Anti-inflammatory Properties of *Ruellia tuberosa.*" Taylor and Francis online, *Pharmaceutical Biology.* 2009. www.tandfonline.com/doi/full/10.1080/138802008024 34575.

"*Ruellia tuberosa* (Acanthaceae)." Dr. Duke's Phytochemical and Ethnobotanical Database. USDA. https://phytochem.nal.usda.gov/ethnobotanical-plant-ruellia -tuberosa.

Ukwubile, Cletus Anes, Henry Nettey, Troy Salvia Malgwi, et al. "*Ruellia simplex* C. Wright (Acanthaceae): Antinociceptive, Anti-inflammatory, and Antidiabetic Activities of a Novel Fatty Acid Isolated from Its Leaf Extract." *International Journal of Plant Based Pharmaceuticals.* July 10, 2022. https://ijpbp.com/index.php/ijpbp /article/view/57.

YARROW

Books

Bokelman, Jean M., M.D. *Medicinal Herbs in Primary Care: An Evidence-Guided Reference for Health Care Providers.* New York: Elsevier, 2022.

Carpenter, Jeff, and Melanie Carpenter. *The Organic Medicinal Herb Farmer, Revised Edition.* White River Junction, VT: Chelsea Green, 2023.

Perrin, Mary B., and Beverly Fusilier. *Healing Traditions of South Louisiana: Prayers, Plants and Poultices.* Opelousas, LA: Andrepont, 2022.

Weed, Susun S. *Abundantly Well: The Complementary Integrated Medicine Revolution.* Woodstock, NY: Ash Tree, 2020.

Online

"*Achillea millefolium.*" Dr. Duke's Phytochemical and Ethnobotanical Databases. USDA. https://phytochem.nal.usda.gov/ethnobotanical-plant-achillea-millefolium.

Far, Bahareh Farasati, Golnaz Behzad, and Hasti Khalili. "*Achillea millefolium:* Mechanism of Action, Pharmacokinetic, Clinical Drug-Drug Interactions and Tolerability." NIH PubMed Central. November 30, 2023. www.ncbi.nlm.nih.gov/pmc/articles/PMC10703637.

Saeidnia, S., A. R. Gohari, N. Mokhber-Dezfuli, et al. "A Review on Phytochemistry and Medicinal Properties of the Genus *Achillea.*" NIH PubMed, *DARU Journal of Pharmaceutical Sciences* 19, no. 3 (2011): 173–86. www.ncbi.nlm.nih.gov/pmc/articles/PMC3232110/.

RECOMMENDED RESOURCES

BOOKS

Allen, Charles M., Andrew W. Allen, and Harry H. Winters. *Edible Plants of the Gulf South.* Pitkin, LA: Allen's Native Ventures, 2005

Allen, Charles M., Dawn Allen Newman, and Harry H. Winters. *Trees, Shrubs, and Woody Vines of Louisiana.* Pitkin, LA: Allen's Native Ventures, 2002.

Allen, Charles M., Kenneth A. Wilson, and Harry H. Winters. *Louisiana Wildflower Guide.* Pitkin, LA: Allen's Native Ventures, 2010.

Bennett, Chris. *Southeast Foraging: 120 Wild and Flavorful Edibles from Angelica to Wild Plums.* Portland, OR: Timber Press, 2015.

Bokelman, Jean M., M.D. *Medicinal Herbs in Primary Care: An Evidence-Guided Reference for Health Care Providers.* New York: Elsevier, 2022.

Boyd, Eddie, and Leslie A. Shimp. *African American Home Remedies: A Practical Guide with Usage and Application Data.* Lafayette: University of Louisiana at Lafayette Press, 2014.

Bryson, Charles T., and Michael S. DeFelice, eds. *Weeds of the South.* Athens: University of Georgia Press, 2009.

Carpenter, Jeff, and Melanie Carpenter. *The Organic Medicinal Herb Farmer, Revised Edition.* White River Junction, VT: Chelsea Green, 2023.

English, Camper. *Doctors and Distillers: The Remarkable Medicinal History of Beer, Wine, Spirits and Cocktails.* New York: Penguin, 2022.

Foster, Steven, and James A. Duke. *Peterson Field Guide to Medicinal Plants and Herbs of Eastern and Central North America.* 3rd ed. Boston: Houghton Mifflin Harcourt, 2014.

Gladstar, Rosemary. *Rosemary Gladstar's Herbal Recipes for Vibrant Health: 175 Teas, Tonics, Oils, Salves, Tinctures, and Other Natural Remedies for the Entire Family.* North Adams, MA: Storey, 2008.

Howell, Patricia Kyritsi. *Medicinal Plants of the Southern Appalachians.* Clayton, GA: Botanologos, 2006.

Johnson, Rebecca L., Steven Foster, Tieraona Low Dog, M.D., and David Kiefer, M.D. *National Geographic Guide to Medicinal Herbs: The World's Most Effective Healing Plants.* Washington, DC: National Geographic, 2012.

Light, Phyllis D. *Southern Folk Medicine: Healing Traditions from the Appalachian Fields and Forests.* Berkeley, CA: North Atlantic Books, 2018.

Martin, Corinne. *Louisiana Herb Journal: Healing on Home Ground.* Baton Rouge: Louisiana State University Press, 2022.

McGuffin, Michael, John F. Kartez, Albert Y. Leung, and Arthur O. Tucker. *Herbs of Commerce.* Silver Spring, MD: American Herbal Products Association, 2000.

Mellichamp, Larry. *Native Plants of the Southeast: A Comprehensive Guide to the Best 640 Species for the Garden.* Portland, OR: Timber Press, 2014.

Moerman, Daniel E. *Native American Ethnobotany.* Portland, OR: Timber Press, 1998.

Perrin, Mary B, and Beverly Fusilier. *Healing Traditions of South Louisiana: Prayers, Plants and Poultices.* Opelousas, LA: Andrepont, 2022.

Shane, CoreyPine. *Southeast Medicinal Plants: Identify, Harvest, and Use 106 Wild Herbs for Health and Wellness.* Portland, OR: Timber Press, 2021.

Telkes, Nicole A. *Medicinal Plants of Texas: Materia Medica and Wildcrafting Ethics.* Cedar Creek, TX: Wildflower School of Botanical Medicine Publishing, 2014.

Touchstone, Samuel J. *Herbal and Folk Medicine of Louisiana and Adjacent States.* Princeton, LA: Folk-Life Books, 1983

Van Dyke, Lucretia. *African American Herbalism: A Practical Guide to Healing Plants and Folk Traditions.* New York: Simon and Schuster, 2023.

Weed, Susun S. *Abundantly Well: The Complementary Integrated Medicine Revolution.* Woodstock, NY: Ash Tree, 2020.

ONLINE AND OTHER RESOURCES

One important way to learn about plants in your area is to join a native/wild plant or medicinal herb identification group in your area. Louisiana botanist Charles Allen in Pitkin offers numerous plant ID and wild edible classes, and you can sign up for his daily plant reports or check his website for ongoing events (https.allenacresbandb.com). The Louisiana Audubon Society offers classes in local plant information (la.audubon.org), and the Vermilionville Healing Garden in Lafayette offers on-site classes and demonstrations as well as a comprehensive website (bayouvermiliondistrict.org/vermilionville). The Acadiana Native Plant Project has numerous identification, propagation, and wild-walks classes as well as an informative website (greauxnative.org). Another helpful online group is Louisiana Wild Edibles, Foraging, and Wild Medicinal Plants and Mushrooms (www.facebook.com/groups/193083031481346).

A great resource for plant identification is the U.S. Geological Survey, *Guide to the Plants of Louisiana* (https://warcapps.usgs.gov/PlantID).

In addition, several herb/plant-related organizations have excellent online information. These include the American Botanical Council (abc.herbalgram.org), the American Herbalists Guild (americanherbalistsguild.com), James Duke's Ethnobotanical Databases (phytochem.nal.usda.gov/phytochem/search/list), the Louisiana Herbal Events calendar (herbrally.com/events/Louisiana), the Herb Society of Louisiana, Baton Rouge Unit (hsabr.org), the Acadiana Native Plant Project (greauxnative.org), and the Louisiana State University Agricultural Center in Baton Rouge (lsuag-center.com). To learn more about the changes and challenges affecting southern Louisiana lands, cultures, and tradition bearers, check out the Louisiana Folklife Society programs, including the Bayou Culture Collaborative (www.crt.state.la.us/cultural-development/arts/folklife/bayou-culture-collaborative/).

INDEX OF COMMON USES